NURSES and
FAMILIES

A Guide to
Family Assessment
and Intervention

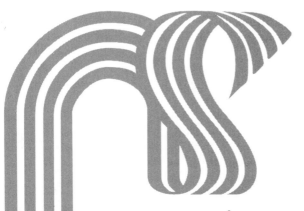

Lorraine M. Wright, RN, PhD

Director, Family Nursing Unit
Professor, Faculty of Nursing
University of Calgary
Calgary, Alberta, Canada

Maureen Leahey, RN, PhD

Manager, Psychiatric/Mental Health Outpatient Program
Calgary Regional Health Authority
Adjunct Associate Professor
Faculties of Nursing and Medicine (Psychiatry)
University of Calgary
Calgary, Alberta, Canada

NURSES and FAMILIES

FAMILIES

A Guide to Family Assessment and Intervention

third edition

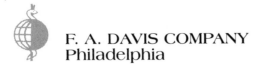

F. A. DAVIS COMPANY
Philadelphia

F. A. Davis Company
1915 Arch Street
Philadelphia, PA 19103

Printed in the United States of America

Last digit indicates print number: 10 9 8 7 6 5

Managing Publisher, Nursing: Lisa A. Biello
Acquisitions Editor: Joanne P. DaCunha, RN, MSN
Production Editor: Jessica Howie Martin
Cover Designer: Louis J. Forgione

As new scientific information becomes available through basic and clinical research, recommended treatments and drug therapies undergo changes. The authors and publisher have done everything possible to make this book accurate, up to date, and in accord with accepted standards at the time of publication. The authors, editors, and publisher are not responsible for errors or omissions or for consequences from application of the book, and make no warranty, expressed or implied, in regard to the contents of the book. Any practice described in this book should be applied by the reader in accordance with professional standards of care used in regard to the unique circumstances that may apply in each situation. The reader is advised always to check product information (package inserts) for changes and new information regarding dose and contraindications before administering any drug. Caution is especially urged when using new or infrequently ordered drugs.

Library of Congress Cataloging-in-Publication Data

Wright, Lorraine M., 1944-
    Nurses and families : a guide to family assessment and intervention/Lorraine M. Wright, Maureen Leahey.—3rd ed.
      p. cm.
    Includes bibliographical references and index.
    ISBN 0-8036-0371-1 (pbk.)
    1. Family nursing. 2. Family assessment. I. Title. II. Leahey, Maureen, 1944-
    [DNLM: 1. Nursing Assessment. 2. Family Health—Nurses' Instruction. 3.
    Interviews—methods—Nurses' Instruction. WY 100 W95ln 2000]
    RT120.F34 W75 2000
    610.73 21—dc21   99-042916

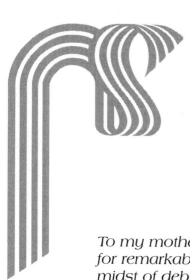

*To my mother, Hazel Jean Schollar Wright,
for remarkable graciousness in the
midst of debilitating illness, and
to my father, James William Wright,
for exemplary honoring of the
vow "in sickness and in health."*

Lorraine M. Wright

*To Donald Neus, my brother,
who courageously "plays the hand he's been dealt,"
and
to my sister-in-law, Marion, who cares so well.*

Maureen Leahey

Acknowledgments

We are grateful to our friends, families, and students for their nudging, support, interest, and encouragement throughout the writing (and procrastination of writing) of this third edition.

In particular, we are grateful to:

- Bob Martone, publisher, F. A. Davis, for his long-term interest and wonder about this book
- Joanne DaCunha, acquisitions editor, F. A. Davis, for her persistent encouragement
- Jessica Howie Martin, production editor, F. A. Davis, for guiding the manuscript through production
- Darlene Pederson and Diane Blodgett, developmental editors, for their care in readying the manuscript for production
- Marg Osborne, for sharing her personal knowledge and generously loaning us books and articles about diversity issues
- Anne Marie Levac, friend and colleague, who has diligently taught and practiced family nursing and has so willingly and enthusiastically offered articles, evaluations, and professional experiences of what is useful and what is not in family nursing practice

For each of us there have been other individuals to whom we would like to express special thanks and appreciation:

LMW

- Dr. Janice Bell for sustained and supportive colleagueship throughout the writing of this book and always asking that wonderful question: "Is there anything I can do to help?"
- Ryan Timothy Wright, my nephew, who so willingly agreed to share his illness experiences on videotape and

consequently has touched the hearts and minds of numerous nurses and hopefully influenced their practice

- Thelma Midori, treasured friend, who has honored me by sharing her illness story, suffering, triumphs, and spiritual journey

ML

- "Dougie" Leahey for his abiding interest, delight, encouragement, and cooking
- Stephen and Dennice Leahey for making available the use of "The Shore" to write; Greta Dow for cooking me dinners and pies, letting me use her computer and play with Chum; Helen Shirley for bringing me fresh mackerel and tomatoes

Finally, we are grateful to each other. We've continued to share innumerable and varied experiences:

- Wonderful meals in numerous places and "upscale fish restaurants"
- E-mails (long and short), telephone calls, and answering machine messages
- Trips, parties, movies, committee meetings, conferences, articles and stock tips

We appreciate witnessing and supporting each other's struggles, delights, sufferings, and joys. We celebrate that we've given up the dream of having balanced lives and now share the dream of becoming athletes!

LMW and ML

Contents

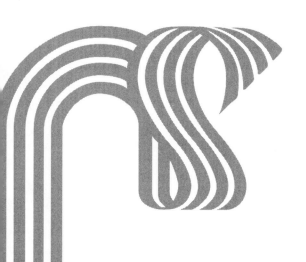

Introduction

▪▪▪ A DEFINING MOMENT

This is the third edition of *Nurses and Families.* The publication of this edition is evidence of our own continuing evolution as family nurse clinicians, teachers, researchers, and authors. It also attests to the ongoing evolution and developments in the field of family nursing. We consider it a great privilege to collaborate and consult with families, whether it be to promote health or to diminish or alleviate emotional, physical, and spiritual suffering from illness. We are also grateful for opportunities to teach professional nurses and undergraduate and graduate nursing students about involving, caring for, and learning from families in healthcare. Through our own clinical practice and teaching of health professionals for over 25 years and our personal family experiences with illness, we recognize the extreme importance of nurses possessing sound family assessment and intervention knowledge and skills to assist families. We also acknowledge the profound influence that the families have on our own lives and relationships.

▪▪▪ LOOKING BACK IN FAMILY NURSING: CHANGES, DEVELOPMENTS, AND INFLUENCES

Over the 15 years since the publication of the first edition of *Nurses and Families,* we have seen developments and changes in family nursing that are highly worthy of celebration and also areas where we need to put our "shoulders to the wheel." Bell (1996) offers a fascinating listing of publications and meetings of what she calls "signal events"—significant events that distinguished development in family nursing from 1981 through an international conference then scheduled for 1997. We believe that one of the most far-reaching signal events, and one that offers the greatest opportunity for uniting family nurses and disseminating family nursing knowledge, is the publication of the *Journal of Family Nursing* in 1995 under the editorship of Dr. Janice M. Bell. Another signal event, the Fourth International Family Nursing Conference (IFNC) held in Valdivia, Chile in 1997, was an important development in the field. For the

3

first time in the history of the IFNC, the conference was held outside of North America, which enabled a further appreciation of the global expansion of family nursing.

The changes and developments within family nursing in North America over the past 15 years are, of course, also influenced by larger societal changes. Massive healthcare restructuring and downsizing in Canada, the growth of managed care in the United States, and the movement to reduce the length of hospitalizations have expanded and enlarged community-based nursing practice in both countries. This movement has directly and indirectly placed more responsibility on families for the care of their ill members. Perhaps as a result of these dramatic changes, there is an expanded consumer movement and more collaboration with families about their healthcare needs. Adding to this consumer movement is an increase in technology, particularly the use of computers. Access to the Internet and e-mail enables family members to be more proactive and knowledgeable about their health problems through an ability to obtain current knowledge about these problems, options for treatment, and traditional and alternative healthcare resources.

The face of families is also changing as our demographics indicate an ever-increasing aging population. "Baby boomers" are approaching retirement with significantly reduced numbers in generation X to care for them. Diversity in North American populations is clearly evident, demanding ever-increasing recognition of a wide array of cultural differences in our healthcare system. Increased globalization invites the possibility of better healthcare practices worldwide but also allows universal transmission of diseases, making it much more difficult for healthcare providers to isolate, control, and segregate the origins of disease.

Amid all the changes in demographics, technology, healthcare delivery, and diversity, profound changes are also occurring in our world views, from modernism to postmodernism and from secularism to spiritualism. Family nursing has not been immune to these changes, nor have we.

■ ■ ■ THE IMPACT OF CHANGE ON US AND ON *NURSES AND FAMILIES*

The first edition of *Nurses and Families* was published in 1984 and the second in 1994. Now, just at the turn of the century, the third edition appears. The effect of some of the changes and developments in family nursing and the influence of larger societal differences in the past 15 years on us and our text are obvious and apparent; others are more subtle and perhaps tenuous.

One example of the palpable globalization of family nursing is the fact that our text has been translated into French, Japanese, Korean, and Swedish. Also, educational videotapes have been produced (Watson, 1988a, 1988b, 1988c, 1989a, 1989b) that describe the application of the Calgary Family Assessment Model (CFAM), family interventions, and family interviewing skills to actual clinical work with families. They have been purchased by faculties and schools of nursing worldwide.

Further tangible evidence of the expansion of family nursing assessment models worldwide is the fact that the CFAM continues to be widely adopted in undergraduate and graduate nursing curricula and by practicing nurses. We are aware that the CFAM is used in curricula throughout North America, Australia, Brazil, Chile, England, Japan, Taiwan, Finland, Scotland, Spain, and Sweden. With this expansion, we have had to revisit and revise our thinking about the CFAM to acknowledge, recognize, and embrace the evolving importance of certain dimensions of family life that influence health and illness, such as class, gender, ethnicity, race, family development, and beliefs.

A significant amplification in our text was the development of a framework and model for interventions, namely the Calgary Family Intervention Model, which was introduced in the second edition. This was done to recognize the need for emphasis on intervention equal to that placed on assessment of families and to provide a framework within which to capture family interventions. This change was clearly influenced by the advances in family nursing research, education, and practice from a primary emphasis on assessment to an expanding and equal emphasis on intervention.

Perhaps a more subtle but equally significant development is our ever-changing and evolving relationship with the families with whom we work. This change is reflected in our choice of language used to describe the nurse-family relationship that we deem most desirable. Our preferred stance or posture with families has drifted toward a more collaborative, consultative, nonhierarchical relationship over the past 15 years. When we adopt this stance, we notice that greater equality, respect, and status are given to the family's expertise. Therefore the combined expertise of the nurse and the family forms a new and effective synergy in the context of therapeutic conversations that otherwise did not and could not exist.

Another subtle development evolving throughout our three editions has been the movement toward a postmodernist world view. We embrace the notion that there are multiple realities in and of "the world," that each family member and nurse sees a world that he or she brings forth through interacting between themselves and with others in language. We encourage openness in ourselves, our students, and the families with whom we work to the many "worlds," differences, and diversity between and among family members and among the healthcare providers.

We have also been influenced by the dramatic restructuring in healthcare that has occurred over the past 5 years in Canada and the United States. Many practicing nurses inform us that the massive restructuring in healthcare institutions and community clinics, budgetary constraints, and managed care do not afford them the opportunity to become involved with or attend to the needs of families in healthcare settings. Nurses, particularly those in acute care hospital settings, have expressed their frustration at the substantially reduced time they have to attend to families' needs and concerns because of increased caseloads, heightened acuity of patients, and short-term stays. To recognize and respond to this change, we have developed ideas for how to conduct a 15-minute (or shorter) family interview. These ideas have been presented at nursing workshops and to our own nursing students with enthusiastic and encouraging responses. More importantly, based on anecdotal reports, the implementation of these ideas shows great promise. We have been encouraged by nurses' reports of reduced suffering by family members and enhanced health promotion in families in their care. Equally gratifying are reports of increased job satisfaction by practicing nurses when collaborating with families, if only for 15 minutes or less.

THE THIRD EDITION: WHAT IT IS AND WHAT IS NEW AND UNIQUE

This revised third edition of *Nurses and Families* continues to be a "how-to" basic text for undergraduate, graduate, and practicing nurses. It is the only textbook of which we are aware that provides specific how-to guidelines for family assessment and intervention. This practical guide for clinical work offers the opportunity for nursing students, practitioners, and educators to deliver better healthcare to families. Students and practitioners of community and public health nursing, maternal and child nursing, pediatric nursing, mental health nursing, gerontologic nursing, and family systems nursing will find it most useful. Nurse educators who presently teach a family-centered approach and those who will be introducing the concept of the "family as the client" will find it a valuable resource. Educators involved in continuing education courses or nurse practitioner programs will be able to use this book to update nurses' clinical skills in family-centered care.

Our text provides specific guidelines for nurses to consider when preparing for, conducting, and documenting family meetings from the first interview through discharge or termination. Actual clinical case examples are given throughout the book. These case examples reflect ethnic, cultural, racial, and sexual orientation diversity in conjunction with various family developmental life-cycle stages and transitions. Special attention is given to the variety of family forms and structures prevalent in today's society. Issues in a variety of practice settings are addressed. The clinical practice ideas are based on solid theory, research, and our own 25 years of clinical experiences with families.

The major purposes of this book are to (1) provide nurses with a sound theoretical foundation for family assessment and intervention; (2) provide nurses with clear, concise, and comprehensive family assessment and intervention models; (3) provide a guideline for beginning family interviewing skills; and (4) offer detailed ideas and suggestions with clinical examples of how to prepare, conduct, document, and terminate family interviews.

In this third edition, the following features are new and unique:

1. The Calgary Family Assessment Model (CFAM) has been thoroughly updated and expanded. Increased attention is given to diversity issues, including ethnicity, race, culture, sexual orientation, gender, and class. The CFAM is an easy-to-apply, practical, and relevant model for busy nurses working with a variety of family structures and encountering various developmental stages. In addition, helpful hints for constructing genograms and ecomaps have been added.

2. The Calgary Family Intervention Model (CFIM) has been updated and revised to make it more user friendly and expanded to include more clinical examples for crisis intervention. It remains, to our knowledge, the only family intervention model for nurses by nurses. It offers new interventions to assist with improving or sustaining family functioning and coping with illness.

3. A new chapter has been added on how to conduct a 15-minute (or shorter) family interview. This will help nurses working in time-pressured environments to offer valuable assistance to families.

4. Specific suggestions for fostering collaborative nurse-family relationships have been added throughout this third edition. Sample questions for nurses to ask themselves and the family are also offered.

▪▪▪ TOUR OF THE CHAPTERS

The first five chapters provide the conceptual base for collaborating and consulting with families. To be able to interview families, identify strengths and concerns, and intervene to diminish suffering, it is first necessary to have a sound conceptual framework. The specific how-to section of the book is included in Chapters 6 through 10, with numerous clinical examples in a variety of practice settings.

Chapter 1 establishes a rationale for family assessment and intervention. It describes the conceptual shift required in considering the family system, rather than the individual, as the unit of healthcare. It outlines the indications and contraindications for family assessment and intervention.

Chapter 2 addresses the major concepts of systems, cybernetics, communication, biology of knowing, and change theory that underpin the two models offered in this text, namely the CFAM and CFIM. It also presents a brief description of some of the major world views that influence our models, such as modernism and postmodernism, as well as gender sensitivity. Clinical examples of the application of these concepts are offered.

Chapter 3 presents the CFAM, a comprehensive, three-pronged structural, developmental, and functional family assessment framework. This widely adopted model has been thoroughly updated and expanded to reflect the current range of family forms in North American society, with increased emphasis on diversity issues such as ethnicity, race, culture, sexual orientation, gender, and class. Ideas of specific questions that the nurse may ask the family are provided. Two structural assessment tools, the genogram and ecomap, are delineated, and instructions and helpful hints are given for how to use them when interviewing families. Excerpts from actual family interviews are presented to illustrate the use of the model in clinical practice.

Chapter 4 describes the updated and revised CFIM. The revisions enable nurses to move beyond assessment and have easier access to a repertoire of family interventions that will effect or sustain changes in family functioning in cognition, affect, and behavior. Actual clinical examples of family work are presented, along with a variety of interventions. Traditionally, nurses have primarily focused on family assessment because there have been no family nursing intervention models within nursing to draw on.

Chapter 5 describes the family interviewing skills and competencies necessary in family-centered care. Specifically, perceptual, conceptual, and executive skills necessary for family assessment and intervention are presented. The skills are written in the form of training objectives, and clinical examples are given to help broaden the nurse's understanding of how to use these skills. Nurse educators, in particular, may find this chapter useful in focusing their evaluation of students' family interviewing skills. Ethical considerations in family interviewing are addressed.

Chapter 6 presents guidelines that are useful when preparing for family interviews. Ideas are given for developing hypotheses, choosing an appropriate interview setting, and making the first telephone contact with the family.

Chapter 7 delineates the various stages of the first interview and the remaining stages of the entire interviewing process: engagement, assessment, intervention, and termination. Actual clinical case examples in a variety of healthcare settings illustrate the practice of conducting interviews.

Chapter 8 is new. It offers clear, specific suggestions on how to conduct 15-minute (or shorter) family interviews in a manner that enhances the possibilities for healing or health promotion. These ideas respond to the realities facing many nurses in this era of managed care and health restructuring. It also encourages nurses to adopt the belief that any time spent with families is better than no time.

Chapter 9 presents ideas on how to document in a manageable fashion the vast amounts of data generated during family assessment and intervention meetings. Suggestions are given for how to develop a strength and problems list, assessment summary, progress record, and discharge synopsis.

Chapter 10 highlights how to terminate with families in a therapeutic manner, whether it is after only one very short meeting or several meetings. Ideas are given for family-initiated and nurse-initiated termination, as well as for discharges determined by the healthcare system.

The major difference between this book and other books on family nursing is that this book's primary emphasis is on how to meet and interview families. We wish to emphasize, however, that this text does not offer a "cookbook" approach to family meetings and interviews. The real development of skills results from actual clinical practice and supervisory feedback. We envision this book as a springboard for nursing students, nursing educators, and practicing nurses. With a solid conceptual base and practical how-to ideas for family assessment and intervention, we hope that more nurses will gain confidence and a commitment to engage in the nursing of families. In so doing, they will be reclaiming some aspects of nursing that have been directly or inadvertently given to other health professionals. In the process, nurses will continue to regain an important and expected dimension of nursing practice and be instrumental in the health promotion and healing of families with whom they collaborate.

▮▮▮ REFERENCES

Bell, J.M.(1996). Signal events in family nursing. *Journal of Family Nursing, 2* (4), 347–349.

Watson, W. L. P. (1988a). *A family with chronic illness: A "tough" family copes well* (Videotape). Calgary, AB: University of Calgary.

Watson, W. L. P. (1988b). *Aging families and Alzheimer's disease* (Videotape). Calgary, AB: University of Calgary.

Watson, W. L. P. (1988c). *Fundamentals of family systems nursing* (Videotape). Calgary, AB: University of Calgary.

Watson, W. L. P. (1989a). *Families and psychosocial problems* (Videotape). Calgary, AB: University of Calgary.

Watson, W. L. P. (1989b). *Family systems interventions* (Videotape). Calgary, AB: University of Calgary.

CHAPTER **1**

Family Assessment and Intervention: An Overview

Nursing has a commitment and an obligation to involve families in healthcare. The theoretical, practical, and research evidence of the significance of the family to the health and well-being of individual members as well as the influence of the family on illness compels nurses to consider family-centered care an integral part of nursing practice. However, family-centered care will be achieved responsibly and respectfully only by the enlistment of sound family assessment and intervention practices.

A rich tradition of nursing literature about the involvement of families in nursing care is developing. Some of the classic and newer texts in family nursing have enabled a new language to emerge through naming, describing, and communicating about the involvement of families in healthcare. Such terms as "family centered care" (Cunningham, 1978); "family focused care" (Janosik & Miller, 1979); "family interviewing" (Wright & Leahey, 1984; 1994); "family health promotion nursing" (Bomar, 1989); "family health care nursing" (Hanson & Boyd, 1996); "family nursing" (Bell, Watson, & Wright, 1990; Friedman, 1997; Gilliss, 1989; Gilliss, 1991; McFarlane, 1986; Hanson, 1991, Leahey & Wright, 1987a, 1987b; Wegner & Alexander, 1993; Wright & Leahey, 1987; Wright & Leahey, 1990; Broome, Knafl, Pridham, & Feetham, 1998), "family systems nursing" (Wright & Leahey, 1990; Wright, Watson, & Bell, 1990) and "nursing of families" (Feetham, Meister, Bell, & Gilliss, 1993) have all helped to bring forth the awareness and emergence of a crucial aspect of nursing practice heretofore overlooked, neglected, or minimized.

As nurses theorize about, conduct research on, and involve families more in healthcare, they are altering or modifying their usual patterns of clinical practice. The implication for this change in practice is that nurses need to become competent in assessing and intervening with families through collaborative nurse-family relationships. The knowledge and clinical skills required to conduct family interviews can be most efficiently learned by nurses who embrace the belief that illness is a family affair (Wright, Watson, & Bell, 1996). This belief will lead nurses to thinking interactionally or reciprocally about families. The dominant focus of family nursing assessment and intervention must be the reciprocity between health and illness and the family, and between the patient and family and the nurse. It is most helpful and enlightening for nurses to assess the impact of illness on the family and the influence of family interaction on the "cause," "course," and "cure" of health and illness. Health and illness, families, and nurses have each been studied as separate elements by a variety of disciplines. However, it is the reciprocity or relationships between the elements that are often new or startling to nurses. Therefore, it is our belief that nursing of families must focus on relationships, not on discrete elements. Fortunately, nursing is making strides in shifting toward a systemic understanding of families experiencing health problems.

■ ■ ■ EVOLUTION OF THE NURSING OF FAMILIES

A significant part of nursing history is that the involvement of families has always been part of nursing but has not always been labeled as such. Because nursing originated in patients' homes, it was natural to involve family members and to provide family-centered care. With the transition of nursing practice from homes to hospitals during the Depression and World War II, families became excluded not only from involvement in caring for ill members but from major family events such as birth and death.

Hanson and Boyd (1996) express a much bolder belief that "family nursing has existed since prehistoric times" (p. 21). They suggest that the primary responsibility of caring for ill family members has fallen to women and that women have traditionally made efforts to provide a clean and safe environment for the maintenance of health and wellness. From these very early beginnings of being a natural part of family life, nursing has undergone many developmental changes, even to excluding family members from the major family events mentioned previously. Nursing has now come full circle, with emphasis on inviting families "back" to participate in healthcare. However, this invitation is being made with much more knowledge, sophistication, respect, and collaboration than at any other time in nursing history.

The history, evolution, and theory development of the nursing of families has been discussed in depth in the literature (Feetham, Meister, Bell, & Gilliss, 1993; Friedman, 1992; Gilliss, 1991; Gilliss, Highley, Roberts, & Martinson, 1989; Lansberry & Richards, 1992; Whall & Fawcett, 1991). These authors have made a significant contribution to the advancement of family nursing knowledge with families by contextualizing nursing care with families. A landmark work synthesizing the research literature in nursing of children and their families, particularly in the areas of health promotion, acute illness, chronic illness, and the healthcare system, is an incredible contribution to the family nursing literature by Broome, Knafl, Pridham, and Feetham (1998). This text methodically reviews the assessment and intervention models used in the research reports.

Despite the ever-growing contribution of family nursing texts, a significant gap remains between theory and research and actual clinical practice. Friedman (1997) contends that a "family-centered approach remains a stated ideal rather than a prevailing practice—not only in inpatient but also community and clinic settings" (p. xv). We believe that the most significant variable that promotes or impedes family-centered care is how a nurse conceptualizes health and illness problems. It is the ability to "think interactionally" that raises the delivery of healthcare from an individual to a family (interactional) level. In an older but classic article, Sluzki (1974) suggests that the ability "to conceive [of] the individual as constantly defining and being defined by his relationships to his family and to other meaningful members of his milieu and by his insertion in the community at large" (p. 484) is perhaps more difficult for those who are already knowledgeable and well trained in intrapersonal, psychological, or medical models.

Robinson (1995) offers the thought-provoking idea that "distinctions between individual and family nursing have been framed as dichotomies and so have become separations rather than simply perceptions of difference" (p. 2). She proposes conceptualizing nursing as including *both* individuals and families, with distinctions made about the focus of practice. Robinson's (1995) ideas emerged from her application of Maturana's (1988) notion that not only are persons and families different kinds of systems but that they exist in different domains. Learning to make the transition from a more traditional individualistic perspective toward "thinking interactionally" or "thinking family" can be facilitated by providing nurses with a clear framework for assessing families and the necessary interventions to treat families.

▪ ▪ ▪ FAMILY ASSESSMENT

There have been many attempts to define and conceptualize the family from multiple perspectives by numerous disciplines. Duvall (1977) lists a series of 15 of the social sciences and disciplines conducting research on one or more aspects of family life. These include anthropology, counseling, economics, human development, psychology, public health, religion, social work, and sociology. Each discipline has its own point of view or frame of reference for viewing the family, and all have an ever-increasing appreciation of diversity issues. Economists, for example, have been concerned with how the family works together to meet material needs. Sociologists, on the other hand, are concerned with the family as a specific group in society. Nursing authors such as Liefson (1987), Mischke-Berkey, Warner, and Hanson (1989), and Hanson and Boyd (1996) have identified and described several family assessment models and instruments developed by both nurses and non-nurses. Hartwick, Lindsey, and Hills (1994) are encouraging a health-promoting family nursing assessment rather than the traditional illness-care models. This compilation of family assessment models and instruments is a very useful and worthwhile effort to make distinctions between models and the variables emphasized in each. There is no one assessment model, however, that explains *all* family phenomena.

In any clinical practice setting, it is useful for nurses to adopt a clear conceptual framework or a map of the family. This encourages the synthesis of data so that family strengths and problems can be identified and a useful management plan devised. When a conceptual framework is absent, it is extremely difficult for the nurse to group disparate data or to examine the relationships among the multiple variables that have an impact on the family. Use of a family assessment framework helps to organize this massive amount of seemingly disparate information. It also provides a focus for intervention.

CALGARY FAMILY ASSESSMENT MODEL: AN INTEGRATED FRAMEWORK

The Calgary Family Assessment Model (CFAM) is a multidimensional framework consisting of three major categories: structural, developmental, and functional (see Chap. 3). The model is based on a theory foundation involving systems, cybernetics, communication, and change. It has been adapted from Tomm and Sanders' (1983) family assessment model and substantially embellished since our first edition of this textbook in 1984. The model is also embedded within larger world views of postmodernism, feminism, and biology of cognition. Diversity issues are also emphasized and appreciated within our particular model.

INDICATIONS AND CONTRAINDICATIONS FOR A FAMILY ASSESSMENT

It is important to identify some guidelines for determining *which* families will automatically be considered for family assessment. It is not yet a common practice in our society to have families present themselves as a family unit for assistance with particular *family* health and illness problems, difficulties, or suffering. Rather, the illness is more frequently presented as isolated within a particular family member. Therefore, with each illness situation a judgment must be made about whether that particular problem should be approached within a family context.

The following indications for a family assessment are offered:

1. A family is experiencing emotional, physical, and/or spiritual suffering or disruption caused by a family crisis (e.g., acute illness, injury, or death).
2. A family is experiencing emotional, physical, and/or spiritual suffering or disruption caused by a developmental milestone (e.g., birth, marriage, or youngest child leaving home).
3. A family defines a problem as a family issue and there is motivation for family assessment (e.g., the impact of chronic illness on the family).
4. A child or adolescent is identified by the family as having difficulties (e.g., school phobia or fear of treatment for cancer).
5. The family is experiencing issues that are serious enough to jeopardize family relationships (e.g., terminal illness or sexual/physical abuse).
6. A family member is about to be admitted to the hospital for psychiatric treatment.
7. A child is about to be admitted to the hospital.

Conducting and completing a family assessment does not absolve nurses from assessing serious risks such as suicide and homicide nor serious illnesses in individual family members. Family assessment is neither a panacea nor a substitute for an individual assessment. In advanced nursing practice, particularly family systems nursing, assessment of individuals and assessment of the whole family system occurs simultaneously (Wright & Leahey, 1990).

Some contraindications for family assessment are:

• Individuation of a family member would be compromised by the family assessment. For example, if a young adult has recently left home for the first time, a family interview may not be desirable.
• The context of a family situation permits little or no leverage. That is, the family might have the fixed belief that the nurse is working as an agent of some other institution (e.g., the court).

During the engagement process, nurses need to be quite explicit in presenting the rationale for family assessment. Suggestions for how to do this are given in Chapters 6 and 7. In deciding whether or not to do a family assessment, the nurse should be guided by sound clinical principles and judgment. The nurse can take advantage of opportunities to consult with peers and supervisors if there are any questions about the suitability of such an assessment.

Once the nurse has completed the family assessment, he or she must decide whether or not to intervene with the family. In the next section of this chapter, we will discuss our general ideas about intervention. Specific ideas for nurses to consider when making clinical decisions about interventions with particular families are presented in Chapters 4 and 8.

■ ■ ■ NURSING INTERVENTIONS: A GENERIC DISCUSSION

Numerous terms are used to distinguish and ultimately label the treatment portion of nursing practice: intervention, treatment, therapeutics, action, and activity (Bulechek & McCloskey, 1992b). In our clinical practice and research with families, we prefer the designation of *intervention*. The most rigorous efforts to contribute to a standardized language for nursing interventions is the work of Bulechek and McCloskey (1992a&b) and their colleagues at the University of Iowa. More recently, they have done further work in standardizing language and building taxonomies such as the Nursing Interventions Classification based on nurses' reports of their practice (McCloskey & Bulechek, 1994; 1996). We applaud their ambitious and needed efforts to develop and validate nursing intervention labels. Because we perceive them as clearly providing leadership in this much-neglected area of nursing, we will use their conceptualization and findings as our base of reference, from which we will agree and disagree.

First, however, we wish to present a brief overview of the evolutionary process of identifying, defining, and describing nursing interventions. In 1980, the American Nurses' Association (ANA) published *Nursing: A Social Policy Statement,* which stated that "nursing is the diagnosis and treatment of human responses to actual or potential health problems" (p. 9). Although the ANA accepted the activity of nursing diagnoses, much debate and controversy continue within the nursing profession about the nature and labels of nursing diagnoses (Bulechek & McCloskey, 1992a; Wright & Levac, 1992). At the Ninth North American Nursing Diagnosis Association (NANDA) conference, the following definition was accepted: "A nursing diagnosis is a clinical judgment about individual, family or community responses to actual or potential health problems/life processes. Nursing diagnoses provide the basis for selection of nursing interventions to achieve outcomes for which the nurse is accountable" (Carroll-Johnson, 1990, p. 50).

Bulechek and McCloskey (1992a) prefer to define a nursing diagnosis as "the identification of a patient's problem that the nurse can treat" (p. 5). This definition comes closest to the way we prefer to label difficulties experienced by families. That is, after assessing a family, we prefer to generate a list of strengths and problems rather than diagnoses. We conceptualize the list as one observer's perspective, not the "truth" about a family. We view the problem list as presenting problems that nurses can treat. It has been our experience that nursing diagnoses have unfortunately become too rigid and do not include enough consideration of ethnic and cultural issues. We agree with Bulechek and McCloskey (1992a) that wellness diagnoses are not necessary, but for different reasons. We prefer to identify the strengths of the family and list them alongside their problems (see Chap. 9). The advantage of this type of classification is that it gives a balanced view of a family. It also asks us as nurses not to be blinded by a family's problems but to realize that every family has strengths, even in the face of potential or actual health problems.

DEFINITION OF A NURSING INTERVENTION

Bulechek and McCloskey (1989) define a nursing intervention as "any direct care treatment that a nurse performs on behalf of a client which includes nurse-initiated treatments, physician-initiated treatments and performance of daily essential functions." Wright, Watson, and Bell (1996) offer an alternate definition: "any action or response of the clinician, which includes the clinician's overt therapeutic actions and internal cognitive-affective responses, that occurs in the context of a clinician-client relationship offered to effect individual, family, or community functioning for which the clinician is accountable" (120). Wright, Watson, and Bell (1996) expand on their definition of "intervention" and suggest that an intervention "usually implies a onetime act with clear boundaries, frequently offering something or doing something to someone else" (p.154). Interventions are normally purposeful, conscious, and usually involve observable behaviors of the nurse.

CONTEXT OF A NURSING INTERVENTION

The focus of concern with a nursing intervention should be the nurse's behavior *and* the family response. This differs from nursing diagnosis and nursing outcome, in which the focus is client behavior (Bulechek & McCloskey, 1992a). We believe that nurse behaviors and client behaviors are contextualized in the nurse-client relationship. Therefore, an interactional phenomenon occurs whereby the responses of a nurse (interventions) are invited by the responses of clients (outcome) which, in turn, are invited by the responses of a nurse. To focus on only client behaviors *or* nurse behaviors does not take into account the relationship between nurses *and* clients. Haller (1990) makes an important point when she comments that interactional research is the study of relationships and states that "many of our nursing interventions are interactional; that is, not doing to or for the patient, but with the patient" (p. 272). We believe that *all* nursing interventions are interactional. Nursing interventions are actualized only in a relationship.

INTENT OF NURSING INTERVENTIONS

The intent of any nursing intervention is to effect change. Therefore, effective nursing interventions are those to which clients and families respond because of the "fit," or meshing, between the intervention offered by the nurse and the biopsychosocial-spiritual structure of family members (Wright & Levac, 1992). Gottlieb and Feeley (1995) offer a very useful discussion of the issues of change and timing related to nursing intervention studies. They pose some interesting questions to consider when embarking on nursing intervention research, such as: What is the nature of the phenomenon that is being targeted for change? Does the intervention seek to develop the phenomenon, change it, or maintain it? Whom are we trying to change? How can we know that the intervention contributed to the observed change? Who will assess the change? These questions are useful within the domain of research that follows a modernist philosophy and uses a standardized intervention with a specific population for a desired outcome. One example of the application of these questions was a randomized control trial study to evaluate the effectiveness of a yearlong home-based nursing intervention to enhance the psychosocial adjustment of children with a chronic condition (Pless, Feeley, Gottlieb, Rowat, Dougherty, & Willard, 1994).

However, postmodernist practices in working with families would not have a predetermined standardized intervention to use across a number of families. Rather, the nurse, in collaboration with the specific family, would determine what interventions are most useful for families experiencing a particular illness. Indeed, both approaches are needed and useful at a time when we are so deficient in our understanding and implementation of nursing interventions in family nursing.

▉▉▉▉ NURSING INTERVENTIONS WITH FAMILIES: A SPECIFIC DISCUSSION

There are numerous ways in which to intervene with families. This section discusses some specific aspects of interventions with families. It also presents indications and contraindications for family intervention.

CONCEPTUALIZATION OF INTERVENTIONS WITH FAMILIES

Notions and ideas about reality gleaned from postmodernism and social constructionism are helpful when conceptualizing ideas about interventions. It is unwise to attempt to ascertain what is "really" going on with a particular family or what the "real" problem is; rather, we should recognize that what is "real" to us as nurses, whether it be the problem or the intervention, is always a consequence of our social construction of the world (Keeney, 1982). Keeney further states that, because family clinicians join their clients in the social construction of a therapeutic reality, the clinician is also responsible "for the universe of experience that is created" (p. 165). Maturana (1988) presents another twist on this critical notion of reality by submitting that individuals (living systems) bring forth reality—they do not construct it, nor does it exist independent of them. This has implications for nurses' clinical work with families in that what we perceive about particular situations with families is influenced by how we behave (our interventions) and how we behave depends on what we perceive.

Therefore, one way to change the "reality" that family members have drawn forth is to assist them in developing new ways of interacting in the family. The interventions that we use in this endeavor are focused on changing cognitive, affective, or behavioral domains of family functioning. As family members' perceptions about each other and their illness change, so will their behavior. Clinical experience indicates that interventions normally directed at challenging the meanings or beliefs that families give to behavioral events or their experience of illness tend to have the most sustaining changes (Watson & Nanchoff-Glatt, 1990; Watson, Bell, & Wright, 1992; Wright, Bell, & Rock, 1989; Wright & Nagy, 1993; Wright & Simpson, 1991; Wright & Watson, 1988; Wright, Watson, & Bell, 1996).

We must also keep in mind the element of time with regard to interventions. Interventions do not begin just with the intervention stage of family work. Rather, they are an integral part of family interviewing, spanning engagement to termination. Normally, interventions used during the specific intervention stage of family interviewing are based on the nurse's and family's influence on the issue, problem, or illness. If engagement and assessment have been adequate, this will generally increase the effectiveness of the interventions. For example, if a nurse working with a Latino family perpetually addresses family members other than the father first, the family may disengage. The opportunity to intervene further will be eliminated. In this example, one needs not only to possess family interviewing skills but also to possess sensitivity to ethnic issues before embarking on specific goal-oriented interventions.

INDICATIONS AND CONTRAINDICATIONS FOR FAMILY INTERVENTIONS

After a family assessment, nurses have to decide whether or not to intervene with a family. They need to consider the family's level of functioning, their own skill level, and the resources available. Leahey and Wright (1987) have drawn up some indicators for family intervention beyond the initial interviews. We have recommended intervention under the following circumstances (pp. 66–67):

- A family member presents with an illness that has an obvious detrimental impact upon the other family members. For instance, a grandfather's Alzheimer's disease may cause his grandchildren to be afraid of him, or a young child's acting-out behavior may be related to his mother's deterioration from multiple sclerosis.
- Family members contribute to an individual's symptoms or problems, for example, when lack of visitation from adult children exacerbates hypochondriasis in an elderly parent.
- One family member's improvement leads to symptoms or deterioration in another family member, for example, when decreased asthma symptoms in one child correlate with increased abdominal pain in a sibling.
- A child or adolescent develops an emotional, behavioral, or physical problem in the context of a family member's illness. Perhaps a diabetic adolescent suddenly requests that his mother give him his daily insulin injections when he has been injecting himself for the past 6 months.

- Illness is first diagnosed in a family member. If a family has no previous knowledge or experience with a particular illness, they will require information and may also require reassurance and support.
- A family member's condition deteriorates markedly. Whenever there is deterioration, family patterns will need restructuring and intervention is indicated.
- A chronically ill family member moves from a hospital or rehabilitation center back into the community.
- An important individual or family developmental milestone is missed or delayed, such as when an adolescent is unable to move out of the home at the anticipated time.
- A chronically ill patient dies. Although the patient's death may be a relief, the family can be faced with a tremendous void where the caregiving role used to be.

After the nurse and family have decided that intervention is indicated, they must then collaboratively decide on the duration and intensity of the family sessions. If sessions occur too frequently, there may be insufficient time for the family to recalibrate and process the change. The optimal number of days, weeks, or months between sessions is difficult to state categorically. We recommend that nurses ask the family when they would like to have another meeting. In our clinical experience, families are much better judges than nurses of how frequently they need to be seen to resolve a particular problem. Furthermore, nurses should be aware that the duration and intensity of sessions depend on the context in which the family is seen. For example, if a hospital nurse is working with a family, he or she may have the opportunity for only one or two meetings before discharge, whereas a community health nurse may be able to schedule a series of meetings. Often the context in which the nurse encounters families dictates the frequency and number of family meetings. Whether the nurse has 1 or 10 meetings with a family for assessment or intervention, there are important considerations for terminating with families. Additional information on termination is discussed in Chapter 10.

Family intervention is not always required, and the question arises about the *contraindications* for family intervention. These include:

1. All family members state that they do not wish to pursue family meetings or treatment even though it is recommended.
2. The family states that they agree with the recommendation for family meetings or treatment but would prefer to work with another professional.

These contraindications are generally evident to the nurse immediately after the family assessment. Sometimes during the course of intervention, however, families indicate a desire to stop treatment. We will discuss this situation more fully in Chapter 10.

It is evident that nurses working with patients and families in a variety of healthcare settings need to have a good understanding of when family involvement is indicated and when it is contraindicated. Not only for their own benefit but also for the family's benefit, nurses should make a distinction between family assessment and family intervention. Families are often willing to come for an assessment when they can see the nurse face to face and make *their* own assessment of the nurse's competence. If a nurse does a careful, credible assessment, he or she will have an easier time in doing family intervention work.

DEVELOPMENT AND IDENTIFICATION OF NURSING INTERVENTIONS WITH FAMILIES

Craft and Willadsen (1992) state that "the development of nursing interventions with families has been hampered by the lack of nursing theory of family" (p. 517). They further suggest that specification, validation, and testing of interventions related to the family is relatively novel in nursing. We concur with these thoughts, but we also believe that the lack of specific interventions with families has been caused by the lack of nurse educators who are skilled family clinicians. Because interventions related to the family are independent nursing interventions for which nurses are accountable (Wright, Watson, & Bell, 1990), nurse educators and researchers must begin specifying and testing interventions related to the family (Craft & Willadsen, 1992). It is not surprising that there have been very few tested nursing interventions with families when our profession is at a very early stage of even identifying and describing family interventions.

In a review of the nursing literature on families, chronic illness, and interventions, Robinson (1994) identified three distinct orientations to nursing interventions with families: traditional, transitional, and nontraditional. She also described how these orientations varied, particularly with respect to ideas about objectivity and the merits of a systemic orientation. This article highlights the importance of knowing the beliefs and assumptions underpinning different intervention approaches that target desirable family responses to chronic illness.

Chesla (1996) also concurs that the articulation and testing of nursing interventions with families lags behind other research and theory development. Family nursing interventions are even more deficient within hospital settings, particularly in critical care units (CCUs). In Chesla's study, 130 nurses caring for families in a variety of CCUs participated in an interpretive phenomenologic study resulting in 100 examples of care of the family in CCUs. These examples served as text for interpretation. The results of this study are both disheartening and encouraging. Some CCU nurses are "less caring and helpful in order to focus on technologic biomedical care" (p.202). However, stories of family care were more evident when the patients were infants and children and when death was imminent, whereas family care was less evident in acute phases of a patient's illness or when patients were slow to recover. This valuable study led Chesla to conclude that working with families in CCUs needs to be documented in order to legitimize expert family care. She also recommended that consultants or educators who are skilled in family care be introduced into CCUs to reduce the tremendous gap between the daily practice of the nurse at the bedside and theory of family interventions. These recommendations are in response to the startling comments from nurses who indicated that they learned most of their family practice by trial and error. We wonder if feeling incompetent or inadequate in family nursing care is the trigger that causes nurses to use strategies to distance themselves from families and maintain the focus on technological care (Chesla, 1996; Chesla & Stannard, 1997; Hupcey, 1998).

The recent efforts by Craft and Willadsen (1992) are a major contribution to assisting nursing practice to specify and validate family interventions and eventually test them. They conducted a study that surveyed 130 nurse experts in the United States, of whom 54 (41 percent) responded. From their findings, Craft and Willadsen (1992) conclude that "nursing intervention levels related to family can be specified in a manner that has common meaning to experts in family nursing" (p. 524). Specifically, this study labeled, defined, and gave critical and supporting activities for nine interventions related to family. These nine interventions were as follows: family support, family process maintenance, family integrity promotion, family involvement, family mobilization, caregiver support, sibling support, parent education and family therapy.

Craft and Willadsen's (1992) study is an important beginning. Efforts now need to be made to validate these identified interventions through both clinical and empirical means. We suggest that it would be useful in future studies attempting to label family interventions to specify the amount of clinical contact the experts have with families. We believe that nurses in direct clinical contact with families perceive family interventions differently from nurses who predominantly conduct research or engage in theory development. We found Craft and Willadsen's labeling, defining, and citing of specific activities of nine interventions to be useful. However, we found some of the descriptions of critical and supporting activities of each intervention to be more congruent with activities describing family assessment than intervention (e.g., "determine how patient behavior affects family; identify family member's perceptions of the situations and precipitating events"). We agree with the identification and descriptions of all but one of the interventions cited. We disagree with the labeling of family therapy as an intervention. We believe this to be a conceptual error.

Family therapy is *not* an intervention; it is much more. "It is a world view that involves a conceptual shift from linear to systems (systemic) thinking" (Watson, 1992, p. 379). Family therapy is not only a particular type of clinical practice with families but also a distinct profession with licensure or certification in 40 states in the United States. Since 1978, the American Association for Marriage and Family Therapy's Commission on Accreditation has been recognized by the United States Department of Education as the professional body that defines the practice and the profession of family therapy. At the same time, specialization in family therapy can and does occur within nursing, social work, psychology, and psychiatry.

The education and training of undergraduate students in clinical work with families primarily focuses on the family as context (Wright & Leahey, 1990). Nursing students specializing in family systems nursing (Wright & Leahey, 1990; Wright, Watson, & Bell, 1990) are at the graduate or advanced practice level. Thus, it is extremely important that our efforts to label interventions be consistent within a particular practice framework, for example, interventions within family as context, interventions within family systems nursing, or interventions within family therapy. However, it is possible that some interventions labeled as being in one domain of clinical practice with families will be identifiable in another domain of clinical practice.

■■■ CALGARY FAMILY INTERVENTION MODEL: AN ORGANIZING FRAMEWORK

The Calgary Family Intervention Model (CFIM) is an organizing framework for conceptualizing the relationship between families and nurses that helps change to occur and healing to begin. Specifically, the model highlights the family-nurse relationship by focusing on the intersection between family member functioning and interventions offered by nurses (see Chap. 4). It is at this intersection that healing may take place. CFIM is a collaborative, nonhierarchical model that recognizes the expertise of family members experiencing illness and the expertise of nurses in managing illness and promoting health. The model is embedded in notions from postmodernism and the biology of cognition. It can be applied and used with clients and families from diverse cultures because it emphasizes fit versus treatment for change from a particular cultural viewpoint. It remains, to the best of our knowledge, the only family nursing intervention model that is currently documented.

FAMILY RESPONSES TO INTERVENTIONS

Our discussion of interventions in family nursing practice has primarily focused on the behaviors of the nurse. However, interventions are actualized only in a relationship. Therefore, it is equally important to ascertain the responses of family members to interventions that are offered. A study by Robinson (Robinson & Wright, 1995) found that families who were experiencing difficulty managing a member's chronic condition and sought assistance in an outpatient nursing clinic could readily identify interventions that alleviated or diminished their suffering. The family nursing interventions that made a difference for these families were within two stages of the therapeutic change process. Specifically, the first useful intervention, within the stage of "creating the circumstances for change," was bringing the family together to engage in new and different conversations. The second useful intervention was establishing a therapeutic relationship between the nurse and family, particularly in the areas of providing comfort and demonstrating trust.

Within the stage of "moving beyond and overcoming problems," four interventions were identified as healing by families. These were: inviting meaningful conversation; noticing and distinguishing family and individual strengths and resources; careful attention and exploration of concerns; and putting illness problems in their place.

The identification of these interventions offers incredibly useful ideas for improving our care of families experiencing illness. Many more studies are needed to ascertain families' responses to the interventions offered.

▩▩▩ NURSING PRACTICE LEVELS WITH FAMILIES: GENERALIST AND SPECIALIST

Lansberry and Richards (1992) emphasize that nursing practice with families is directed by whether the concept of the family is family as context or family as client. They offer the interesting notion that different belief systems inform each type of practice with families. One way to alleviate any potential confusion of practice levels is to have a clear distinction of two levels of *expertise* in nursing with regard to clinical work with families: generalists and specialists (Wright & Leahey, 1988). Typically, generalists are nurses at the baccalaureate level who predominantly use the concept of the family as context (Wright & Leahey, 1990). Specialists, on the other hand, are nurses at the graduate (master or doctoral) level who predominantly use the concept of the family as the unit or client of care. This requires specialization in "family systems nursing" (Wright & Leahey, 1990). Family systems nursing specialization requires that "the focus is always on interaction and reciprocity. It is not 'either/or' but rather 'both/and.' Family systems nursing is the integration of nursing, systems, cybernetics and family therapy theories" (Wright & Leahey, 1990, p. 149). It requires familiarity with an extensive body of knowledge: family dynamics, family systems theory, family assessment, family intervention, and family research. It also requires accompanying competence in family interviewing skills. Family systems nursing focuses on *both* the family system and individual systems simultaneously (Wright & Leahey, 1990). A unique effort has been made by Forchuk and Dorsay (1995) to combine family systems nursing theory with Hildegard Peplau's theory. The authors suggest that a combined theoretical perspective offers several advantages, such as providing grounding for family work in an articulated nursing theory. All nurses should be knowledgeable and competent about how to involve families in healthcare as well as knowledgeable about ethics or pharmacology, which also cut across all domains of nursing practice. Consequently, the emphasis in the practice of family nursing at the generalist level is the family as context.

In contrast, the practice of family systems nursing at the specialist level emphasizes the family as the unit of care. However, we admit that these boundaries may and can become blurred, with upper level baccalaureate students recognizing the importance of a focus on interaction and reciprocity. These students often develop nursing competence and are able to deal with individual and family systems simultaneously.

▪▪▪ CONCLUSIONS

We consider it a great privilege to work with families experiencing health problems. We are also grateful for opportunities to teach professional nurses and nursing students how to involve families in healthcare. Through this process, we recognize the extreme importance of nurses having sound family assessment and intervention knowledge and skills. The remainder of this textbook is our effort to help nurses to help families.

▪▪▪ REFERENCES

Bell, J. M., Watson, W. L., & Wright, L. M. (Eds.). (1990). *The cutting edge of family nursing.* Calgary, Alberta, Family Nursing Unit Publications.

Bomar, P. J. (Ed.). (1989). *Nurses and family health promotion: Concepts, assessment and interventions.* Baltimore: Williams & Wilkins.

Broome, M. E., Knafl, K., Pridham, K., & Feetham, S. (Eds.) (1998) *Children and families in health and illness.* Thousand Oaks: Sage Publications.

Bulechek, G. M., & McCloskey, J. C. (Eds.). (1992a). Defining and validating nursing interventions. *Nursing Clinics of North America, 27*(2), 289–297.

Bulechek, G. M., & McCloskey, J. C. (Eds.). (1992b). *Nursing interventions: Essential nursing treatments.* Philadelphia: W. B. Saunders Company.

Bulechek, G. M., & McCloskey, J. C. (1989). Nursing interventions: Treatments for potential nursing diagnoses. In R. M. Carroll-Johnson (Ed.), *Current issues in nursing,* (3rd ed., pp. 23–28). St. Louis: C. V. Mosby.

Carroll-Johnson, R. M. (1990). Reflections on the ninth biennial conferences. *Nursing Diagnosis, 1,* 50.

Chesla, C. A. (1996). Reconciling technologic and family care in critical-care nursing. *Image: Journal of Nursing Scholarship, 28*(3), 199–203.

Chesla, C. A., & Stannard, D. (1997). Breakdown in the nursing care of families in the ICU. *American Journal of Critical Care, 6,* 64–71.

Cousins, N. (1979). *Anatomy of an illness as perceived by the patient.* New York: Bantam Books.

Craft, M. J., & Willadsen, J. A. (1992). Interventions related to family. *Nursing Clinics of North America, 27*(2), 517–540.

Cunningham, R. (1978). Family-centered care. *Canadian Nurse, 2,* 34–37.

Doherty, W. J. (1985). Family interventions in health care. *Family Relations, 34,* 129–137.

Duvall, E. (1977). *Marriage and family development* (5th ed.). New York: Harper & Row.

Feetham, S. L., Meister, S. B., Bell, J. M., & Gilliss, C. L. (1993). *The nursing of families: Theory, research, education and practice.* Newbury Park: Sage Publications.

Forchuck, C., & Park Dorsay, J. (1995). Hildegard Peplau meets family systems nursing: Innovation in theory-based practice. *Journal of Advanced Nursing, 21,* 110–115.

Friedman, M. M. (1997). *Family nursing: Research, theory and practice.* East Norwalk, Connecticut: Appleton & Lange.

Gilliss, C.L. (1991). Family nursing research, theory and practice. *Image: Journal of Nursing Scholarship, 23*(1), 19–22.

Gilliss, C. L., Highley, B. L., Roberts, B. M., & Martinson, I. M. (Eds.) (1989). *Toward a science of family nursing.* Menlo Park, CA: Addison-Wesley.

Gottlieb, L. N., & Feeley, N. (1995). Nursing intervention studies: Issues related to change and timing. *Canadian Journal of Nursing Research, 27(1),* 13–29.

Haller, K. B. (1990). Characteristics of interactional research. *MCN, 15,* 272.

Hanson, S. (1991). *Pocket guide to family assessment and intervention.* St. Louis: Mosby Year Book.

Hanson, S. M. H., & Boyd, S. T. (1996a). *Family health care nursing: Theory, practice, and research.* Philadelphia: F. A. Davis.

Hanson, S. M. H., & Boyd, S. T. (1996b). *Family nursing: An overview.* In S. M. H. Hanson & S. T. Boyd (Eds.). *Family health care nursing: Theory, practice, and research.* Philadelphia: F. A. Davis.

Hartwick, G., Lindsey, A. E., & Hills, M. (1994). Family nursing assessment: Meeting the challenge of health promotion. *Journal of Advanced Nursing, 20,* 85–91.

Hupcey, J. E. (1998). Establishing the nurse-family relationship in the intensive care unit. *Western Journal of Nursing Research, 20(2),* 180–194.

Janosik, E., & Miller, J. (1979). Theories of family development. In D. Hymovich & M. Barnard (Eds.), *Family health care—General perspectives* (vol.1, 2nd ed.) (pp. 3–16). New York: McGraw-Hill.

Keeney, B. (1982). What is an epistemology of family therapy? *Family Process, 21,* 153–168.

Lansberry, C. R., & Richards, E. (1992). Family nursing practice paradigm perspectives and diagnostic approaches. *Advances in Nursing Science, 15(2),* 66–75.

Leahey, M., & Wright, L. M. (1987). Families and chronic illness: Assumptions, assessment and intervention. In L.M. Wright & M. Leahey (Eds.), *Families and chronic illness* (pp. 55–76). Springhouse, PA: Springhouse Corp.

Leifson, J. (1987). Assessing families of infants with congenital defects. In L. M. Wright & M. Leahey, (Eds.) *Families and chronic illness.* Springhouse, PA: Springhouse Corporation.

Maturana, H. (1988). Reality: The search for objectivity or the quest for a compelling argument. *The Irish Journal of Psychology, 6(1),* 25–83.

McFarlane, J.M. (1986). *The clinical handbook of family nursing.* New York: John Wiley & Sons.

Mischke-Berkey, K., Warner, P., & Hanson, S. (1989). Family health assessment and intervention. In P.J. Bomar (Ed.) *Nurses and family health promotion: Concepts, assessment, and interventions.* Baltimore: Williams & Wilkins.

McCloskey, J. C., & Bulechek, G. M. (1994). Standardizing the language for nursing treatments: An overview of the issues. *Nursing Outlook, 42(2),* 56–64.

McCloskey, J. C. & Bulechek, G. M. (1996). *Nursing intervention classification (NIC)* (2nd ed.). St. Louis: C. V. Mosby.

Pless, L. B., Feeley, N., Gottlieb, L., Rowat, K., Dougherty, G., & Willard, B. (1994). Randomized control trial of a nursing intervention to promote the adjustment of children with chronic physical disorders. *Pediatrics, 94(1),* 70–75.

Robinson, C. (1995). Beyond dichotomies in the nursing of persons and families. *Image, 27*(2), 116–120.

Robinson, C.A., & Wright, L.M. (1995). Family nursing interventions: What families say makes a difference. *Journal of Family Nursing, 1*(3), 327–345.

Sluzki, C. (1974). On training to think interactionally. *Social Science and Medicine, 8*, 483–485.

Tomm, K., & Sanders, G. (1983). Family assessment in a problem oriented record. In J. C. Hansen & B. F. Keeney (Eds.), *Diagnosis and assessment in family therapy* (pp. 101–122). London: Aspen Systems Corporation.

Watson, W. L. (1992). Family therapy. In G. M. Bulechek & J. C. McCloskey (Eds.), *Nursing interventions: Essential nursing treatments,* Philadelphia: W. B. Saunders Company.

Watson, W. L., Bell, J. M., & Wright, L. M. (1992). Osteophytes and marital fights: A single case clinical research report of chronic pain. *Family Systems Medicine, 10*(4), 423–435.

Watson, W. L., & Nanchoff-Glatt, M. (1990). A family systems nursing approach to premenstrual syndrome. *Clinical Nurse Specialist, 4*, 3–9.

Wegner, G. D., & Alexander, R. J. (Eds.) (1993). *Readings in family nursing.* Philadelphia: J. B. Lippincott Company.

Whall, A.L., & Fawcett, J. (Eds.) (1991). *Family theory development in nursing: State of the science and art.* Philadelphia: F. A. Davis.

Wright, L. M., & Bell, J. M. (1994). The future of family nursing research: Interventions, interventions, interventions. *The Japanese Journal of Nursing Research, 27*(2–3), 4–15.

Wright, L. M., Bell, J. M., & Rock, B. L. (1989). Smoking behavior and spouses: A case report. *Family Systems Medicine, 7*(2), 158–171.

Wright, L.M., & Leahey, M. (1990). Trends in the nursing of families. *Journal of Advanced Nursing, 15*, 148–154.

Wright, L. M., & Leahey, M. (1988). Nursing and family therapy training. In H. A. Liddle, D. C., Breunlin, & R. C Schwartz (Eds). *Handbook of family therapy training and supervision.* New York: The Guilford Press.

Wright, L. M., & Leahey, M. (1987a). Families and life-threatening illness: Assumptions, assessment and intervention. In M. Leahey & L. Wright (Eds.), *Families & life-threatening illness* (pp. 45–58). Springhouse, PA: Springhouse Corp.

Wright, L. M., & Leahey, M. (1987b). Families and psychosocial problems: Assumptions, assessment and intervention. In M. Leahey & L. M. Wright (Eds.), *Families & psychosocial problems* (pp. 17–34). Springhouse, PA: Springhouse Corp.

Wright, L. M., & Leahey, M. (1984). *Nurses and families. A guide to family assessment and intervention.* Philadelphia: F. A. Davis Co.

Wright, L. M., & Levac, A. M. (1992). The non-existence of non-compliant families: The influence of Humberto Maturana. *Journal of Advanced Nursing, 17*, 913–917.

Wright, L. M., & Nagy, J. (1993). Death: The most troublesome family secret of all. In E. Imber Black (Ed.), *Secrets in families and family therapy* (pp. 121–137). New York: W.W. Norton & Co.

Wright, L. M., & Simpson, P. (1991). A systemic belief approach to epileptic seizures: A case of being spellbound. *Contemporary Family Therapy: An International Journal, 13*(2), 165–180.

Wright, L. M., & Watson, W. L. (1988). Systemic family therapy and family development. In C. J. Falicov (Ed.), *Family transitions: Continuity and change over the life cycle* (pp. 407–430). New York: Guilford Press.

Wright, L. M., Watson, W. L., & Bell, J. M. (1990). The Family Nursing Unit: A unique integration of research, education and clinical practice. In J. M. Bell, W. L. Watson, & L. M. Wright (Eds.) *The cutting edge of family nursing* (pp. 95–109). Calgary, Alberta: Family Nursing Unit Publications.

Wright, L. M., Watson, W. L., & Bell, J. M. (1996). *Beliefs: The heart of healing in families and illness.* New York: Basic Books.

CHAPTER 2

Theoretical Foundations of the Calgary Family Assessment and Intervention Models

Models are useful ways to bring clusters of ideas, notions, and concepts into our awareness. However, models cannot stand alone. They are built on a foundation of many world views, theories, beliefs, premises, and assumptions that influence and inform the models that arise. Models in nursing practice are more comprehensible and meaningful if the underlying theories are articulated and made known. Therefore, to comprehend and use the Calgary Family Assessment Model (see Chap. 3) and the Calgary Family Intervention Model (see Chap. 4) in nursing practice with families, it is important to know the theoretical assumptions underlying these models. Underlying theoretical assumptions of any family assessment and intervention models are important to declare because they are the foundation of the way in which those models are operationalized. The six theoretical foundations and world views that inform the models and eventual family nursing practice presented in the rest of this textbook are postmodernism (see next section), systems theory, cybernetics, communication theory, change theory, and a biology of cognition. Each theory, or world view, with some of the distinguishing concepts, will be presented and related to families.

▓▓▓▓ POSTMODERNISM

We humans seem to delight in rethinking, reexamining, reconstructing, and deconstructing our history and culture. One popular way to do this is through the lens of postmodernism. Anything before this present "enlightened" world view is considered modernist and therefore less desirable. Consequently, the influence of the ideas, conditions, and beliefs of postmodernism has been demonstrated in art, literature, architecture, science, culture, religion, philosophy, and, more recently, nursing (Kermode & Brown, 1996; Lister, 1991, 1997; Mitchell, 1996; Moules, 1998; Parsons, 1995; Reed, 1995; Tapp & Wright, 1996; Watson, 1995).

We too have been influenced by and have embraced many of the notions of postmodernism. These ideas have proved useful in our clinical nursing practice with families. However, we do not wish to imply that we have been able to successfully distance ourselves from all modernist ideas, nor would we want to. We cannot deny our history and culture and how it is a function of who we were and are. Therefore, we acknowledge the previous and continuing influences of both modernist and postmodernist paradigms on our lives, our relationships, and our practice of family nursing.

> **Concept 1**
> **Pluralism is a key focus of postmodernism.**

Postmodernism offers the "end of a single world view and, by extension, 'a war on totality,' a resistance to single explanations, a respect for difference and a celebration of the regional, local and particular" (Jencks, 1992, p.11). One of the major notions of postmodern thinking is the idea of pluralism, or a belief in multiplicity; that is, that there are as many ways to understand and experience the world as there are people who experience it (Moules, 1998). In family nursing practice, this idea becomes operational by recognizing that there are as many ways to understand and experience illness as there are families experiencing illness.

> **Concept 2**
> **Postmodernism is a debate about knowledge.**

Postmodernism is partly a reaction to the modernist claim that knowledge primarily emerges from science and technology (Lyotard, 1992). The belief that progressive technology will necessarily lead to a better world has become open to reexamination, questioning, and doubt (Tapp & Wright, 1996). Therefore an intense critique is being made of our metanarratives and grand belief systems that have formed the foundation of many of our scientific, religious, and political movements and institutions. As these grand narratives have been questioned, opportunities have been provided to uncover certain "taken-for-granted" beliefs and practices, to hear voices of marginal groups, and to value knowledge from a variety of domains heretofore not legitimized (Tapp & Wright, 1996). In encounters with families experiencing illness, much more emphasis is now given to the illness narratives and experiences of family members within their particular cultural context, not just to medical narratives. Collaboration and consultation between nurses and families honor the knowledge and expertise of both nurses and family members.

Other offshoots of postmodernism have been constructivism, social constructionism, and "bring forthism" (a biology of cognition) (Maturana & Varela, 1992; Moules, 1998). The latter, the biology of cognition, is the offshoot that we have found most useful in our clinical work and therefore will discuss later in this chapter.

There have been some strong critiques of the postmodern movement by feminists, who claim that women's voices continue to be diminished or ignored because of the grand narrative of patriarchy and oppression (Kermode & Brown, 1996). This has not been our experience in working with families. The most recent evidence for acknowledging women's voices and their illness burden in family systems nursing practice was in Robinson's (1998) study. She discovered that women in families experiencing chronic illness are vulnerable to the demands of illness responsibility, illness work, and illness problems. As a more equitable balance of illness demands was sought by the nurse and family members, the women in this study found a life for themselves beyond illness and the problems they experienced as they took on new views of their situation and thus behaved differently. In this study, hearing women's voices as distinct and different and not part of a collective "family voice" seems in keeping with the best that the postmodern movement has to offer.

▪▪▪▪ SYSTEMS THEORY

General systems theory, introduced in 1936 by von Bertalanffy, has been applied to the understanding of families for a number of years by health professionals. In addition to the original writings on systems theory by von Bertalanffy (1968, 1972, 1974), numerous articles and chapters in books have also been written on systems theory and its concepts. This proliferation of systems information is also evident within nursing literature.

One of the most useful analogies that highlights systems concepts as applied to families is offered by Allmond, Buckman, and Gofman (1979). They suggest that, when thinking of the family as a system, it is useful to compare it to a mobile:

> Visualize a mobile with four or five pieces suspended from the ceiling, gently moving in the air. The whole is in balance, steady yet moving. Some pieces are moving rapidly; others are almost stationary. Some are heavier and appear to carry more weight in the ultimate direction of the mobile's movement; others seem to go along for the ride. A breeze catching only one segment of the mobile immediately influences movement of every piece, some more than

others, and the pace picks up with some pieces unbalancing themselves and moving chaotically about for a time. Gradually the whole exerts its influence in the errant part(s) and balance is re-established but not before a decided change in direction of the whole may have taken place. You will also notice the changeability regarding closeness and distance among pieces, the impact of actual contact one with another, and the importance of vertical hierarchy. Coalitions of movement may be observed between two pieces. Or one piece may persistently appear isolated from the others; yet its position of isolation is essential to the balancing of the entire system (p. 16).

Keeping the analogy of the mobile in mind, some of the most useful concepts of systems theory, which have frequent application in clinical practice with families, are highlighted in the following paragraphs. These systems concepts provide a theoretical foundation for understanding the family as a system. A system can be defined as a complex of elements in mutual interaction. When this definition is applied to families, it allows us to view the family as a unit and thus focus on observing the interaction among family members rather than studying family members individually. However, remember that each individual family member is both a subsystem and a system in its own right. An individual system is *both* a part and a whole, as is a family.

> *Concept 1*
> **A family system is part of a larger suprasystem and in turn is composed of many subsystems.**

The concept of hierarchy of systems is very useful when applied to families. A family is composed of many subsystems such as parent-child, marital, and sibling subsystems. These subsystems are also composed of subsystems of individuals. Individuals are very complex systems composed of various subsystems, physical (e.g. cardiovascular, reproductive), or psychological (e.g., cognitive, affective). At the same time, the family is also one unit nested in larger suprasystems such as neighborhoods, organizations, or church communities. It is helpful to visualize a system by drawing a large circle and placing the elements, parts, or variables inside the circle. Then, inside the circle, lines can be drawn among the component parts. Outside of the circle is the larger context, where all other factors impinging on the system may be placed. Thus, a nurse can draw a circle to visualize a family and then place the individual family members within it (Fig. 2–1).

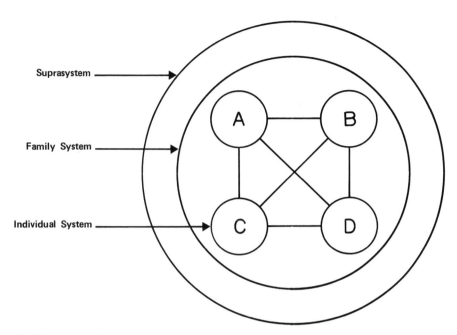

FIGURE 2–1. The family as it relates to other systems.

Systems are arbitrarily defined by their boundaries, which aid in specifying what is inside or outside the system. Normally, boundaries are associated with living systems of a physical nature, such as the number of people in a family or the skin of an individual. It is also possible to construct a boundary and, therefore, create a system around ideas, beliefs, expectations, or roles. For example, there could be a system of multiple roles for a person such as daughter, wife, sister, nurse, and mother.

When working with families, it is most useful to initially consider:

- Who is in *this* family system?
- What are some of the important subsystems?
- What are some of the significant suprasystems to which the family belongs?

From time to time, however, it may be useful to draw a boundary (in one's mind) and create, for example, a system of parental beliefs about the use of corporal punishment with children.

In addition, within family systems and their subsystems it is useful to assess the amount of permeability of the boundaries. In family systems, the boundary must be both permeable and limiting. If the family boundary is too permeable, the system loses identity and integrity (e.g., too open to ideas and input from the outside environment) and therefore does not allow the family to use its own resources in decision making. However, if it is too closed or impermeable, necessary interaction with the larger world is shut off (e.g., an immigrant family from Bosnia relocated in Pennsylvania may inadvertently remain closed initially because of great differences in language and culture largely defined by the information or communication that crosses over).

The concept of hierarchy of systems and the boundaries that create systems is a most useful concept to apply when working with and attempting to conceptualize the uniqueness of each particular family. In certain ethnic groups, it is essential to honor hierarchy and boundaries, for example, in Iranian families.

Concept 2
The family as a whole is greater than the sum of its parts.

This concept of systems theory applied to families emphasizes that the family's "wholeness" is more than simply the addition of each family member. It also emphasizes that individuals are best understood within their larger context, which is normally the family. To study individual family members separately does not equate to studying the family as a unit. By studying the whole family, it is possible to observe interaction among family members, which often explains more fully individual family member functioning. For example, a young Filipino mother complains to the community health nurse (CHN) that her 3-year-old child has temper tantrums, which she is not able to control, and she is asking for guidance. The CHN could intervene in a variety of ways:

- See the mother individually and discuss some behavioral methods that could be used to assist in controlling her child's temper tantrums.
- See the child individually and do an individual assessment.
- See the whole family (mother, father and child) and do a child-and-family assessment (see Chap. 3) in order to understand the child, the child's behavior in the family context, and the Filipino family's beliefs about discipline.

The CHN chose to see the whole family because the CHN understood the importance of Concept 2. During the first session with the family, the child was very well behaved in the interview for the first half hour. Then the child had a temper tantrum, in response to which the mother became annoyed and the father withdrew. The CHN was astute enough to observe the sequence of interaction before the temper tantrum. When the child had the temper tantrum, the parents were in a heated argument about their parenting styles. When the temper tantrum started, the parents stopped arguing and focused on the child. This child was most likely responding to the tension between the parents, and thus the temper tantrums invited the parents to stop their conflict. Thus, the temper tantrums were understood quite differently in the context of the family than they would have been if the child had been assessed in isolation.

Therefore, it is important that nurses see *whole* families when possible to more fully understand family member functioning by observing family interaction. This enables an appreciation of the relationships existing among family members as well as individual family member functioning. Ranson (1984) emphasizes this point by stating that "we cannot understand the parts of a body, a family, a practice, a theory, unless we know how the whole works, for the parts can be understood only in relation to the whole; conversely, we cannot grasp how the whole works unless we have an understanding of its parts" (p. 231).

Concept 3
A change in one family member affects all family members.

This concept aids the recognition that any significant event or change in one family member will affect all family members in varying degrees, as illustrated in the analogy of the mobile. The concept can be most useful to nurses when thinking of the impact of illness on the family. For example, the father of a Malaysian family experienced a coronary, which affected all family members and various family member relationships. The father and mother were unable to continue their active interest in sports together, and the mother increased her employment from part-time to full-time to assist with the substantially reduced income during the father's convalescence. The eldest daughter, who had been more remote from the family since her marriage, began visiting her father more often. The youngest daughter, by providing emotional support, became closer to her mother. Thus all family members were affected and the usual organization and functioning of the family were changed.

This concept can also be used to understand the impact of the nurse and family coconstructing interventions to change the family system. That is, if one family member begins to change, other family members will be unable to respond as previously because one family member is now behaving differently.

> **Concept 4**
> **The family is able to create a balance between change and stability.**

Over the past few years, there has been a shift away from the belief that families tend toward maintaining equilibrium. Instead, there is now a trend toward the belief that families are really in a constant state of flux and are always changing. The pendulum has now swung to the other end of the continuum. However, von Bertalanffy (1968) warned us some years ago to avoid this polarized view of families. He suggested that systems, in this case family systems, are able to achieve a balance among the forces operating within them and on them and that change and stability can coexist in living systems (see Change Theory later in this chapter).

However, when change occurs in a family, there is a shift to a new position of balance after a disturbance. The family reorganizes or recalibrates in a way that is different from any previous organization of the family. For example, if a family member has a diagnosis of multiple sclerosis, the entire family will have to reorganize itself in ways that are totally different from before the diagnosis. However, the balance between change and stability will constantly shift in periods of remission and exacerbation, but more often there will be a balance between change and stability.

The concept of change and stability coexisting is perhaps one of the most difficult concepts of systems theory for nurses to understand. This is partly because, in actual clinical practice, families frequently present themselves "as if" they are in total equilibrium or "as if" they are constantly changing rather than manifesting an observable balance between the two. However, the more experienced one becomes in family nursing, the greater appreciation one has for the complexity of families. When families are "stuck" or experiencing severe difficulties, frequently they are polarized in maintaining rigid equilibrium or are in a phase of too much change. Eventually, the family will need to find solutions to obtain a more equal balance between the phenomena of stability and change.

> **Concept 5**
> **Family members' behaviors are best understood from a view of circular rather than linear causality.**

One method of dealing with the massive amounts of data presented in a family interview is to observe for patterns. Tomm (1981) offers a very useful discussion of the differences between linear and circular patterns.

> One major difference between linear and circular patterns lies in the overall structure of the connections between elements of the pattern. Linear patterns are limited to sequences (e.g. A→ B → C) whereas circular patterns form a closed loop and are recursive (e.g. A → B → C → A → . . . or A → B, B → C, C → A). A less obvious but more significant difference lies in the relative importance usually given to *time* and *meaning* when making the connections or links in the pattern. Linearity is heavily rooted in a framework of a continuous progression of time . . . *Circularity* . . . is more heavily dependent on *a framework of reciprocal relationships based on meaning* (p. 85).

Linear causality, defined as one event causing another, can serve a useful and helpful function for individuals and families. For example, when the clock strikes 6 PM, a family will routinely eat supper. This is an example of linear causality because event A (the clock striking 6 PM) is seen as the cause of event B (the eating of supper (A → B), whereas event B, does not affect event A.

However, circular causality occurs when event B *does* affect event A. For example, if a spouse takes an interest in his wife's ostomy care (event A) and the wife responds by explaining the daily procedures (event B), then it is likely to result in the husband continuing to take an interest and offer support regarding his wife's ostomy care and his wife feeling supported, and thus the cycle continues. (A → B → A). Each individual's behavior has an effect on and influences the other. A method for diagramming these circular interactional patterns will be discussed in Chapter 3.

The application of these concepts in clinical practice affects the nurse's style of questioning during a family interview. Linear questions tend to explore *descriptive* characteristics (e.g., "Is the father fearful of another heart attack?"), whereas circular questions may explore interactional characteristics. Types of circular questions include: difference questions (e.g., "Who's the most worried about Sunil having another heart attack?"), behavioral effect questions (e.g., "What do you do when your wife's pain becomes unbearable for you?"), hypothetical or future-oriented questions (e.g., "What might you do in the future to prevent your elderly father from falling?"), and triadic questions (e.g., "When your Dad shows support to your sister Manisha, how does your Mom feel?") (Selvini-Palazzoli, Boscolo, Cecchin, & Prata, 1980; Loos and Bell, 1990; Tomm, 1984, 1985, 1987a, 1987b, 1988). Bateson (1979) offers the idea that "information consists of differences that make a difference" (p. 99). Tomm (1981) connects the idea of "differences" to relationships:

> Differences between perceptions/objects/events/ideas/etc. are regarded as the basic source of all information and consequent knowledge. On closer examination, one can see that such *relationships are always reciprocal or circular.* If she is shorter than he, then he is taller than she. If she is dominant, then he is submissive. If one member of the family is defined as being bad, then the others are being defined as being good. Even at a very simple level, a circular orientation allows implicit information to become more explicit and offers alternative points of view. A linear orientation on the other hand is narrow and restrictive and tends to mask important data (Tomm, 1981, p. 93).

Various types of assessment and interventive questions that could be asked during a family interview are highlighted in Chapters 3, 4, 6, 7, and 8.

With regard to family member interaction, the assumption is made that each person contributes to adaptive as well as maladaptive interaction. For example, a common problem presented in geriatric healthcare facilities is an elderly parent complaining that the adult children don't visit enough and therefore frequently withdrawing, whereas the adult children complain that their elderly parent constantly nags them when visiting. Each is "correct" in the perception of the other but does not recognize how each person's behavior influences the behavior of the other.

Normally, families and individual family members need to be helped to move from a linear perspective of their situation to a more interactional, reciprocal, and systemic view. This is possible only if the nurse doesn't become caught in linear thinking when attempting to understand family dynamics.

These five concepts are by no means inclusive of all systems concepts, but reflect those deemed the most significant and important to serve as a theoretical foundation when working with families.

▦▦▦ CYBERNETICS

Cybernetics is the science of communication and control theory. The term cybernetics was originally coined by a mathematician, Norbert Weiner. We believe it is important to differentiate between general systems theory and cybernetics, and we do not use the terms synonymously, although some regard each as a branch of the other. Systems theory is primarily concerned with changing our conceptual focus from parts to wholes, whereas, cybernetics changes focus from substance to form.

Concept 1
Family systems possess self-regulating ability.

Interpersonal systems, particularly family systems, "may be viewed as feedback loops, since the behavior of each person affects and is affected by the behavior of each other person" (Waltzlawick, Beavin, & Jackson, 1967, p. 31). For any substantial change to occur in a relationship the regulatory limits must be adjusted so that a new range of behaviors is possible or an entirely new pattern can emerge (transformation) (Tomm, 1980, p. 8). Tomm (1980) has offered a useful method of applying cybernetic regulatory concepts in actual clinical interviewing. His method of diagramming circular patterns of communication will be discussed in Chapter 3.

Concept 2
Feedback processes can simultaneously occur at several systems levels with families.

Initially, the application of cybernetic concepts in family work began by observations of simple phenomena (e.g., wife criticizes, husband withdraws), which is generally referred to as simple cybernetics. However, as cyberneticians began examining more complex orders of phenomena, they developed a recognition of different orders of feedback (e.g., feedback of feedback, change of change). "Margaret Mead suggested that the field call this perspective of higher-order process 'cybernetics of cybernetics'" (Keeney, 1982, p. 158). Maturana and Varela (1980) suggest a higher-order cybernetics that links the organization of living process and cognition. A further labeling by von Foerester (1974) makes the distinction between first-order cybernetics or the cybernetics of simple feedback and second-order cybernetics or the cybernetics of cybernetics.

Therefore, the simple feedback phenomenon observed in the interactional pattern of criticizing wife-withdrawing husband may also be understood to be part of a larger feedback loop involving the couple's relationship to their families of origin, which may recalibrate the lower-order loop of the couple's interaction. Thus, cybernetics of cybernetics moves into a larger context that includes both the observer and the observed. There is a recursive analysis that emphasizes the internal structure of the system and the mutual connectedness of the observer and the observed (Varela, 1979).

▩▩▩ COMMUNICATION THEORY

The focus of the study of communication is how individuals interact with one another. One of the most significant contributions to our understanding of interpersonal processes is the classic book *Pragmatics of Human Communication* (1967) by Waltzlawick, Beavin, and Jackson. The concepts presented here are primarily drawn from this important book on communication and have been updated by the recent research studies of Janet Beavin Bavelas (1992).

Concept 1
All nonverbal communication is meaningful.

This concept helps us to realize that there is no such thing as *not* communicating because all nonverbal communication carries a message in the presence of another (Waltzlawick, Beavin, & Jackson, 1967). In personal communication with Dr. Janet Beavin Bevelas, and in her 1992 publication, she states that she now makes a distinction between nonverbal behavior (NVB) and nonverbal communication (NVC). NVC is viewed as a subset of NVB. With NVB there is an "inference-making observer," whereas with NVC there is a "communicating person" (encoder). In the original text, the concept was presented that all NVB is meaningful.

A significant component of this concept is context. Behavior is relevant and meaningful only when the immediate context is considered.

A mother complains to the CHN that she has been experiencing insomnia for 2 months and finds herself very irritable because of the prolonged sleep deprivation. This behavior of the mother needs to be understood in her immediate context. On further exploration, the nurse discovered that this mother has a child on an apnea monitor and that the father sleeps soundly. Also, the family apartment is very close to a subway. Therefore the mother's insomnia will be understood and treated more fully by the CHN with this additional context information.

Concept 2
All communication has two major channels for transmission: digital and analogical.

Digital communication is what is normally referred to as verbal communication. It consists of the actual content of the message or the brute facts. For example, a man may say, "I have lost 15 pounds this past month," or a 10-year-old girl may say, "I can now give myself my own insulin." However, when the analogical communication is also taken into account, the meaning of these facts may change dramatically.

Analogical communication consists not only of the usual types of nonverbal communication such as body posture, facial expression, and tone but also of music, poetry, and painting. It can be seen that a man who is quite obese and states that he has lost 15 pounds in a month will give a more positive message, both digitally and analogically, than a man who is very emaciated and states that he has lost 15 pounds.

In discussing the two channels of communication, we do not wish to imply that there are separate verbal and nonverbal channels dedicated to different uses. Bavelas (1992) has accumulated "a great deal of data in favor of an alternative, 'whole message model' in which verbal and nonverbal acts are completely integrated and often interchangeable" (p. 23). Based on our clinical experience, we agree with her research experience that nonverbal communication is an integrated part of language.

If there are discrepancies between analogical and digital communication (e.g., when a teenager states, "It doesn't bother me" regarding being in a cumbersome cast but the teenager's eyes are filled with tears) then the analogical mode of communicating is considered more pertinent to the nurse's observing eye. To the teenager's friend, the digital communication may be the most relevant.

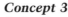

> **Concept 3**
> **A dyadic relationship has varying degrees of symmetry and complementarity.**

The terms symmetry and complementarily are very useful in identifying typical family interaction patterns. Jackson (1973) discussed these terms:

> A complementary relationship consists of one individual giving and the other receiving. In a complementary relationship, the two people are of unequal status in the sense that one appears to be in the superior position, meaning that he initiates action and the other appears to follow that action. Thus the two individuals fit together or complement each other. The most obvious and basic complementary relationship would be the mother and infant. A symmetrical relationship is one between two people who behave as if they have equal status. Each person exhibits the rights to initiate action, criticize the other, offer advice and so on. This type of relationship tends to become competitive; if one person mentions that he has succeeded in some endeavor the other person mentions that he has succeeded in an equally important endeavor. The individuals in such a relationship emphasize their equality or their symmetry with each other. The most obvious symmetrical relationship is a pre-adolescent peer relationship (p. 189).

There are many situations in which complementary and symmetrical relationships are appropriate and healthy. For example, an employee needs to be able to take a one-down position to the employer most of the time. If the employee is unable to do this, it could result in increasing conflict and eventually a relationship that is predominantly symmetrical. This symmetrical escalation could have the end result of the employer dismissing the employee or the employee quitting on unpleasant terms. An example of a healthy symmetrical relationship could be two individuals involved in a tennis match.

In family relationships, the *predominance* of complementary *or* symmetrical behavior usually results in problems. In some cultural groups there may be a preference for one style over another. Couples, especially, need to experience a balance between situations and experiences where symmetry and complementarity exist. Parent-child relationships however, need to experience a gradual shift from a predominantly complementary relationship as the child moves into the teenage and young adult years to a more symmetrical relationship.

> **Concept 4**
> **All communication has two levels: content and relationship.**

Communication consists not only of what is being said (content) but also of giving information that defines the nature of the relationship between those interacting. For example, a father may say to his son, "Come over here, son; I want to tell you something," or "*Get* over here; I've got something to *tell you!*" These statements are similar in content, but each implies a very different relationship. The first statement could be viewed as part of a loving relationship; the second statement implies a conflictual relationship. In this instance, it is the tone of the content that gives evidence to a particular kind of relationship.

CHANGE THEORY

The process of change is a fascinating phenomenon with a variety of ideas about how and what constitutes change in family systems. An extensive review of the literature will be synthesized and presented with the most profound and salient points followed by our own beliefs about change and the conditions that affect the change process.

Systems of relationships appear to possess a tendency toward progressive change (Bateson, 1979). However, there is a French proverb that states, "the more something changes, the more it remains the same." This beautifully highlights the dilemma frequently faced in working with families. The nurse must learn to accept the challenge of the paradoxical relationship between persistence (stability) and change. Maturana (1978) explains the recursiveness of change and stability in this way: change is an alteration in the family's structure that occurs as compensation for perturbations and has the purpose of maintaining structure (i.e., stability). Change itself is experienced as a perturbation to the system so change generates further change and also stability. A change in state is seen as behavior and therefore differences in family interactional patterns must be explored. Changes in behavior may or may not be accompanied by insight. However, "the most profound and sustaining change will be that which occurs within the family's belief system (cognition)" (Wright & Watson, 1988, p. 425).

Watzlawick, Weakland, and Fisch (1974) suggest that persistence and change need to be considered together despite their opposing natures. They have offered a widely accepted notion of change and have suggested that there are two different types or levels of change. One type they refer to as change occurring within a given system that remains unchanged itself. In other words, the system itself remains unchanged while its elements or parts undergo some type of change. This type of change is referred to as *first-order change*. It is a change in quantity, not quality. First-order change involves using the same problem-solving strategies over and over again. Each new problem is approached mechanically. If a solution to the problem is difficult to find, more old strategies are used and are usually more vigorously applied. An example of first-order change is the learning of a new behavioral strategy to deal with a misbehaving child. A parent who formerly disciplined his child by restricting the child's access to the computer is said to have undergone first-order change when he now limits the child's spending money.

The second type of change is one that changes the system itself. This type of change is referred to as *second-order change.* Second-order change is thus a "change of change." It appears that the French proverb is applicable only to first-order change. Regarding second-order change, there are actual changes in the rules governing the system, and therefore the system is transformed structurally or communicationally. It is also important to note that second-order change is always in the nature of a discontinuity or logical jump and tends to be sudden and radical. This type of change represents a quantum jump in the system to a different level of functioning. Second-order change can be said to occur, for example, when parents begin to treat their 16-year-old as an adolescent instead of as a child.

Watzlawick, Weakland, and Fisch (1974) also refer to the most obvious source of change. This is *spontaneous* change, by which they mean the type of problem resolution that occurs in daily living without the input of professionals or sophisticated theories. For example, an anorexic young woman suddenly and apparently spontaneously begins to eat regularly after 2 years of not doing so, or a man suffering from shingles (herpes zoster) reports that his chronic pain disappeared overnight.

Bateson (1979) offers a most thought-provoking statement with regard to change when he suggests that we are almost always unaware of changes. He suggests that changes in our social interactions and in our environment around us are occurring dramatically and constantly, but that we become accustomed to the "new state of affairs before our senses can tell us that it is new" (p. 98). Bateson further offers the idea that, with regard to the perception of change, the mind can only receive news of difference. Therefore, change can be observed, as Bateson (1972) states, as "difference which occurs across time" (p. 452). These ideas also concur with those of Maturana and Varela (1992), who offer the idea that change is occurring in humans from moment to moment.

This change is either triggered by interaction(s) or perturbations coming from the environment in which the system (family member) exists or is a result of the system's (family member's) own internal dynamics.

Our own view of change in family work has been drawn from the above authors as well as our own clinical experience in working with families. In summary, we believe with Bateson and Maturana and Varela that change *is* constantly evolving in families and that frequently we are unaware of it. This is the type of continuous or spontaneous change that occurs with everyday living and progression through individual and family stages of development. These changes may or may not occur with professional input.

We also believe that major transformation of an entire family system can occur and can be precipitated by major life events such as illness, divorce, unemployment, or death of a family member; or by interventions from professionals such as nurses. Change within a family may occur within the cognitive, affective, or behavioral domains, but change in any one domain will have an impact on the other domain. Interventions can be aimed at any or all three domains. Interventions will be discussed further in Chapter 4, in which the Calgary Family Intervention Model is presented. We believe that it is impossible to know what interventions result in what changes, and therefore it is impossible to predict outcome or the type of change that will occur within families.

An important role for nurses (operating from a systems perspective) is to carefully observe the connections between systems. To effect change within the original system (e.g., individual), it is necessary to intervene at a higher systems level or the metalevel (e.g., family system [see Fig. 2–1]). In other words, if nurses wish to effect change within a family system, they need to be able to maintain a metaposition to the family. They must simultaneously conceptualize both the family system interactions and their own interactions with the family. However, if a problem arises between the nurse and the family, this problem will need to be resolved at a higher level (e.g., nurse-family system), preferably by a supervisor, who can examine the problem from a further metaposition.

> *Concept 1*
> **Change is dependent on the perception of the problem.**

In a now-famous statement, Alfred Korzybski proclaimed that "the map is not the territory." In other words, the name is different from the thing named and the description is different from what is described. In applying this to family interviewing, our "mapping" of a particular situation or our perception of a problem or problems follows from how we, as nurses, choose to see it. How we perceive a particular problem has profound implications for how we will intervene and, therefore, how change will occur and whether it will be effective.

One of the most common traps for nurses working with families is acceptance of one family member's perception as the "truth" or deciding who is "right." Of course there is no one "truth" or "reality," or perhaps it is more accurate to say that there are as many "truths" or "realities" as there are members of the family (Maturana & Varela, 1992). The important task for the nurse is to accept all family members' perceptions and offer the family another view of their problems. Individual family members draw forth their own reality of a situation based on their history of interactions with persons throughout their lives and their genetic history (Maturana & Varela, 1992). Maturana, in an interview with Simon (1985), offered an even more radical idea with regard to different family members' perceptions:

> Systems theory first enabled us to recognize that all the different views presented by the different members of a family had some validity. But, systems theory implied that these were different views of the same system. What I am saying is different. I am *not* saying that the different descriptions that the members of a family make are different views of the *same* system. I am saying that there is no one way which the system is; that there is no absolute, objective family. I am saying that for each member there is a different family; and that each of these is absolutely valid (p. 36).

Although Maturana and Varela (1992) emphasize that human systems "bring forth" reality, constructivists, be they radical constructivists (von Glaserfeld, 1984) or social constructionists, emphasize that reality is constructed or is invented (Watzlawick, 1984). One example of the constructivist view from Furth (1987) is that "(the world) is patently not a fixed reality and even less a particular physical environment, but most definitely a world of ever-changing individual constructions, or better . . . a world of social co-constructions" (p. 86).

We concur that there are indeed very different, yet valid perceptions of problems. However, as nurses, we are part of a larger societal system and thus are bound by moral, legal, cultural, and societal norms that require us to act in accordance with these norms regarding illegal or dangerous behaviors (Wright, Watson, & Bell, 1990; 1996).

If a nurse does not conceptualize human problems from a systems/cybernetics perspective, the nurse's perceptions of problems will be based on a completely *different* conception of "reality" based on *different* theoretical assumptions. We wish to emphasize *different* theoretical assumptions as opposed to more correct or "right" views of problems.

> **Concept 2**
> **Change is determined by structure.**

Changes that occur in a living system are governed by the present structure of that system. The concept of structural determinism (Maturana & Varela, 1992) offers the notion that each individual's biopsychosocial-spiritual structure is unique and is a product of the individual's genetic history (phylogeny) as well as his or her history of interactions over time (ontogeny).

The implication for nursing practice is that an individual's present structure specifies the interpersonal, intrapersonal, and environmental influences that will be experienced as "perturbations," that is, which interactions will trigger structural changes. Therefore, we cannot say beforehand which family nursing interventions will be useful in promoting change for this particular family member at this time and which will not. Individuals, therefore, are selectively "perturbed" by the interventions that are offered by nurses according to what fits or does not fit their own unique biopsychosocial-spiritual structures. We cannot predict which family nursing interventions will fit for a particular person and which, therefore, will disturb that person's structure and which will not.

A deep respect for and curiosity about family members develops in nurses who are cognizant of the notion of structural determinism. When Maturana and Varela's concept of structural determinism is applied to clinical work with families, Wright and Levac (1992) suggest that the description of families as noncompliant, resistant, or unmotivated is not only "an epistemological error but a biological impossibility" (p. 913). This concept has made a dramatic difference in the way in which we think about families and the interventions that are offered by nurses.

> **Concept 3**
> **Change is dependent on context.**

Efforts to promote change in a family system must always take into account the important variable of context. Interventions must be planned with sufficient knowledge of the contextual constraints and resources. This is particularly important considering the emphasis in the healthcare industry on accountability, cost-effectiveness, efficiency, and time-effective intervention. Nurses need to be aware of their position in the healthcare delivery system vis-à-vis the family. For example, are other professionals involved with the family, and if so, what is their role with the family? How does this differ from the nurse's role and how are the nurse and family influenced by and influencing the context in which they find themselves? We find it particularly useful to underscore the positive contributions each healthcare stakeholder can make to the family's care rather than attributing or assuming self-serving motives to stakeholders who have different vested interests in family care (e.g., limiting costs).

Larger systems (e.g., schools, mental health agencies, hospitals, and public service delivery systems) frequently impose certain "rules" on families that ultimately serve to maintain the larger system's stability and impede change (Imber Coppersmith, 1983; Imber-Black, 1991). The first is the "rule" of linear blame. That is, institutions tend to blame families for difficulties (e.g., unmotivated family) and tend to make referrals for family treatment in order to "cure" the family. This is a process similar to that used by families in sending the identified patient to be "cured."

Because members of some larger systems, particularly hospital staff, become intensely involved in a patient or family member's life, they frequently have a tendency to go beyond the immediate concerns. The end result is that patients in hospitals and their families find themselves inundated with services that frequently usurp the family's own resources. This then places the family in a one-down position in terms of articulating what *they* perceive their present needs to be. When a nurse decides or is asked to complete a family assessment, the nurse may become one more irritant in the life of this family and can be hamstrung before even beginning because of the number of professionals involved. This is another reason why nurses should carefully assess the larger context in which the family and the staff find themselves. In some of these cases, the more serious problem(s) is at the interface of the family with other professionals rather than *within* the family itself. Thus, interventions would need to be targeted at the family-professional system *before* addressing problems at the family system level.

Another situation that can arise is unclear expertise and leadership. Families may find themselves in a larger system, such as an outpatient drug assessment and treatment clinic. Families may receive varying ideas on how to deal with a particular problem (e.g., cocaine addiction), depending on whether they are seen at the clinic, at home, or in a class. Usually this occurs because no one clinic or educational program offered within a hospital setting has any more decision-making power than another regarding a particular family's treatment plan.

Conflicts can also occur between larger systems or between families and larger systems. Unacknowledged or unresolved conflicts often result in triads, which inhibit healthy behavior. For example, if the family wishes to send their adolescent to a drug rehabilitation center but the nurse and rehab director have been in conflict over rehab policies, the family is placed in a situation in which pressure from the larger system (nurse-rehab director system) leads them to align or take sides with *either* the nurse or the rehab director.

How the family is being influenced and is influencing their involvement with these suprasystems is important information. Change within a family can be thwarted, sabotaged, or impossible if the issue of context is not addressed.

Concept 4
Change is dependent on coevolving goals for treatment.

Change requires that goals be coevolved between nurses and families within a realistic time frame. Frequently, one of the main reasons for failure in working with families is either the nurse's or family's setting of unrealistic or inappropriate goals. Frank and open discussions with family members regarding treatment goals can often avoid misunderstanding and disappointments on both sides.

Because one of the primary goals in family intervention is to change or alter the family's view or beliefs of the problem or illness, nurses can help family members to search for alternative behavioral, cognitive, and affective responses to problems. Therefore, one of the goals of the nurse is to help the family discover its own solutions to problems.

The task of setting specific goals for treatment is accomplished in collaboration with the family. Part of the assessment process is to identify the problems that the family is most concerned with at present and the changes they would like to see in relation to these problems. This provides the baseline for the goals of family interviews and becomes the therapeutic contract.

Contracts with families can be either verbal or written. In our own clinical practice and in the practice of our nursing students, we normally make verbal contracts with families stating which specific problems will be tackled during what specified period of time or sessions.

At the end of that period, progress is evaluated and either contact with the family is terminated or a new contract made if further therapeutic work is required.

In most instances, clear goals in the form of a contract will be set with families with obtained verbal commitments by family members to work on the problems outlined. On conclusion of the contract, evaluation should consist of assessing changes in the family system in addition to changes in the identified patient.

In summary, family assessment and intervention are often more effective and successful if based on clear therapeutic goals. However, it is very uncommon for families to come to family interviews with the understanding that *family* change is required. Therefore, in addition to setting goals, the nurse must help the family to obtain a different view of their problems. First the nurse needs to engage the family, and this can most easily be accomplished by focusing on the presenting problem *first* and the changes the family desires in relation to it. More information about goal setting is given in Chapter 7.

> **Concept 5**
> **Understanding alone does not lead to change.**

Changes in family work rarely occur by increasing a family's understanding of problems but rather through changes in their beliefs and behavior. Too often, health professionals engaged in family work assume that *understanding* a problem will bring about a solution by the family. From a systems perspective, however, we believe that solutions to problems come about as beliefs about problems and patterns change, whether or not this is accompanied by insight.

There has been a tendency in nursing to believe that, to solve a problem, one has to understand *"why."* Thus, nurses with good intentions spend many hours attempting to obtain masses of data (usually historical) that will lead them to understand the "why" of a problem. Often the patient, the family, or both will encourage the nurse in this quest and even participate in it. For example, a patient might ask: "Why did I have my heart attack?" "Why won't my son give up crack?" or "Why did my wife have to die so young?" We strongly *discourage* searching for the answers because we do not feel that this is a precondition for change; rather, it steers one away from effective efforts at change. We strongly suggest that the prerequisite or precondition for change is not understanding the *"why"* of a situation but rather understanding the *"what!"* Therefore, we recommend that nurses ask, *"What* is the effect of the father's heart attack on him and his family?" *"What* are the implications of the father's heart attack on his employment?" These serve a much more useful purpose in paving the way for possible interventions than wasting time on the "why" of the situation.

"Why" questions seem to be entrenched in psychoanalytic roots that bring forth psychopathologies. This is not congruent with a systems or cybernetic foundation of understanding family dynamics that focuses on human problems as interpersonal escalations or dilemmas. Even if the "why" of a problem *is* occasionally understood, it rarely contributes toward its solution. Therefore, it is more useful to explore what is being *done* in the here and now that serves to perpetuate the problem and what can be done in the here and now to effect a change (Watzlawick, Weakland, & Fisch, 1974). We need to avoid the search for causes because we are then invited to view problems from a linear rather than a systemic perspective. In other words, we prefer to think that problems reside *between* persons rather than *within* persons.

> **Concept 6**
> **Change does not necessarily occur equally in all family members.**

Remembering the analogy of the mobile presented previously in this chapter, imagine the mobile *after* a wind has passed on it. Some pieces would turn or react more rapidly or energetically than others. This is similar to change in family systems, in that one family member may begin to respond or change more rapidly than others and by this very process set up an opportunity for change throughout the rest of the family. This is so because other family members will not be able to respond in the same way to the family member who is changing and, therefore, there will be a ripple effect of change through the system.

Change depends on the recursive (cybernetic) nature of a family system. Therefore, a small intervention can lead to a variety of reactions, with some family members changing more dramatically or quickly than others.

> **Concept 7**
> **Facilitating change is the nurse's responsibility.**

It is our belief that it is the nurse's responsibility to facilitate change in collaboration with each family. Facilitating change doesn't presuppose that a nurse can predict the outcome, nor should the nurse be invested in a particular outcome. However, there is a distinct difference between facilitating change and being an expert in resolving family problems. We believe that families possess expertise and nurses have expertise. It is also crucial for nurses to avoid making value judgments about how families *should* function. Otherwise, the changes or outcomes in a family system may not be satisfying to the nurse if they are incongruent with how the *nurse* perceives a family should function. It is more important that the *family* be satisfied with their new level of functioning than that the nurse be satisfied.

From time to time, nurses need to evaluate the level or degree of responsibility they feel for treatment. The level of responsibility is out of proportion if the nurse feels more concerned, more worried, or more responsible for family problems than the families themselves. The opposite response can be a detachment involving lack of concern or responsibility on the part of the nurse for facilitating change within families. Both of these extreme responses are indicators for obtaining clinical supervision.

How much change nurses should expect themselves to be able to facilitate in family work depends on their own competence, the context of family treatment, and the response of the family. Nurses need to be cognizant that they are not change agents; they cannot and do not change anyone (Wright & Levac, 1992). Changes in family members are determined by the members' own biopsychosocial structures, not by those of others (Maturana & Varela, 1992). Therefore, it is the nurse's responsibility to facilitate a context for change.

> **Concept 8**
> **Change occurs by means of a "fit" or meshing between the therapeutic offerings (interventions) of the nurse and the biopsychosocial-spiritual structures of family members.**

The concept of fit arises from the notion of structural determinism (Maturana & Varela, 1992). It is the family member's structure, not the nurse's therapeutic offering, that determines whether or not the intervention is experienced as a perturbation that triggers change.

The concept of fit is aligned with the guiding principle that the nurse is not a change agent (Wright & Levac, 1992) but is rather one who, among other things, creates a context for change. In our clinical experience, family members who respond to particular therapeutic offerings do so because of the fit or meshing between their current biopsychosocial-spiritual structures and the family nursing intervention offered (see Chap. 4). This includes a nurse being sensitive to the family's race, ethnicity, and social class.

The concept of "fit" allows us to be nonblaming of clients and ourselves when "nonfit" and, therefore, "nonadherence" and "nonfollow-through" occur (Wright, Watson, & Bell, 1996). Nurses operating from a therapeutic stance appreciative of fit can be highly curious about ways to increase the fit for these family members at this time. When the concept of fit is overlooked, neglected, or not appreciated, nurses operate with more lecturing, prescribing behaviors, and often label family members as noncompliant, not ready for change, or challenging the professional system.

Concept 9
Change can have a myriad of causes.

Change is influenced by so many different variables that most often it is difficult to know what *specifically* precipitated or triggered the change. It is not always a result of some well-thought-out intervention. Frequently, it can be the result of the method of inquiry into family problems. Asking interventive questions (see Chap. 4) may in and of itself promote change. It is more important to attribute change to the family than to concern oneself about what the *nurse* did to create change (see Chap. 10). To search for or take undue credit for change is inappropriate at this stage of our knowledge of the change process in families.

■■■ BIOLOGY OF COGNITION

The biology of cognition has been described and articulated by two neurobiologists, Maturana and Varela (1992), in their landmark publication *The Tree of Knowledge: The Biological Roots of Human Understanding.* They offer the idea that humans bring forth different views to their understanding of events and experiences in their lives. This idea is not new, but their perspective on how we humans make and claim observations is much more radical: it is based on biology and physiology, not philosophy (Wright & Levac, 1992). If a nurse adopts a particular view of reality, it follows that a nurse now encompasses a particular view of persons and their functioning, relationships, and illness.

> **Concept 1**
> **Two possible avenues for explaining our world are objectivity and objectivity-in-parentheses (Maturana & Varela, 1992; Wright & Levac, 1992).**

The view of objectivity assumes that there is one ultimate domain of reference for explaining the world. Within this domain, entities are assumed to exist independent of the observer. Such entities are as numerous and broad as imagination might allow and may be explicitly or implicitly identified as mind, knowledge, truth, and so on. Within this avenue of explanation, we come to believe we have access to a true and correct view of the world and its events, an objective reality. From this "objectivist" view, "a system and its components have a constancy and a stability that is independent of the observer that brings them forth" (Mendez, Coddou, & Maturana, 1988, p.154). Nursing diagnoses, emotional conflict, pride, and politics are all products of an "objective" view of reality.

When objectivity is placed in parentheses, persons recognize that objects do exist but are not independent of the living system that brings them forth. The only "truths" that exist are those brought forth by observers, such as nurses and family members. Each person's view is not a distortion of some presumably correct interpretation. Instead of one objective universe waiting to be discovered or correctly described, Maturana has proposed a "multiverse," where many observer "verses" coexist, each valid in its own right. To increase options and possibilities for families to cope with illness or improve their well-being, nurses need to help family members to drift toward objectivity-in-parentheses. When nurses are able to maintain an (objectivity) stance, they are increasingly able to invite family members to resist the sin of certainty.

> **Concept 2**
> **We bring forth our realities through interacting with the world, ourselves, and others through language.**

Reality does not reside "out there" to be absorbed; rather, persons exist in many domains of the realities that we bring forth to explain our experiences (Maturana & Varela, 1992). The ability to bring forth personal meaning and to respond and interact with the world and with each other, but always with reference to a set of internal coherences, can be seen as the essential quality of living. Maturana and Varela (1980) assert that this statement applies to all organisms, with or without a nervous system. They further suggest that it is best to think of cognition as a continual interaction between what we expect to see (i.e., our unconscious premises or beliefs) and what we bring forth. In a telephone interview, Maturana (1988) embellished this notion of reality as follows:

> We exist in many domains of realities that we bring forth . . . What I'm saying in the long run is that there is no possibility of saying absolutely anything about anything independent from us. So whatever we do is always our total responsibility in the sense that it depends completely on us and all domains of reality that we bring forth are equally legitimate although they are not equally desirable or pleasant to live in. But they are always brought forth by us in our coexistence with other human beings. So if we bring forth a community in which there is misery, well, this is it. If we bring forth a community in which there is well-being, this is it. But it is us always in coexistence with others that . . . are bringing forth reality. Reality is indeed an explanation of the world that we live [in] with others.

In sum, the world everyone sees is not the world but a world that we bring forth with others (Maturana & Varela, 1992).

■■■ CONCLUSIONS

Nursing is striving to articulate and describe more clearly the theories that inform clinical practice models. This chapter is our effort to be more transparent about the theories that we know provide the foundations of the CFAM and CFIM. It is hoped that our practice models will have more relevancy, more meaning, and of course more usefulness in clinical practice with families because of this transparency.

■■■ REFERENCES

Allmond, B.W., Buckman, W., & Gofman, H.F. (1979). *The family is the patient.* St. Louis: C.V. Mosby.

Bateson, G. (1979). *Mind and nature.* New York: E.P. Dutton.

Bavelas, J.B. (1992). Research into the pragmatics of human communication. *Journal of Strategic and Systemic Therapies, 11*(2), 15–29.

Becvar, D.S., & Becvar, R.J. (1992). *Family therapy: A systemic integration.* Boston: Allyn and Bacon, Inc.

Fisch, R., Weakland, J.H., & Segal, L. (1982). *The tactics of change.* San Francisco: Jossey-Bass.

Furth, H.G. (1987). *Knowledge as desire: An essay on Freud and Piaget.* New York: Columbia University Press.

Imber-Black, E. (1991). The family-larger-system perspective. *Family Systems Medicine, 9*(4), 371–396.

Imber Coppersmith, E. (1983). The place of family therapy in the homeostasis of larger systems. In M. Aronson & R. Wolberg (Eds.), *Group and family therapy: An overview* (pp. 216–227). New York: Brunner/Mazel.

Jackson, D. (1973). Family interaction, family homeostasis and some implications for conjoint family psychotherapy. In D. Jackson (Ed.), *Therapy, communication and change* (4th ed.) (pp. 185–203). Palo Alto: Science & Behavior Books.

Jencks, C. (1992). The post-modern agenda. In C. Jencks (Ed.), *The post-modern reader* (pp. 10–39). London: Academy Editions.

Kermode, S., & Brown, C. (1996). The postmodernist hoax and its effect on nursing. *International Journal of Nursing Studies, 33*(4), 375–384.

Lister, P. (1991). Approaching models of nursing from a postmodernist perspective. *Journal of Advanced Nursing, 16,* 206–212.

Lister, P. (1997). The art of nursing in a 'postmodern' context. *Journal of Advanced Nursing, 25,* 38–44.

Loos, F., & Bell, J.M. (1990). Circular questions: A family interviewing strategy. *Dimensions in Critical Care Nursing, 9*(1), 46–53.

Lyotard, J.F. (1992). *The inhuman: Reflections on time.* Stanford: Stanford University Press.

Maturana, H. (1978). Biology of language: The epistemology of reality. In G. Millar and E. Lenneberg (Eds.), *Psychology and biology of language and thought,* (pp. 27–63). New York: Academic Press.

Maturana, H.R. (1988). Telephone conversation: Calgary/Chile coupling [Telephone transcript]. Calgary, Canada: University of Calgary.

Maturana, H., & Varela, F. (1992). *The tree of knowledge: The biological roots of human understanding.* Boston, MA: Shambhala Publications, Inc.

Maturana, H., & Varela, F. (1980). *Autopoiesis and cognition: The realization of the living.* Dordrecht, Holland: D. Reidl.

Mendez, C.L., Coddou, F., & Maturana, H.R. (1988). The bringing forth of pathology. *Irish Journal of Psychology, 9*(1), 144–172.

Mitchell, D.P. (1996). Postmodernism, health, and illness. *Journal of Advanced Nursing, 23,* 201–205.

Moules, N.J. (1998). Postmodernism and the sacred: Reclaiming meaning in our greater than human worlds. Unpublished manuscript, University of Calgary, Faculty of Nursing., Calgary.

Parsons, C. (1995). The impact of postmodernism on research methodology: implications for nursing. *Nursing Inquiry 2,* 22–28.

Ranson, D. C. (1984). Random notes: The patient is not a dirty window. *Family Systems Medicine, 2*(2), 230–233.

Reed, P.G. (1995). A treatise on nursing knowledge development for the 21st century: Beyond postmodernism. *Advances in Nursing Science, 17,* 70–84.

Robinson, C.A. (1998). Women, families, chronic illness, and nursing interventions: From burden to balance. *Journal of Family Nursing, 4*(3), 271–290.

Selvini-Palazzoli, M., Boscolo, L., Cecchin, G., & Prata, G. (1978). A ritualized prescription in family therapy: Odd days and even days. *Journal of Marriage and Family Counseling, 4*(3), 3–9.

Simon, R. (1985). Structure is destiny: An interview with Humberto Maturana. *Family Therapy,* May-June, 32–43.

Tapp, D.M., & Wright, L.M. (1996). Live supervision and family systems nursing: Postmodern influences and dilemmas. *Journal of Psychiatric and Mental Health Nursing, 3,* 225–233.

Tomm, K. (1984). One perspective on the Milan systemic approach: Part II. Description of session format, interviewing style and interventions. *Journal of Marital and Family Therapy, 10*(3), 253–271.

Tomm, K. (1981). Circularity: A preferred orientation for family assessment. In A. S. Gurman (Ed.), *Questions and answers in the practice of family therapy* (Vol. 1) (pp. 874–87). New York: Brunner/Mazel.

Tomm, K. (1995). Circular interviewing: A multifaceted clinical tool. In D. Campbell & R. Draper (Eds.), *Applications of systemic family therapy: The Milan approach* (pp. 33–45). London: Grune & Stratton.

Tomm, K. (1980). Towards a cybernetic-systems approach to family therapy at the University of Calgary. In D.S. Freeman (Ed.), *Perspectives on family therapy* (pp. 3–18). Toronto: Butterworths.

Tomm, K. (1987a). Interventive interviewing: Part I. Strategizing as a fourth guideline for the therapist. *Family Process, 26*(6), 167–183.

Tomm, K. (1987b). Interventive interviewing: Part II. Reflexive questioning as a means to enable self-healing. *Family Process, 26*(6), 167–183.

Tomm, K. (1988). Interventive interviewing: Part III. Intending to ask lineal, circular, strategic, or reflexive questions? *Family Process, 27*(1), 1–15.

Varela, F.J. (1979). *Principles of biological autonomy.* New York: Elsevier North Holland.

von Foerester, H. (1974). Notes for an epistemology of living things. In E. Morin & M. Piatelli (Eds.), *L'unite de l'homme.* Paris, Seuil.

von Bertalanffy, L. (1974). General systems theory and psychiatry. In S. Arieti (Ed.), *American handbook of psychiatry* (pp. 1095–1117). New York: Basic Books.

von Bertalanffy, L. (1972). The history and status of general systems theory. In G. Klir (Ed.) *Trends in general systems theory.* New York: John Wiley & Sons.

von Bertalanffy, L. (1968). *General systems theory: Foundations, development, applications.* New York: George Braziller.

von Glaserfeld, E. (1984). An introduction to radical constructivism. In P. Watzlawick (Ed.), *The invented reality: Contributions to constructivism* (pp. 17–40). New York: W.W. Norton.

Watson, J. (1995). Postmodernism and knowledge development in nursing. *Nursing Science Quarterly 8,* 60–64.

Watzlawick, P. (Ed.). (1984). *The invented reality: Contributions to constructivism.* New York: W.W. Norton.

Watzlawick, P., Weakland, J., & Fisch, R. (1974). *Change: Principles of problem formulation and problem resolution.* New York: W.W. Norton & Co.

Watzlawick, P., Beavin, J.H., & Jackson, D.D. (1967). *Pragmatics of human communication.* New York: W.W. Norton & Co.

Wright, L.M., & Levac, A.M. (1992). The non-existence of noncompliant families: The influence of Humberto Maturana. *Journal of Advanced Nursing, 17,* 913–917.

Wright, L.M., & Watson, W.L. (1988). Systemic family therapy and family development. In C.J. Falicov (Ed.), *Family transitions: Continuity and change over the life cycle* (pp. 407–430). New York: Guilford Press.

Wright, L.M., Watson, W.L., & Bell, J.M. (1996). *Beliefs: The heart of healing in families and illness.* New York: Basic Books.

Wright, L.M., Watson, W.L., & Bell, J.M. (1990). The Family Nursing Unit: A unique integration of research, education and clinical practice. In J.M. Bell, W.L. Watson, & L.M. Wright (Eds.) *The cutting edge of family nursing* (pp. 95–109). Calgary, Alberta: Family Nursing Unit Publication.

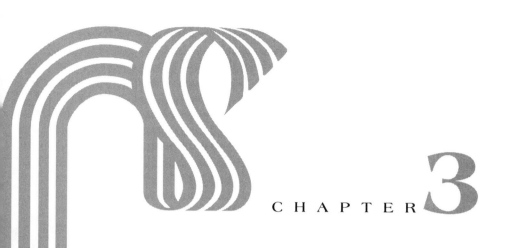

CHAPTER 3

The Calgary Family Assessment Model

The Calgary Family Assessment Model (CFAM) is an integrated, multidimensional framework based on the systems, cybernetics, communication, and change theoretical foundations. This third edition includes a discussion of postmodern and biology of cognition influences. CFAM has received wide recognition since the first edition of this book in 1984. It has been adopted by many faculties and schools of nursing in Australia, Great Britain, North America, Brazil, Japan, Finland, Sweden, Korea, and Taiwan. It has been referenced frequently in the literature, especially the *Journal of Family Nursing*. We originally adapted a family assessment framework developed by Tomm and Sanders (1983). However, CFAM was substantially revised in 1984 and 1994. The present version is embellished in this chapter.

CFAM consists of three major categories:

1. Structural
2. Developmental
3. Functional

Each category contains several subcategories. It is important for *each* nurse to decide which subcategories are relevant and appropriate to explore and assess with *each* family at *each* point in time. That is, not all subcategories need to be assessed at a first meeting with a family, and some subcategories need never be assessed. If nurses use too many subcategories, they may become overwhelmed by all the data. If they and the family discuss too few subcategories, each may have a distorted view of the family situation.

It is useful to conceptualize the three assessment categories (structural, developmental, and functional) and the many subcategories as a branching diagram (Fig. 3–1 and inside back cover).

As nurses use the subcategories on the right of the branching diagram, they collect more and more microscopic data. It is important for nurses to be able to move back and forth on the diagram to draw together all of the relevant information into an integrated assessment.

It is also important for nurses to recognize that a family assessment is based on the nurse's personal and professional life experiences, beliefs, and relationship with those being interviewed. "It should not be considered as 'the truth' about the family, but rather one perspective at a particular point in time" (Levac, Wright, &Leahey, 1997, p. 5).

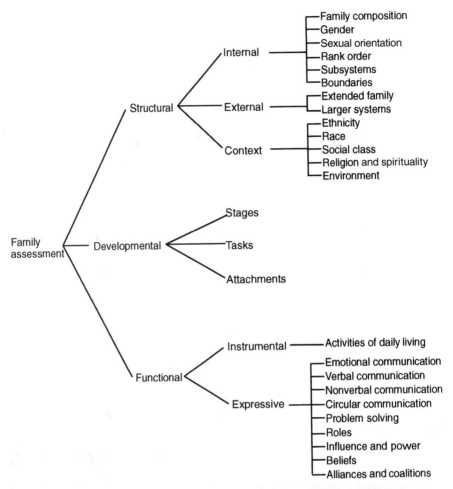

FIGURE 3–1. Branching diagram of CFAM.

In this chapter, each assessment category is discussed separately. Terms are defined and sample questions are proposed for the nurse to ask family members. Various types of assessment questions are presented and examples given. The use of assessment and interventive questions will be discussed in Chapter 4, The Calgary Family Intervention Model (CFIM). Again, we wish to emphasize that not all questions about various subcategories of the model need to be asked at the first interview, and questions about each subcategory are not appropriate for every family. Families are obviously composed of individuals, but the focus of a family assessment is less on the individual and more on the interaction *among* all of the individuals within the family.

■■■ STRUCTURAL ASSESSMENT

In assessing a family, the nurse needs to examine its structure, that is, who is in the family, what is the connection among family members vis-à-vis those outside the family, and what is the family's context. Three aspects of family structure can most readily be examined: internal structure, external structure, and context. Each of these dimensions of family structural assessment are addressed separately.

INTERNAL STRUCTURE

This aspect includes six subcategories:

1. Family composition
2. Gender
3. Sexual orientation
4. Rank order
5. Subsystems
6. Boundaries

Family Composition

This subcategory has many meanings because of the many definitions given to family. Wright, Watson, and Bell (1996) define family as a group of individuals who are bound by strong emotional ties, a sense of belonging, and a passion for being involved in one another's lives. Families can be portrayed as long-term committed relationships in which persons organize themselves in relationship to each other (Tomm, 1994). Stuart (1991) concludes that there are five critical attributes to the concept of family:

1. The family is a system or unit.
2. Its members may or may not be related and may or may not live together.
3. The unit may or may not contain children.
4. There is commitment and attachment among unit members that include future obligation.
5. The unit caregiving functions consist of protection, nourishment, and socialization of its members (p. 40).

Using these ideas, the nurse can include the various family forms that are prevalent in society today, such as the biological family of procreation, the nuclear family that incorporates one or more members of the extended family (family of origin), the single-parent family, the stepfamily, the communal family, and the homosexual couple or family. Designating a group of people with a term such as "couple," "nuclear family," or "single-parent family" specifies attributes of membership, but these distinctions of grouping are not more or less "families" by reason of labeling. Rather, attributes of affection, strong emotional ties, a sense of belonging, and durability of membership determine family composition.

Nurses need to find a definition of family that moves beyond the traditional boundaries of limiting membership using the criteria of blood, adoption, and marriage. We have found the following definition of family to be most useful in our clinical work: the family is who they say they are. With this definition, nurses can honor individual family members' ideas about which relationships are significant to them and their experience of health and illness. Research has shown that a powerful and reciprocal connection exists between health and the nature of a person's long-term relationships (Radley & Green, 1986; Ross & Cobb, 1990). Although we recognize the dominant North American type of separately housed nuclear families, our definition allows us to address the emotional past, present, and anticipated future relationships within the family system. We know that "gays and lesbians often refer to their friendship network as 'family,' and that for many gays and lesbians this 'family' is often as crucial and influential as their family of origin and at times, even more so" (Long, 1996, p. 385). Our definition is based on the family's beliefs about *their* conception of family rather than on who lives in the household.

Changes in family composition are important to note. These changes could be permanent as a result of the loss of a family member or the addition of a new person. Changes in family composition can also be transient. For example, stepfamilies often have different family compositions on weekends or during vacation periods when children from previous relationships cohabit. Losses tend to be more severe in relation to how recently they have occurred, the younger family members are when loss occurs, the smaller the family, the greater the numerical imbalance between male and female members of the family resulting from the loss, the greater the number of losses, and the greater the number of prior losses (Toman, 1976). The serious illness or death of a family member, especially by violence, can lead to disruption in the family. The extent of the impact of a death on the family depends on the social and ethnic meaning of death, the history of previous losses, the timing of the death in the life cycle, and the nature of the death (Walsh & McGoldrick, 1991). The position and function of the person who died in the family system and the openness of the family system must also be considered. We have found it useful to note the family's losses and deaths during the structural assessment process, but do not immediately assume that these losses are of major significance to the family. By taking this stance, we disagree with the position taken by McGoldrick (1991), who asserts that "it is important to track patterns of adaptation to loss as a routine part of family assessment even when it is not initially presented as relevant to chief complaints" (p. 52).

In our clinical practice with families we have found it useful to ask ourselves, Who is in *this* family? Who does the family consider to be "family"?

Questions to Ask the Family. Could you tell me who is in your family? Does anyone else live with you, for example, grandparents, boarders? So, there are yourself and your 60-year-old son—anyone else? Has anyone recently moved out? Is there anyone else whom you think of as family who does not live with you? Anyone not related biologically?

Gender

This subcategory is a basic construct, a "fundamental organizing principle of all family systems" (Goldner, 1988, p. 17). Since the first edition of our book, there has been an explosion of interest in the subject of gender. We believe in the constructivist "both . . . and" position, that is, we view gender as both a universal "reality" operational in hierarchy and power and a reality constructed by ourselves from our particular frame of reference. We recognize gender as both a fundamental basis for all human beings and as an individual premise. Gender is important for nurses to consider because the difference in how men and women experience the world is at the heart of the therapeutic conversation. Often in couple relationships the problems described by men and women include unspoken conflicts between their perceptions of gender—that is, how their family and society or culture tell them that men and women should feel, think, or behave—and their own experiences.

We agree with Sheinberg and Penn (1991), who argue on behalf of the integration of male and female attributes in each person. Human development is a process of increasingly complex forms of relatedness and integration rather than a progression from attachment to separation. Gender is, in our view, a set of beliefs about or expectations of male and female behavior and experiences. These beliefs have been developed by cultural, religious, and familial influences as well as by class and sexual orientaton. They are in some ways more important than anatomical differences. Sheinberg and Penn (1991) define maturity as "an alternating of both connections and differentiation within the context of ongoing relationships" (p. 35). This definition supports a developmental model based not solely on male norms but rather representative of both genders.

Gender plays an important role in family healthcare, especially child healthcare. Differences in parental roles in caring for the ill child may be significant sources of family stress. For example, the majority of help seeking is initiated by the mother when the child is ill. Robinson's research (1998) found role strain for families in which chronic illness became an unwelcome, dominant, powerful family member. She asserts that "it became clear that the women—the wives and mothers in these families—were responsible for day-to-day, 24 hour, day in, day out protection" (p. 277). The women carried both the burden of responsibility and the majority of the workload. Levac, Wright, and Leahey (1997) recommend that assessment of the influence of gender is especially important when there are societal, cultural, or family beliefs about male and female roles that are creating family tension. Box 3–1 outlines some characteristics of equal relationships.

In our clinical supervision with nurses we have found it useful to have them consider their own ideas about masculinity and femininity. For example, how do you believe men should behave toward ill family members? What ways have you noticed that men express emotion? What are your thoughts about couples who choose a child's gender?

Questions to Ask the Family. What effect did your parents' ideas have on your own ideas of masculinity and femininity? If your parents had had different ideas about male or female behavior, how might it have changed your relationship with them? How might it have changed your relationship with your partner? Would you like your child to feel differently than you do about his or her masculinity or femininity? If your arguments with your child were about how to stay connected rather than how to separate, would they be different? If you would show the feelings you keep hidden, would your wife think more or less of you? How did it come to be that Mom assumes more responsibility for the dialysis than Dad does?

Sexual Orientation

This subcategory includes gay, lesbian, heterosexual, and bisexual orientations. Heterosexism is a form of multicultural bias that has the

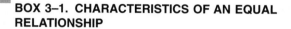

BOX 3–1. CHARACTERISTICS OF AN EQUAL RELATIONSHIP

I. **Partners hold equal status, as evidenced by:**

Equal entitlement of each partner to personal goals, needs, and wishes

Open expression of own goals, needs, and wishes by each partner

Collaborative and direct conflict resolution

Low-status tasks such as housework shared equally

Conscious negotiation of relationship roles and patterns

Equal power of each partner to influence the relationship

II. **Accommodation in the relationship is mutual, as evidenced by:**

Schedules organized equally around each partner's need

Equal priority given to work or career regardless of income

No latent, invisible power on part of one to which the other accommodates

Boundaries that respect the individuality of each mutually established

III. **Attention to the other in the relationship is mutual, as evidenced by:**

Displays of interest in the other's needs and desires by both partners

Attunement to other's perspective and experience is equally shared

Responsiveness to other's state is equally demonstrated

Each taking initiative toward the care and well-being of the other

Each recognizes and respects the other from the perspective of the other

IV. **Mutual well-being of partners, as evidenced by:**

The relationship supporting psychological health of each equally (one partner's sense of competence, optimism, and well-being does not come at the expense of the other's depression or low self-esteem)

The relationship supporting the economic viability of each equally

Relationship patterns equally supporting the physical health of each (structure of relationship does not cause one partner to be more physically stressed or fatigued than the other over the long term)

Source: Knudson-Martin, C., & Mahoney, A. R. (1996). Gender dilemmas and myth in the construction of marital bargains: Issues for marital therapy, *Family Process, 35,* 137–153. Reprinted with permission of Family Process, Inc., PO Box 23980, Rochester, NY 14692. *Characteristics of an Equal Relationship* (Table), Knudson-Martin & Mahoney. Family Process 1996, No. 35, p. 140. Reproduced by permission of the publisher via Copyright Clearance Center, Inc.

potential to harm both families and healthcare providers. Discrimination, lack of knowledge, stereotyping, and insensitivity about sexual orientation have more recently been addressed in North American society. Nonetheless, the topic of sexual orientation is one that nurses approach with varying levels of acceptance, comfort, and knowledge. "Lesbians, gay men, and heterosexual women and men live in partially overlapping but partially separate cultures, and their gender role development often follows distinctive trajectories leading to different outcomes"(Green, 1996, p. 394). In our clinical supervision, we have found it useful to reflect critically on attitudes about sexual orientation. We like Long's (1996) suggestion to watch our language when working with families. We do not assume that what applies to gay relationships can be applied to lesbian relationships or that a patient is heterosexual if the patient says that he or she is dating.

Questions to Ask the Family. At what age did you first engage in sexual activity (rather than at what age did you first have intercourse)? When Sarah told your Mom that she was lesbian, what effect did it have on your Mom's caretaking of her? When your brother announced that he was homosexual and leaving his marriage, how did your parents respond?

Rank Order

This subcategory refers to the position of the children in the family with respect to age and gender. Birth order, gender, and distance in age between siblings are important factors to consider when doing an assessment. Toman (1988) has been a major contributor to research about sibling configuration. His main thesis is the duplication theorem. He asserts that the more new social relationships resemble earlier intrafamilial social relationships, the more enduring and successful they are. For example, the marriage between the older brother (of a younger sister) and the younger sister (of an older brother) has good potential for success because the relationships are complementary. If the marriage is between two firstborns, there might be a symmetrical competitive relationship, each one vying for the position of leadership.

McGoldrick and Gerson (1985) suggest that the following factors also influence sibling constellation: the timing of each sibling's birth in the family history, the child's characteristics, the family's idealized "program" for the child, and the parental attitudes and biases regarding sex differences. Although we believe that sibling patterns are important to note, we urge nurses to remember that different child-rearing patterns have also emerged as a result of the increased use of birth control, the women's movement, and the large number of women in the workforce. We agree with Simon's (1988) position that sibling position is an organizing influence on the personality but is not a fixed influence. Each new period of life seems to bring a reevaluation of these influences. An individual transfers or generalizes familial experiences to social settings outside the family, such as kindergarten, schools, and clubs. As an individual is influenced by the environment, his or her relationships with colleagues, friends, and spouses are also generally affected. With the passage of time, there are multiple influences on personality organization in addition to sibling constellation.

Before meeting with a family, we encourage nurses to hypothesize about the potential influence of rank order on the reason for the family interview. For example, nurses could ask themselves, "If this child is the youngest in the family, could this be influencing the parents' reluctance to allow him to give his own insulin injection?" The nurse could also consider the influence of birth order on motivation, achievement, and vocational choice. For example, is the firstborn child under pressure to achieve academically? If the youngest child is starting school, what influence might this have on the couple's persistent attempts with in vitro fertilization?

   Questions to Ask the Family. How many children do you have? Who is the eldest? How old is he or she? Who comes next in line? Have there been any miscarriages or abortions?

Subsystems

This subcategory is a term used to label or mark the family system's level of differentiation. A family carries out its functions through its subsystems. Dyads, such as husband-wife or mother-child, can be seen as subsystems. Subsystems can be delineated by generation, sex, interest, function, or history.

Each person in the family belongs to several different subsystems. In each, that person has a different level of power and uses different skills. A 65-year-old woman can be a grandmother, mother, wife, and daughter within the same family. An eldest boy child is a member of the sibling subsystem, the male subsystem, and the parent-child subsystem. In each of the subsystems, he behaves according to his position. He has to concede the power that he exerts over his younger brother in the sibling subsystem when he interacts with his stepmother in the parent-child subsystem. An only girl child living in a single-parent household will have different subsystem challenges when she lives on alternate weekends with her father, his new wife, and their two daughters. The ability to adapt to the demands of different subsystem levels is a necessary skill for each family member.

In our clinical practice we have found it useful to consider whether clear generational boundaries are present in the family. If there are, does the family find them helpful or not? For example, we ask ourselves whether one child behaves like a parent or husband surrogate. Is the child a child or is there a surrogate-spouse subsystem? By generating these hypotheses before and during the family meeting, we will be able to connect isolated bits of data to either confirm or negate a hypothesis.

Questions to Ask the Family. Some families have special subgroups; for example, the women do certain things while the men do other things. Are there different subgroups in your family? What effect does it have on your family's stress level? If your family were to have more or fewer subgroups, what effect do you think that might have? When Mom and Ania stay up at night and talk together about Dad's use of crack, what do the boys do? Which subgroup in the family is most affected by this problem and how? Who gets together in the family to talk about Mian's self-mutilating behaviors?

Boundaries

This subcategory refers to the rule "defining who participates and how" (Minuchin, 1974, p. 53). Family systems and subsystems have boundaries, the function of which is to protect the differentiation of the system or subsystem. For example, the boundary of a family system is defined when a father tells his teenage daughter that her boyfriend cannot move into the household. A parent-child subsystem boundary is made explicit when a mother tells her daughter, "You are not your brother's parent. If he is not taking his medication, I'll discuss it with him."

Boundaries can be diffuse, rigid, or permeable. As boundaries become diffuse, the differentiation of the family system decreases. For example, family members may become emotionally close and "richly cross-joined" (Ashby, 1969, p. 208). These family members have a heightened sense of belonging to the family and less individual autonomy. A diffuse subsystem boundary is evident when a child is "parentified," or given adult responsibilities and power in decision making.

When there are rigid boundaries, the subsystems tend to become disengaged. A husband who rigidly believes that "only wives should visit the elderly," and whose wife agrees with him, can become disengaged from or peripheral to the senior adult-child subsystem. Clear, permeable boundaries, on the other hand, allow appropriate flexibility. There are rules, but they can be modified. We agree with Falicov (1998) that "uncritical pathologizing of cross-generational coalitions and the automatic goal of restoring the boundary around the marital couple are based on local constructions that reflect and support the ideology of a particular kind of family: the American middle-class nuclear family" (pp. 37–38). In working with families from different cultures, races, social classes, and rural settings, fostering other central ties may be most beneficial for the family.

Boundaries tend to change over time. Boss (1980) suggests that family boundaries become ambiguous "during the process of reorganization after acquisition or loss of a member" (p. 445). This is particularly evident with families experiencing separation or divorce. Burns (1987) suggests that the involuntarily childless couple may experience infertility as a stress of boundary ambiguity; that is, not knowing whether their unconceived child is in or out of the family system. She hypothesizes that, as infertile couples attempt to make the transition to parenthood, they may experience the desired child as a family member who is psychologically present but physically absent. The opposite phenomenon can be experienced by families caring for a member with Alzheimer's disease. The member can be physically present but psychologically absent. Other variations include the ambiguity experienced by some families when a family member is at war.

Boundary styles can facilitate or constrain family functioning. For example, an immigrant family that moves into a new culture may initially be very protective of its members until it gradually adapts to the cultural milieu. Its boundaries vis-à-vis outside systems will be quite firm and rigid and may gradually become more flexible. "Muslim families' preference for greater connectedness, a less flexible and more hierarchical family structure, and an implicit communication style" is noted by Daneshpour (1998, p. 355).

Green and Werner (1996) discuss another meaning of the term boundary, relating it to interpersonal proximity, intrusiveness, and closeness-caregiving. They agree with Wood (1985) that the relative sharing of territory can be assessed along aspects of contact time (time together), personal space (physical nearness, touching), emotional space (sharing of affects), information space (information known about each other), shared private conversations separate from others, and decision space (extent to which decisions are localized within various individuals or subsystems). The closeness-caregiving dimension of a boundary may be very significant for nurses to assess when dealing with older people with chronic illness and their adult children.

In our clinical supervision with nurses, we encourage them to consider how this family differentiates itself from other families in the neighborhood and in the city. The nurse considers whether there is a parental subsystem, a marital subsystem, a sibling subsystem, and so forth. Are the boundaries clear, rigid, or diffuse? Does the boundary style facilitate or constrain the family?

Questions to Ask the Family. The nurse can infer the boundaries by asking the husband if there is anyone with whom he can talk when he feels stressed by his retirement. The nurse can ask the wife the same question. To whom would you go if you felt happy? If you felt sad? Would there be anyone in your family opposed to your talking with that person? Who would be most in favor of you talking with that person? What impact might it have on your Mom's ability to deal with your Dad's illness if she had more support from your grandparents?

EXTERNAL STRUCTURE

This aspect includes two subcategories:

1. Extended family
2. Larger systems

Extended Family

This subcategory includes the family of origin and the family of procreation as well as the present generation and stepfamily members. Multiple loyalty ties to extended family members can be invisible but may be very influential forces in the family structure. Special relationships and support can exist at great geographical distances. Also, conflictual and painful relationships can seem fresh and close at hand despite the extended family living far away or not in frequent contact. How each member sees himself or herself as a separate individual yet part of the "family ego mass" (Bowen, 1978) is a critical structural area for assessment. Levac, Wright, and Leahey (1997) recommend assessment of the quantity and type of contact with extended family to provide information about the quality and quantity of support.

In our clinical work we consider whether there are many references to the extended family. How significant is the extended family to the functioning of this particular family? Are they available for support in times of need? By telephone? By e-mail? In physical proximity?

Questions to Ask the Family. Where do your parents live? How often do you have contact with them? What about your brothers and sisters? Which family members do you never see? Which of the relatives are you closest to? Who telephones whom? With what frequency? Whom do you ask for help when problems arise in your family? What kind of help do you ask for? Would you be available if they needed your help?

Larger Systems

This subcategory refers to the larger social agencies and personnel with whom the family has meaningful contact. We agree with Doherty and Heinrich (1996) that a number of parties have a legitimate stake in the outcomes of treatment decisions, policy decisions, clinician behavior, and patient-family behavior. "These ethical stakeholders include the patient and family, the clinician or clinical team, the clinical administrator, the managed care organization, the employer/payer, the government, and the broader society or community. Each has a moral claim to due consideration in healthcare decisions" (p. 19). Larger systems generally include work systems, and for some families they include public welfare, child welfare, foster care, courts, and outpatient clinics. There are also larger systems designed for special populations, such as agencies mandated to provide services to the mentally or physically handicapped or the frail elderly. For many families, engagement with such larger systems is not problematic. Imber-Black (1991) states that some families and larger systems, however, may develop difficult relationships that exert a toll on normative development for family members. Some healthcare professionals in larger systems contribute to families being labeled "multiproblem," "resistant," or "uncooperative." These healthcare professionals limit their perspective to include only the family system rather than taking the more complex perspective that includes the family's relationship to larger systems and multiple helpers.

Another larger system relationship that nurses should assess is the computer network. There has been a substantial increase in computer-mediated communication, including electronic bulletin boards, chat rooms, and discussion groups. These can offer families valuable assistance in terms of information, validation, empathy, advice, and encouragement. Miller and Gergen's work (1998) points out that on-line dialogs can be more sustaining than transformative at times. That is, the dialog tends to support the status quo rather than stimulate change. We agree with their urging that vigorous attention should be given to ways that professional expertise and electronic facilitation can be combined in the long run.

In our clinical supervision with nurses, we encourage them to discover whether the *meaningful system* is the family alone or the family *and* its larger-system helpers. Nurses can ask themselves such questions as: "Who are the healthcare professionals involved? What is the relationship between the family and the larger system? How regularly do they interact? Is their relationship symmetrical or complementary? Are the larger systems overconcerned? Overinvolved? Underconcerned? Underinvolved? Is the family blamed for its problems by the larger system? What do the helpers desire for the family? Is the nurse being asked to take responsibility for another system's task? How do the family and helpers define the problem?"

Questions to Ask the Family. What agency professionals are involved with your family? How many agencies regularly interact with you? Has your family moved from one healthcare system to another? Who most thinks that your family needs to be involved with these systems? Who most thinks the opposite? Would there be agreement between your definition of the problem and the system's definition of the problem? How about between the definitions of the solution? What has been the best or worst advice you've been given by professionals for this issue? How is our working relationship going so far? If it weren't going too well, would you tell me?

CONTEXT

Context is explained as the whole situation or background relevant to some event or personality. Each family system is itself nested within broader systems such as neighborhood, class, region, and country, and is influenced by these systems. Because the context permeates and circumscribes both the individual and the family, its consequences are pervasive. Context includes five subcategories:

1. Ethnicity
2. Race
3. Social class
4. Religion
5. Environment

Ethnicity

This subcategory refers to a concept of a family's "peoplehood" derived from a combination of its history, race, social class, and religion. It describes a commonality of overt and subtle processes transmitted by the family over generations and usually reinforced by the surrounding community. Ethnicity is an important factor that influences family interaction. We believe that nurses must be aware of the great variety within as well as between ethnic groups. For example, Cheng-Ham (1989) points out that there are three different classifications of immigrant groups. There are those who are second-, third-, or fourth-generation immigrants with ancestors from a foreign country. There are the "recently arrived" immigrant families, of whom some are refugees. There are also those "immigrant-American" families, in which the parents were born in a foreign country and their children were born in the United States.

For some immigrant families, the impact of cultural adjustment can be seen as a transitional difficulty, with issues such as economic survival, racism, and changes in extended family and support system that need to be addressed. Specific life experiences, such as a college education, financial success in business, or family intermarriage can encourage assimilation into a dominant culture, whereas isolation in a rural area or an urban ghetto tends to foster continuity of ethnic patterns. It is important, though, to recognize that these views of assimilation and isolation are from our "observer perspective." What matters is the family's cultural narrative, how it is deconstructed and co-constructed.

Ethnic differences in family structure and their implications for intervention can be highlighted (McGoldrick, 1982). For example, Italians in North America usually have strong extended family connections and loyalties. African-Americans tend to have flexible family boundaries, and some may include the grandmother in child rearing. Puerto Ricans and members of some Latin American cultures encourage emotionality between relatives and between generations, whereas the Irish in North America have more strictly defined boundaries between generations.

In our clinical work, we have found it essential to recognize the infinite variety and lack of stereotype in families from various ethnic groups. We agree with McGoldrick (1998) that dealing with cultural diversity is a matter of balance between validating the differences among us and appreciating the forces of our common humanity. Laird (1998) reminds us that "our own cultural narratives help us to organize our thinking and anchor our lives but they can also blind us to the unfamiliar and unrecognizable and they can foster injustice" (p. 22). Nurses should sensitize themselves to differences in family beliefs and values and be willing to alter their "ethnic filters." We believe it is important for nurses to recognize their own ethnic blind spots and adjust their interventions accordingly. We are never "expert," "right," or in full possession of the "truth" about a family's ethnicity. Also, if we engage a translator to assist us with family work, we should not assume that the translator is an "expert" on this particular family's ethnicity. Rather, both we and the translator should strive to be informed and curious about ourselves and others' diversity as we collaborate in healthcare.

Some questions that we have found useful to ask ourselves include: What is the family's ethnicity? Is their social network from the same ethnic group? Do they find that helpful or not? If the available economic, educational, health, legal, and recreational services were similar to the family's ethnic values, how would our conversation be different?

Questions to Ask the Family. Could you tell me about your Japanese practices regarding illness? How does being a Japanese immigrant influence your beliefs about when to consult with health professionals? What does health mean to you? How would you know that you are healthy? How would I know that you are healthy? As a second-generation Chilean family, how are your healthcare practices similar to or different from those of your grandparents? Which seem most useful to you at this point in your family's life?

Race

This subcategory is a basic construct and not an intermediate variable. Race influences core individual and group identification. It intersects with such mediating variables as class, religion, and ethnicity. Racial attitudes, stereotyping, and discrimination are powerful influences on family interaction and, if left unaddressed, can be negative constraints on the relationship between the family and the nurse. Only recently has the "myth of sameness" (Hardy, 1990) been challenged and the uniqueness of various family forms emphasized. We agree with Green (1998) that the "multicultural lens . . . (brings) into clearer focus the uniqueness of each race's normative family experience, including problems common to White middle-class families as a distinct cultural group" (p. 95). Family clinicians are now starting to appreciate that the variations in family structure and development of African-Americans, Asians, Hispanics, Whites, and others are potentially strengths in helping families to function under various economic and social conditions. Racial differences, whether intracultural or intercultural, are *not* problems per se. Rather, prejudice, discrimination, and other types of intercultural aggression based on these differences *are* problems. It is important for nurses to understand family health beliefs and behaviors influenced by racial identity, privilege, or oppression.

In our clinical work with families, we have found it very useful to critically reflect on our own ideas about our race, marginalization, invisible and visible minorities, and "the myth of sameness," and to vigorously pursue the differences between and within various racial groups. For example, we ask ourselves how a Jamaican-American family might differ from an African-American family in their beliefs about hospitalization. How might a Vietnamese couple differ from a Japanese couple in their beliefs about whether to institutionalize an aging grandmother?

Questions to Ask the Family. What differences do you notice between, for example, your Hispanic relatives' child-rearing practices and your own? If you and I were the same race, would our conversation be different? How? Would our different type of conversation be more or less likely to assist you in regaining your health? Could you help me to understand what I need to know to be most helpful to you?

Social Class

This subcategory shapes educational attainment, income, and occupation. Each class, whether upper-upper, lower-upper, upper-middle, lower-middle, upper-lower, or lower-lower, has its own clustering of values, lifestyles, and behavior that influences family interaction and healthcare practices. Social class affects how family members define themselves and are defined; what they cherish; how they organize their day-to-day living; and how they meet challenges, struggles, and crises. For example, middle-class older adults are likely to help their adult children, whereas working-class older adults are more likely to receive help.

Social class has been referred to as one of the prime molders of the family value and belief system. Much of the sociological and psychological research has been confounded by social class differences among ethnic groups. We agree with Kliman (1998) that, in a racist and classist society, class and race are not inseparable. Because poverty is disproportionately concentrated among racial minorities, many professionals have considered the African-American statistical subgroup to represent the lower-income class and the white statistical subgroup to represent the middle- or upper-income class group. Furthermore, although Hispanics, including Mexicans, Puerto Ricans, Cubans, and people from South and Central America, have increased substantially in number to become a sizable minority within the United States, until recently data about marriage and family have excluded them. Such data have generally been limited to blacks (African-Americans) and whites, without taking into account Hispanics or Asians. Much of the literature confounds the effects of race and class, not to mention the "myth of sameness" about families within each race or class.

Just as nursing has often been presented as intercultural, it has also been presented as interclass and nonpolitical. We believe that many nurses have pursued sickness in families to the exclusion of obtaining the *meaning* people give to events; their day-to-day living standards; and their access to employment, income, and housing. Social class issues have often been seen to be of little consequence to the "serious talk" about illness. This has enabled nurses to sidestep many class issues associated with inequality and injustice. We agree with Waldegrave (1990) that treatment must take into account the cultural, social, and economic context of the persons seeking help.

Assessment of social class helps the nurse understand in a new way the family's stressors and resources. If nurses recognize differences in social class beliefs between themselves and families, it may encourage new health promotion and intervention strategies. It is important for healthcare delivery that nurses be aware of such influences as the "glass ceiling" and part-time temporary work versus full-time permanent work with benefits. The upward mobility risks of harassment faced by women on entering some male-dominated work environments such as the military should be known to healthcare professionals.

In our clinical work we have often asked ourselves how the family's social class might be influencing their healthcare beliefs, values, utilization of services, and interaction with us. Serious illness can intensify financial problems, diminish the capacity to deal with them, and call for solutions at odds with conventional financial wisdom (Siwolop, 1997). We have wondered about the intrafamilial differences with respect to class and how these might help or hinder a family coping with, for example, chronic illness.

Questions to Ask the Family. How many times have you moved in the past 5 years? Have the moves had a more positive or negative influence on, for example, your ability to deal with your son's having AIDS? How many schools has your daughter Barbara attended? How does your money situation influence your use of healthcare resources? What impact does shift work have on your family's stress level?

Religion and Spirituality

This subcategory influences family values, size, healthcare, and socialization practices. For example, individualism is intricately related to the Protestant work ethic. Community support, on the other hand, is very evident in the Mormon and Jewish religions, which foster intergenerational and intragenerational support. Folk-healing traditions that combine health and religious practices are quite common in some ethnic groups. There are some spiritualistic practices in which a medium is a counselor helping to exorcise the spirits causing illness. For example, *espiritistas* or healers can be found in many Cuban and other Latino communities. Such healers, religious leaders, and clergy can be invaluable resources for families dealing with crises and with long-term needs such as caregiver support (Weaver, Koenig, & Larson, 1997).

Religion influences beliefs about illness and coping. Emotions such as peace, fear, guilt, and hope can be nurtured or tempered by religious beliefs. Levac, Wright, and Leahey (1997) recommend that assessment of the influence of religion is most critical at the time of diagnosis of a chronic or life-threatening illness. Assessment is especially relevant when there are crises such as traumatic death caused by a motor vehicle accident, violence, or abuse. We agree with Walsh (1998) that beliefs, spirituality, and transcendence are keys to family resilience.

Spirituality is a hidden and often underused resource in family work. Anderson and Worthen (1997) define spirituality as "subjective engagement with a . . . transcendent dimension of human experience" (p. 3). Becvar (1997) believes that "the realm of spirituality . . . is that of the soul and its process of growth and development, which may be facilitated both within and without the context of a specific religious perspective" (p. 5). She assumes five guiding principles for her life and work: "acknowledging connectedness, suspending judgment, trusting the universe, creating realities and walking the path with heart" (p. 5). Berenson (1990) writes that "it could be said, spirituality is to conventional religion as systems thinking is to linear, cause and effect thinking" (p. 59). Spirituality has more to do with how people orient their lives in light of an inner awareness. It can be a yearning or desire for contact beyond ordinary life experience. The striking success of Alcoholics Anonymous is one example of the power of a program that incorporates spirituality.

Our clinical experience with families has taught us that the experience of suffering frequently becomes transposed to one of spirituality as family members try to find meaning in their suffering and distress (Wright, 1999). If nurses are to be helpful, we must acknowledge that suffering and, often, the senselessness of it are ultimately spiritual issues (Patterson, 1994). Therefore, in our clinical work we have asked ourselves about the influence of religion and spirituality on the family's healthcare practices. We have noted whether there are signs of religious influence in the home, for example, statues, candles, flags, and religious texts such as the Bible and the Koran. We have been curious about dietary restrictions and habits and traditional or alternative health practices influenced by religious beliefs. We have been cautious, though, not to assume that strong religious beliefs enhance marital happiness or interaction, although they may diminish the possibility of divorce (Booth, Johnson, Branaman, & Sica, 1995).

>   ***Questions to Ask the Family.*** Are you involved with a church, temple, or synagogue? Would talking with anyone in your church or temple be helpful in coping with Pierre's illness? Are your spiritual beliefs a resource for you? For you and other family members? Who among your family members would be most encouraging of your using spiritual beliefs to cope with cancer? Have you found that prayer or other religious practices help you cope with your son's schizophrenia?

Environment

This subcategory encompasses aspects of the larger community, the neighborhood, and the home. Environmental factors such as adequacy of space and privacy and accessibility of schools, day care, recreation, and public transportation influence family functioning. These are especially relevant for older adults, who are more likely to remain in a poor environment even if it has become dangerous to live there. Over the past decade, we have had to adjust our perceptions of homelessness and come to grips with the idea that families with children are the fastest-growing homeless group. Homelessness is neither an urban nor a regional problem, but rather one that is pervasive in North America.

In our clinical work with families, we have asked ourselves and the nurses with whom we work to assess whether the home is adequate for the number of people living there. Does our perception differ from the family's? What health and other basic services are available within the home? Within the neighborhood? How accessible in terms of distance, convenience, and so forth are transportation and recreation services?

>   ***Questions to Ask the Family.*** What community services does your family use? Are there community services you would like to learn about but do not know how to contact? On a scale of 1 to 10, how comfortable are you in your neighborhood? What would make you more comfortable so that you can continue to function independently at home?

STRUCTURAL ASSESSMENT TOOLS

The genogram and the ecomap are two tools that are particularly helpful for the nurse to use in outlining the family's internal and external structures. Each is simple to use and requires only a piece of paper and a pen. The genogram is a diagram of the family constellation. The eco-map, on the other hand, is a diagram of the family's contact with others outside the immediate family. It pictures the important connections between the family and the world. We are aware of the arbitrariness of the distinction for some cultural groups between a genogram and an eco-map. Watts-Jones (1997) suggests the standard genogram is inadequate for African-Americans because of its underlying assumption that "family" is strictly a biological entity. We encourage nurses to develop a fit between these tools to depict specific family compositions. These tools have been developed as family assessment, planning, and intervention devices. They "can be used to reframe behaviors, relationships, and time connections within families, as well as detoxify and normalize families' perceptions of themselves" (Kuehl, 1995, p. 39). By pointing to the future as well as to the past and the present, genograms facilitate alternative interpretations of family experience. They can also be used to foster the training of culturally competent clinicians (Hardy & Laszloffy, 1995) and for nurses to increase their self-awareness (Halevey, 1998). Genograms convey a great deal of information in the form of a visual gestalt. When one considers the number of words it would take to portray the facts thus represented, it becomes clear how simple and useful these tools are. Genograms, when placed on patients' charts, act as constant visual reminders for nurses to "think family."

Genogram

The skeleton of the genogram tends to follow conventional genetic and genealogic charts. It is a family tree depicting the internal family structure. As an engagement tool, it is useful to apply during the first meeting with the family. It provides rich data about relationships over time and may also include data about health, occupation, religion, ethnicity, and migrations. The genogram can be used simultaneously to elicit information helpful to both the family and the nurse about development and other areas of family functioning. It is usual practice to include at least three generations. Family members are placed on horizontal rows that signify generational lines. For example, a marriage or common-law relationship is denoted by a horizontal line. Children are denoted by vertical lines. Children are rank-ordered from left to right beginning with the eldest child. Each individual is represented. A blank genogram is shown in Figure 3–2.

Some authors (McGoldrick, Gerson, & Shellenberger, 1999) differ slightly in the symbols they use to denote the details of the genogram. The symbols in Figure 3–3, however, are generally agreed on.

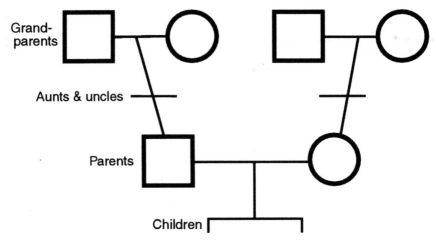

FIGURE 3–2. Blank genogram. (From McGoldrick, M., & Gerson, R. (1988). Genograms and the family life cycle. In B. Carter and M. McGoldrick (Eds)., *The changing family life cycle: A framework for family therapy* (2nd ed.). Boston: Allyn & Bacon. Copyright © 1988 by Allyn & Bacon. Reprinted by permission.)

The person's name and age should be noted inside the square or circle. Outside the symbol, significant data (e.g., travels a lot, depressed, overinvolved in work, and so forth) should be noted. If a family member has died, the year of his or her death is indicated above the square or circle. When the symbol for miscarriage is used, the sex of the child should be identified if it is known.

A sample of a nuclear and an extended family genogram is given in Figure 3–4.

Mike R., age 47, has been married to Karen, age 35, since 1984. They have two children, Ashley, age 14, who is in grade 8; and Jack, age 7, who is repeating grade 1. Mike is employed as a parks department foreman and Karen refers to him as "alcoholic." Karen is a homemaker and states that she has been "depressed" for several years. Both of Mike's parents are deceased. His father died in 1994 and his mother in 1992 of a stroke. Mike's older brother also has a drinking problem. Young Jack was named for his grandfather. Karen's mother, Susan, age 54, has arthritis, which has been getting progressively worse since her husband died in 1991. Karen has two older sisters and a brother.

How to Use the Genogram

At the beginning of the interview, the nurse informs the family that they will be having a conversation so that he or she can gain an over-

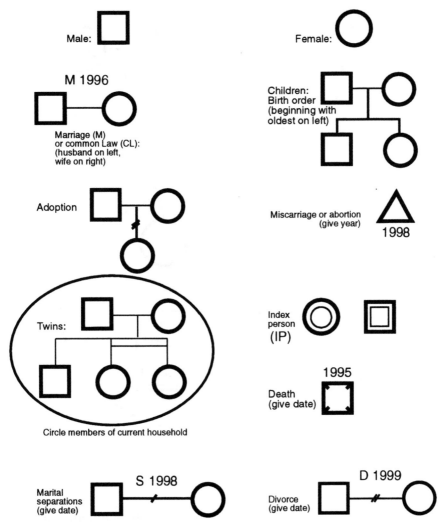

FIGURE 3–3. Symbols used in genograms.

view of who is in the family and their situation. The nurse can then use the structure of the genogram to discern the family's internal and external structures as well as context. Thus, the nurse gains an understanding of the family's composition and boundaries.

Initially, the nurse starts out with a blank sheet of paper and draws a line or circle for the first person in the family to whom a question is directed.

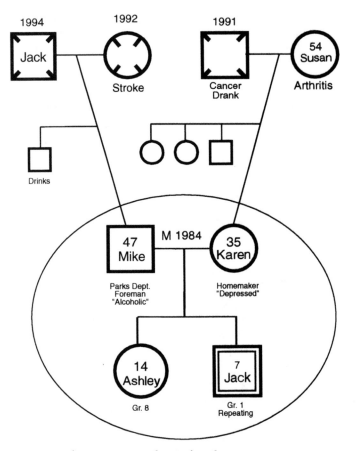

FIGURE 3–4. Sample genogram: The R. family.

Nurse: Hilda, you said you were 23, and Hans, how old are you?

Hans: Thirty-four.

Nurse: How long have you been married?

Hans: This time or the first time?

Nurse: This time. And then the first time.

Hans: Just 2 years for Hilda and me.

Nurse: And the first time?

Hans: Ten years for the first one.

Nurse: And Hilda, have you been married before?

Hilda: (*Laughs nervously*) I'm only 23.

Nurse: Sure, it's just that many people have lived together in common-law marriages or married when they were very young.

Hilda: No. I lived with my parents till I met Hans.

Nurse: Do either of you have children from prior relationships? (*Turns to both Hans and Hilda*)

Hans: Yes, I have two sons.

Hilda: No.

Nurse: In addition to Karine here (*Looks at infant on couch*), do the two of you have any other children?

Hilda: Yes, there's Fred.

Hans: Old stinko, you mean.

Nurse: Old stinko?

Hans: He isn't toilet trained yet.

Nurse: Oh, I see. And he's how old?

Hilda: He's almost 3. I've been trying to train him since I knew I was pregnant with Karine, but he just doesn't seem to want to be trained.

Nurse: (*Nods*) Mm.

Hans: Yeah, old stinko!

Nurse: And Karine is how many weeks now?

Hilda: She'll be 21 days tomorrow (*Smiles at infant*).

Nurse: Does anyone else live with you?

Hans: No. Her parents live next door.

The nurse now has a rudimentary genogram of the family (Figure 3–5). The nurse has gathered information that may or may not be significant depending on the way in which the family has responded to various events in the history of their family:

- Fred was conceived before the marrriage. Fred is unaffectionately called "old stinko" by his father.
- Hilda has been trying to train Fred since he was 24 months old.
- Hilda lived with her family of origin before the marriage. They live next door.
- Hans has been married before and has two sons.

After inquiring about the nuclear family, the nurse can continue to inquire about the extended family. It is generally not very important to go into great detail about these relatives, but clinical judgment should prevail. After questions have been asked about the husband's parents

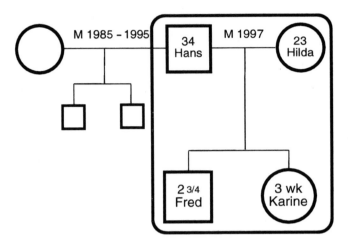

FIGURE 3–5. Genogram of the W. family.

and siblings, the nurse should then inquire about the wife's family of origin. What is important is for the nurse to gain an *overview* of the family structure and to try to avoid getting sidetracked or inundated by a large volume of information. Box 3–2 contains helpful hints for constructing genograms.

The same question format used for nuclear families is used with stepfamilies, with one exception. It is generally easier to ask one spouse about his or her previous relationships before going on to ask the other spouse about her or his relationships. Again, it is unnecessary to gather specific information on all extended family members. It is useful to draw a circle around the current family members to distinguish between the various households. Usually it is easiest to indicate the year of a divorce rather than the number of years ago that it happened. A sample of a genogram showing a stepfamily is given in Figure 3–6.

In this stepfamily, Bill, age 35, has been living in a common-law marriage since 1998 with Lou, age 33, who is a part-time waitress. Also in the household are Lou's two children, Joy, age 11, and Frank, age 9, who is hyperactive and in a special class in grade 3. Bill had been married in 1988 to his first wife, Jean. They were divorced in 1992. Bill and Jean had one son, who is now age 8. Bill was an only child. His father committed suicide in 1995. His mother is still alive. Lou is the youngest of three daughters, and both of her parents are living. Lou was married in 1987 to John, separated in 1995, and divorced in 1998. John, age 36, is a mechanic who is presently living in a common-law marriage with Fran and her three sons.

BOX 3–2. HELPFUL HINTS FOR CONSTRUCTING GENOGRAMS

- Determine priorities for genogram construction based on the family situation.
- A three-generational genogram may be useful when the child's health problem (physical or emotional) is influenced by the third generation.
- A brief two-generational genogram is generally most useful initially, especially for the family that has preventive health care needs (immunizations) or minor health concerns (sports injury). The nurse can always expand to the third generation if needed.
- Engage the family in an exercise to complete the genogram.
- Use the genogram to "break the ice," provide structure, and introduce purposeful conversation.
- Ask family members how an absent significant family member might answer a question.
- Avoid discussion that is hurtful or blameful, especially of absent family members.
- Take an interest in each family member and be sensitive to developmental differences.
- Tailor questions to children's developmental stages so that they become active contributors.
- Notice children's nonverbal and verbal comments.
- If some members are shy or seem uninterested in participating directly (e.g., adolescents), ask other family members about them.
- Begin by asking "easy" questions of individuals followed by exploration of subsystems.
- Ask concrete, easy-to-answer questions of individuals (especially children) about ages, occupations, interests, health status, school grades, and teachers to increase their comfort levels.
- Move the discussion about individuals to subsystems to elicit family relational data. Inquire about parent-child or sibling relationships depending on parenting concerns.
- With stepfamilies, questions about contact with the noncustodial parent, custody, the children's satisfaction with visits, and stepfamily relationships can be asked.
- Observe family interaction.
- During genogram construction, note the content (what's said) and the process (how it's said).
- Move from discussion about present family situation to questions about the extended family if it seems relevant (e.g., are Ruhi's parents able to help with the baby's tracheotomy care? What about babysitting?)
- When discussing generations, the nurse may find it useful to ask about psychosocial family health history (e.g., "Is there a history of alcohol abuse [or violence, learning problems, or mental illness] in your family?") Nurses' questions should be tailored to the family's particular area of concern rather than generic exploration.

Source: Adapted with permission from Levac, A. M., Wright, L. M., & Leahey, M. (1997). Children and families: Models for assessment and intervention. In J. Fox (ed.). *Primary healthcare of children.* Baltimore, MD: Mosby, p 7.

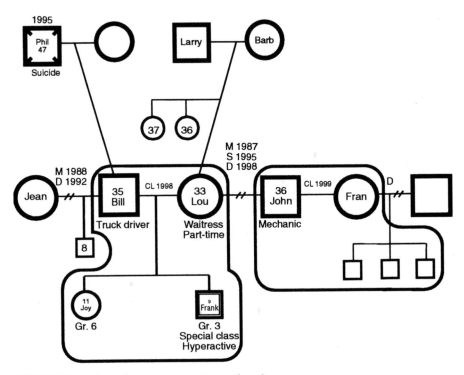

FIGURE 3–6. Sample genogram: A stepfamily.

Most families are extremely receptive to and interested in collaborating with the nurse in completing a genogram. For some, it is the first time that they have ever seen their family life pictured in this manner. Therefore, the nurse needs to be aware that the family may have a reaction to significant events. One family, for example, may express some sensitive material in a very blasé fashion. If divorce is very common in their families of origin, they may not hesitate to discuss their several marriages and those of their siblings. On the other hand, a devout Catholic family may be exquisitely sensitive to seeing the nurse write the word "divorce."

Ecomap

As with the genogram, the primary value of the ecomap is in its visual impact. The purpose of the ecomap is to depict the family members' contact with larger systems. Hartman (1978) notes:

> The eco-map (sic) portrays an overview of the family in their situation; it pictures the important nurturant or conflict-laden connec-

tions between the family and the world. It demonstrates the flow of resources, or the lack of and deprivations. This mapping procedure highlights the nature of the interfaces and points to conflicts to be mediated, bridges to be built, and resources to be sought and mobilized. (p. 467)

How to Use the Ecomap

As with the genogram, family members can actively participate in working on the ecomap during the assessment process.

The family genogram is placed in the center circle labeled family or household. The outer circles represent significant people, agencies, or institutions in the family's context. The size of the circles is not important. Lines are drawn between the family and the outer circles to indicate the nature of the connections that exist. Straight lines indicate strong connections, dotted lines indicate tenuous connections, and slashed lines indicate stressful relations. The wider the line, the stronger the tie. Arrows can be drawn alongside the lines to indicate the flow of energy and resources. Additional circles may be drawn as necessary, depending on the number of significant contacts the family has. An ecomap for the R. family has been drawn in Figure 3–7.

In this family, Mike, Karen, Ashley, and Jack are placed in the center circle. Mike has strong connections with his workplace, where he is foreman and a union representative. He has moderately strong bonds with his "drinking buddies." These relationships, however, are stressful for him. Karen's connections are mainly with her mother and the healthcare system. She sees her family physician every week "for nerves" and sees the community health nurse (CHN) once a week. Karen's mother, Susan, visits Karen every day from 11 AM to 10 PM. There is a strong connection between Karen and her mother, but Karen says she really "doesn't like Mom coming over so often." Jack has a few friends, most of whom are fire setters. He is in a special class for his learning disability and enjoys both the teacher and the school. Ashley is in junior high school, where she maintains an average grade of D. She frequently does not attend school, and when she does attend, she participates little. She spends about 6 hours a day with her boyfriend.

When the CHN completed the ecomap with the R. family, Mrs. R. (Karen) commented, "I seem to spend all my time with medical or health people." Mr. R. (Mike) then said, "You're also so busy with your mother that you don't have time for anybody else." The nurse was able to use this information from the ecomap to discuss further with the family the types of relationships they wanted both with those inside their household and with those outside the immediate family.

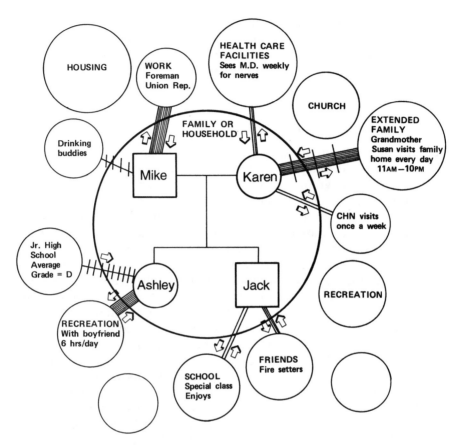

FIGURE 3–7. R. family ecomap.

In summary, the genogram and the ecomap can be used in *all* health-care settings to increase the nurse's awareness of the whole family and the family's interactions with larger systems and their extended family. Box 3–3 gives helpful hints for drawing ecomaps.

▪▪▪ DEVELOPMENTAL ASSESSMENT

In addition to an understanding of the family structure, the nurse requires an understanding of the developmental life cycle for each family. Most nurses are very familiar with stages of child development and the literature in the area of adult development. Many are becoming interested in the burgeoning literature about development in the senior

---

BOX 3–3. HELPFUL HINTS FOR DRAWING ECOMAPS

- Pose questions that explore the family's connections to other individuals or groups outside the family.
  - What community agencies are you involved with now? Which are most and least helpful?
  - How would you describe your relationship with school staff?
  - How did you first become involved with Child Protective Services? What is the nature of your current relationship with them?

Source: Adapted with permission from Levac, A. M., Wright, L. M., & Leahey, M. (1997). Children and families: Models for assessment and intervention. In J. Fox (ed.). *Primary healthcare of children.* Baltimore, MD: Mosby, p 8.

years, an interest that has been fostered by the aging of the baby boomers. But what of family development? It is more than the concurrent development at different phases of children, adults, and seniors who happen to call themselves "family." Carter and McGoldrick (1999) state that "families comprise people who have a shared history and a shared future" (p. 1). We concur with Falicov (1988) that "family development is an over-arching concept, referring to *all* transactional evolutionary processes connected with the growth of a family" (p. 13). Falicov (1988) writes:

> Although there is a regularity and internal logic to many of the processes subsumed under family development . . . each family is different precisely because each can be said to have its own developmental path, which evolves from all the different settings in which development takes place, including each family's construction of its past and present. (p. 13)

There is no single family developmental life cycle or model. In keeping with postmodern ideas, we believe that there are limits to describing family development in precise, absolute, universal ways. Freedman and Coombs (1996) remind us that "postmodernists" differ from modernists in that exceptions interest them more than rules . . . specific, contextualized details more than grand generalizations, difference rather than similarity (pp. 21–22). We are not concerned with authoritative truth, facts, and rules, but rather with the meaning a family gives to its particular story of development over time.

In our clinical supervision with nurses, we have found it useful to distinguish between "family development" and "family life cycle."

The former emphasizes the *unique* path constructed by a family. Family development is shaped by predictable and unpredictable events such as illness, catastrophes (e.g., fires, earthquakes, floods) and societal trends (e.g., the information highway, stock market fluctuations, company mergers, changes in crime and birth rates). Family life cycle refers to the *typical* path most families go through. The typical life cycle events are connected to the comings and goings of family members. For example, most families experience in their life cycle the events of birth, raising of children, departure of children from the household, retirement, and death. Such events generate changes requiring formal reorganization of roles and rules within the family. The life cycle course of families evolves through a generally predictable sequence of stages, despite cultural and ethnic variations. Although individual variations, timing, and coping strategies exist, the biological time clocks and societal expectations for such events as entrance into elementary school and retirement from work are relatively typical in North America.

Given our keen interest in a particular family's specific development over time, it might be questioned why we include a family developmental section in CFAM at all. We take the position that an informed "not-knowing" (Anderson & Goolishian, 1988) stance is useful when working with families. That is, we seek to be informed by the literature, research, and other families' stories of development. Yet, we are "not-knowing" but curious about this particular family's developmental story.

There is a rich history about family development that still pervades clinicians' thinking. We believe that it is useful for nurses to have some understanding of this history. The early proponents of the family life cycle (Duvall, 1977) developed a four-stage model that was subsequently expanded into an eight-stage model featuring successive stages in the progression of primary marriages. With the increase in various family forms, more complex designs were created (Hill, 1986; Carter & McGoldrick, 1988, 1998a). Glick, in 1989, commented that most analyses of the family life cycle began with a discussion of the first marriage, but that it was important also to consider activities that preceded the first marriage such as cohabitation. This is especially important in the late 1990s. In the U.S. in 1996, there were 7 unmarried-couple households for every 100 married-couple households, compared with 1 for every 100 in 1970 (Saluter & Lugaila, 1998). The median age of first marriage has been rising since the mid-1950s to 24.8 years for women and 27.1 years for men in the U.S. in 1996.

In the field of family therapy there were "pioneers" in applying the family development framework. Much was written about the interface between family development, functioning, and therapy. Carter and McGoldrick (1988) believed that the family life cycle perspective viewed symptoms in relation to normal functioning over time and that "therapy" helped to reestablish the family's developmental momentum. Such family therapists as Haley (1977), Minuchin (1974), and the Milan Group (Selvini, Boscolo, Cecchin, & Prata, 1980) noted the frequency of symptom appearance with the addition or loss of a family member. These therapists worked with families that did not move smoothly or automatically from one stage in the family life cycle to another, and they focused on the stressful transition points between stages. In doing an assessment and in planning interventions, these therapists paid considerable attention to life-cycle events as markers of change. Although they differed between themselves, these therapists were similar in seeking to understand the relationship between psychopathology and the family's developmental life cycle stage. For example, Minuchin took normative expectations into account when validating goals, whereas the Milan systemic group purposefully avoided a normative direction (Wright & Watson, 1988). Carter and McGoldrick (1988, 1998a) included the impact of transgenerational stress intersecting with family developmental transitions. They believed that, if vertical (transgenerational) stress was too high, a small amount of horizontal (current) stress would lead to great disruption and symptom formation.

Over the last decade there have been a great many changes in the family life cycle. First, there has been an increase in literature discussing families and their developmental phases (e.g., divorce, remarriage, chronic illness, and so forth). Second, there has been an increased consciousness of differences in male and female development and a rethinking of the trajectory of ethnic minorities in North American society. Third, there has been a lower birth rate, a longer life expectancy, a change in the roles of women and men, an awareness of the "boom, bust and echo" trends (Foot, 1996), and an increasing divorce and remarriage rate. Fourth, the conception of history as an "objective" ordering of the "facts" of the past, has changed. Family development is now seen as an interactive process in which the historian influences which stories of development are told and emphasized. All of these changes have required a critical rethinking of our assumptions about "normality" and the idea of "family" development. The relationship between demographic changes and alterations in the prevalence, timing, and sequencing of some key family transitions also has to be noted.

In our clinical work with families presenting in various forms and at all stages of development, we have found it useful to adopt Falicov's (1988) ideas about family development. She emphasizes culture and gender relativity rather than universality, transitions rather than stages, dimensions and processes rather than markers, and a resource rather than a deficit orientation. We concur with her idea that a systems approach to family development calls for a dialectical integration of two tendencies: stability and change. The emphasis is on both tendencies rather than one or the other. Change and stability must be addressed simultaneously. We do not find it clinically useful to think of families as "stuck" and unable to bring about change. Rather, we find it clinically useful to look for patterns of continuity, identity, and stability that can be maintained while new behavioral patterns are changing.

We believe that there is much evidence to support the position that nurses will find heuristic value in the family development category of CFAM. They should be aware, however, of some of the problems in its indiscriminate adoption and application. We find indefensible such sweeping generalizations as "The family life cycle is genetically determined," or "The family life cycle is culturally universal." We urge nurses to consider carefully the implication of a family's ethnicity, race, and social class in applying the family development category.

We also caution nurses against *indiscriminately* applying the family development category and overemphasizing *smooth progression.* Contradictions and difficulties inherent in progressing through the life cycle are normal. Families are complex systems that need to deal with many different progressions at once. That is, there are biological, psychological, sociological, and cultural progressions. Tensions and continuing change brought about by contradiction between these progressions are normal. Family life is seldom smooth or bland, but rather is zestful and active. We therefore encourage nurses, when using the family development category, to have families discuss their joys and satisfactions as well as their tensions and stresses. The family developmental story told by one family member is from that member's "observer perspective" (Maturana & Varela, 1992).

In addition to delineating stages and tasks implicit in the family life cycle, we have found it useful to assess the attachments between family members. Attachment refers to a relatively enduring, unique emotional tie between two specific persons. Bowlby (1977) notes:

> Affectional bonds and subjective states of a strong emotion tend to go together. . . . Thus many of the most intensive of all emotions arise during the formation, the maintenance, the disruption and renewal of affectional bonds which for that reason are sometimes called emotional bonds. In terms of subjective experience the formation of a bond is described as falling in love, maintaining a bond as loving someone, and losing a partner as grieving over someone.

Similarly the threat of loss arouses anxiety and actual loss causes sorrow, while both situations are likely to arouse anger. Finally the unchallenged maintenance of a bond is experienced as a source of security and renewal of a bond as a source of joy. (p. 203)

Although the terms "bonding" and "attachment" are sometimes used to describe different relationships, we have chosen in this book and in our clinical work to make no distinction between these terms. In assessing a family, we tend to pay the most attention to the reciprocal nature of an attachment and the quality of the affectional tie. We illustrate these bonds between family members by drawing attachment diagrams. The symbols used in these diagrams (Fig. 3–8) are similar to those used in the structural assessment diagrams. Again it is important for us to emphasize that there is no one "right" level of attachment or "best" attachment configuration. We agree with Byng-Hall (1995) that a systemic concept for attachment is needed, one that moves beyond a dyadic relationship, especially that of parent-child. He proposes a concept of a secure family base, "a family that provides a reliable network of attachment relationships in which all family members of whatever age are able to feel sufficiently secure to explore" (p. 46). We like this concept because it expands attachment to include multiple networks, which is especially important as the boomer cohort increases in age.

In the CFAM developmental category, we discuss family life cycle

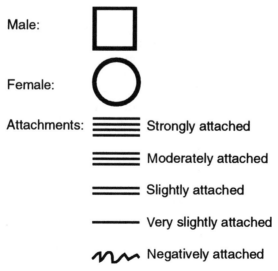

FIGURE 3–8. Symbols used in attachment diagrams.

stages, the emotional process of transition (namely, key principles), and second-order changes—the issues dealt with and tasks often accomplished during each stage. In an effort to emphasize the variability of family development, we discuss five sample types of family life cycles:

1. Middle-class North American family life cycle
2. Divorce and postdivorce family life cycle
3. Remarried family life cycle
4. Comparison of professional and low-income family life cycle stage
5. Adoptive family life cycle

MIDDLE-CLASS NORTH AMERICAN FAMILY LIFE

We are grateful to Carter and McGoldrick (1988,1999) for delineating six stages in the North American middle-class family life cycle (Table 3–1). We highlight the expansion, contraction, and realignment of relationships as entries, exits, and development of family members occur. Although the relationship patterns and family themes may sound familiar, we wish to emphasize that the structure and form of the North American family have changed radically. We believe that it is important for nurses to have a positive conceptual frame for what *is*: dual-career families, permanent single-parent households, unmarried couples, homosexual couples, remarried couples, and sole-parent adoptions. Transitional crises should not be thought of as permanent traumas. We believe it is imperative that the use of language that links us to previous stereotypes be dropped. For example, we try to eliminate such phrases as "children of divorce," "working mother," "out-of-wedlock child," "fatherless home," and so forth from the language we use about families. Also, we urge nurses to critically reflect on how culture, ethnicity, gender, race, and sexual orientation influence a family's development stages and tasks as well as attachments.

Stage One: The Launching of the Single Young Adult

In outlining the stages of the middle-class North American family life cycle, we have chosen to start with the stage of "young adults." The primary task of young adults is to come to terms with their family of origin by remaining connected and yet separate, without cutting off or fleeing reactively to a substitute emotional source. The family of origin has a profound influence on whom, when, how, and whether the young adult will marry. Saluter and Lugaila (1998) report "sharp in-

TABLE 3–1.
THE STAGES OF THE FAMILY LIFE CYCLE

Family Life Cycle Stage	Emotional Process of Transition: Key Principles	Second-Order Changes in Family Status Required to Proceed Developmentally
1. Leaving home: Single young adults	Accepting emotional and financial responsibility for self	1. Differentiation of self in relation to family of origin 2. Development of intimate peer relationships 3. Establishment of self re: work and financial independence
2. The joining of families through marriage: The new couple	Commitment to new system	1. Formation of marital system 2. Realignment of relationships with extended families and friends to include spouse
3. Families with young children	Accepting new members into system	1. Adjusting marital system to make space for child(ren) 2. Joining in childrearing, financial, and household tasks 3. Realignment of relationships with extended family to include parenting and grandparenting roles
4. Families with adolescents	Increasing flexibility of family boundaries to include children's independence and grandparents frailties	1. Shifting of parent-child relationships to permit adolescent to move in and out of system 2. Refocus on midlife marital and career issues 3. Beginning shift toward joint caring for older generation
5. Launching children and moving on	Accepting a multitude of exits from and entries into the family system	1. Renegotiation of marital system as a dyad 2. Development of adult-to-adult relationships between grown children and their parents 3. Realignment of relationships to include in-laws and grandchildren 4. Dealing with disabilities and death of parents (grandparents)

(continued)

TABLE 3–1. *(continued)*
THE STAGES OF THE FAMILY LIFE CYCLE

Family Life Cycle Stage	Emotional Process of Transition: Key Principles	Second-Order Changes in Family Status Required to Proceed Developmentally
6. Families in later life	Accepting the shifting of generational roles	1. Maintaining own and couple functioning and interests in face of physiological decline; exploration of new familial and social role options 2. Support for a more central role of middle generation 3. Making room in the system for the wisdom and experience of elderly people, supporting the older generation without overfunctioning for them 4. Dealing with loss of spouse, siblings, and other peers and preparation for own death; life review and integration

Source: Carter, B., & McGoldrick, M. (1999) Overview: The expanded family life cycle: Individual, family and social perspectives. In B. Carter and M. McGoldrick (Eds.). *The expanded family life cycle: Individual, family and social perspectives* (3rd ed.). Boston: Allyn & Bacon, p 2. Copyright © 1999 by Allyn & Bacon. Reprinted by permission.

creases in the proportion of never married have been primarily seen among men and women in their late twenties and early thirties" (p. 1). The increases are noted for Hispanics, blacks, and whites. The median age of first marriage is increasing.

This stage may last for several years in a family's development. It is an opportunity for young adults to sort out emotionally what they will take along from the family of origin, what they will leave behind, and what they will establish for themselves as they progress through succeeding stages of the family life cycle. For both men and women, this is a particularly critical phase. Men during this stage sometimes have difficulty committing themselves to relationships and form a pseudo-independent identity centered around work. Women may choose to define themselves in relation to a male and postpone or forgo establishing an independent identity. Berliner, Jacob, and Schwartzberg (1998) recommend that clinicians "understand the client's legacies regarding marital status (e.g., the available roles for unmarried men and women, the flexibility of pathways to adulthood, the meaning of marriage as a rite of passage and of family continuity)" (p. 364).

Tasks

1. **Differentiation of self in relation to family of origin.** The young adult's shift toward adult status involves the development of a mutually respectful form of relating with his or her parents in which the young adult's parents can be appreciated for what they are. The young adult adjusts his view of his parents by neither making them into what they are not nor blaming them for what they could not be.
2. **Development of intimate peer relationships.** The emphasis is on the young adult's passing from an individual orientation to an interdependent orientation of self. There is no single mold of social experience for young adults to follow as they develop intimate relationships. During this task, young adults strive to bridge the gap between autonomy and attachment as they share themselves with others rather than using others as the source of self.
3. **Establishment of self in relation to work and financial independence.** In a young adult's 20s, the "trying on" of various identities to test or refine career skills and interest is typical. The young adult who is committed to a career path or occupational choice by his or her mid- to late 20s is less vulnerable to self-doubt or decreased self-esteem than the young adult without direction, and generally functions productively with little anxiety. Issues of competitiveness, expectations, and differences regarding work and financial goals require sorting through by the young adult and his or her family of origin.

Attachments

There are no right or wrong attachments for young adults in stage one. Rather, it is important for the nurse to draw forth from the family its beliefs about attachment to each other and how it regards this attachment. This will be influenced by culture, gender, race, sexual orientation, social class, and whether the young adult lives at home or not. Some sample attachments for stage one are given in Figure 3–9. The first diagram illustrates a young adult who is bonded equally with her father and mother. The second diagram illustrates a young adult who is more closely attached to each parent than the parents are to each other; the parents are negatively bonded. Of significance in the second

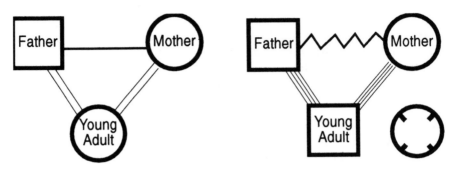

FIGURE 3–9. Sample attachments in stage 1.

diagram is that there was a death during the childhood of the young adult. It could be hypothesized that his difficulties in establishing his own identity are related to the family's hesitancy to come to grips with his deceased sister and the "empty nest."

Questions to Ask the Family. Which of your parents is most accepting of your career plans? How does he or she show this? What does your sister think of your parents' reaction to your career plans? If your father were more accepting of your desire to move into an independent living situation, how do you think your mother would react?

Stage Two: Marriage: The Joining of Families

Many couples believe that when they marry, it is just two individuals who are joining together. However, both spouses have grown up in families that have now become interconnected through marriage. Both spouses, although hopefully differentiated from their families of origin in an emotional, financial, and functional way, carry their whole family into the relationship. Marriage is a two-generational relationship with a minimum of three families coming together: his family of origin, her family of origin, and the new couple. If either new partner comes from a stepfamily, the number of families coming together can increase substantially.

Tasks

1. **Establishment of couple identity.** The new couple must establish itself as an identifiable unit. This requires negotiation of many issues that were previously defined on an individual level. These issues include such routine matters as eating and sleeping patterns, sexual-contact, and use of space and time. The couple must decide about

which traditions and rules to retain from each family and which ones they will develop for themselves. They must develop acceptable closeness-distance styles and recognize individual differences in adult attachment styles.

2. **Realignment of relationships with extended families to include spouse.** A renegotiation of relationships with each spouse's family of origin has to take place to accommodate the new spouse. This can place no small stress on both the couple and each family of origin to open itself to new ways of being. Some couples deal with their parents by cutting off the relationship in a bid for independence. Other couples choose to handle this task of realignment by absorbing the new spouse into the family of origin. The third common pattern involves a balance between some contact and some distance.

3. **Decisions about parenthood.** For most couples, experiencing happiness is highest at the beginning of the life cycle stage of marriage. Although a small but increasing number of married couples are deciding not to have children, most still plan on becoming parents. The question of *when* to conceive is becoming increasingly complex, especially with the changed role of women, the widespread use of contraceptives, the availability of a wide range of fertilization strategies, and the trend toward later marriages. It has been found that couples who have evolved more competent marital structures prenatally are more likely to incorporate the child successfully into the family (Lewis, 1988a; Lewis, 1988b; Lewis, Owen, & Cox, 1988).

Attachments

A sample attachment for a couple in stage two is the development of close emotional ties between the spouses (Fig. 3–10). The first diagram illustrates how they do not have to break ties with their families of origin but rather maintain ties with and adjust to them. A different

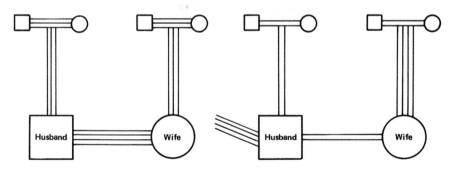

FIGURE 3–10. Sample attachments in stage 2.

type of attachment (illustrated in the second diagram) can occur if both members of a couple do not align themselves together. The wife is more heavily bonded to her family of origin than she is to her husband. The husband is more tied to outside interests (e.g., work, friends) than to his wife.

Questions to Ask the Family. Which family was most in favor of your marriage? How did your siblings show that they supported your marriage? What did your spouse think of your parents' marital relationship? If you two as a couple were to model your marriage on your parents' marriage, what would you incorporate into your marriage? How did the diagnosis of multiple sclerosis influence your bonding as a couple?

Stage Three: Families with Young Children

During this stage, the adults now become caretakers to a younger generation. Issues about taking responsibility and dealing with the demands of dependent children are challenging for most families when financial resources are typically stretched and the parents are heavily involved in career development. The disposition of childcare responsibilities and household chores in dual-career households is a particular struggle. Schnittger and Bird (1990) found that men and women differ significantly in the coping strategies they use to deal with this issue. Women use cognitive restructuring, delegating, limiting avocational activities, and using social support significantly more often than do men. As children progress in age, Schnittger and Bird found that both men and women altered their use of coping strategies; for example, those with children under age 6 reported less use of delegating than those with an oldest child aged 13 to 18. Carter (1999) advocates that clinicians label the work-family problem of juggling accountabilities "as a *social* problem, to be dealt with by the *couple*, not a 'woman's problem' for her to struggle with alone" (p. 253). We concur.

Tasks

1. **Adjusting marital system to make space for child.** The couple must continue to meet each other's personal needs as well as their parental responsibilities. With the introduction of the first child, challenges for personal space, couple sexual and emotional intimacy, and socializing exist. Both mothers and fathers are increasingly aware of the need for emotional integration of the child into the family. Children can be brought into a variety of environments:

there is no space for them, there is space for them, or there is a vacuum that they are expected to fill. If the child has a handicap, there will be more stress on the couple as they adjust their expectations and deal with their emotional reactions.

2. **Joining in childrearing, financial, and household tasks.** The couple must find a mutually satisfying way to deal with childcare responsibility and household chores that does not overburden one partner. Balancing the budget and juggling family and other responsibilities is a major task. The emotional as well as the financial cost of solutions to deal with childcare responsibilities must be addressed. Both mothers and fathers contribute to the child's development and can do so in different or similar ways. Physical and playful stimulation of the child complements verbal interaction. Parents can either support or hinder their children's success in developing peer relationships and achieving at school. Middle-class families, responding to intense pressure from the school system, tend to stress the values of achievement and productivity, whereas some working-class families may respond to this pressure by feelings of alienation.

3. **Realignment of relationships with extended family to include parenting and grandparenting roles.** The couple must design and develop the new roles of father and mother in addition to the marital role rather than replacing it. Members of each family of origin also take on new roles, for example, grandfather or aunt. Frequently, grandparents who perhaps were opposed to the marriage in the beginning become very interested in the young children. For many older adults, this is an especially gratifying time because it allows them to have intimacy without the responsibility required by parenting. It also permits them to develop a new type of adult-adult relationship with their children. Opportunities for intergenerational support or conflict abound as expectations about child-rearing and healthcare practices are expressed.

Attachments

Parents need to maintain a marital bond and continue personal adult-centered conversations in addition to child-centered conversations. Space for privacy and time spent together are important needs. Children require security and warm attachments to adults, as well as the opportunity to develop positive sibling relationships. In Figure 3–11, sample attachment diagrams are given. A competitive, negative relationship (illustrated by the wavy line) exists between the children and between the spouses in the second diagram. The mother is overbonded to the daughter, and the father is underinvolved with the daughter. The

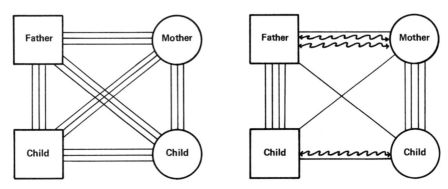

FIGURE 3–11. Sample attachments in stage 3.

father is overattached to the son, and the mother is underinvolved with the son. This is an example of same-sex coalitions existing cross-generationally.

>>**Questions to Ask the Family.** What percentage of your time do you spend taking care of your children? What percentage do you spend taking care of your marriage? Is this a comfortable balance for the two of you? What effect does this pattern have on your children? If your children thought that you should be closer, how might they tell you this? What impact did the miscarriage have on your marriage?

Stage Four: Families with Adolescents

This period has often been characterized as one of intense upheaval and transition, in which biological, emotional, and sociocultural changes occur with great and ever-increasing rapidity.

Tasks

1. **Shift of parent-child relationships to permit adolescents to move in or out of system.** The family must move from the dependency relationship previously established with a young child to an increasingly independent relationship with the adolescent. Growing psychological independence is frequently not recognized because of continuing physical dependence. Conflict often surfaces when a teenager's independence threatens the family. For example, teenagers may precipitate marital conflict when they question who makes the family rules about the car: Mom or Dad? Families frequently respond to an adolescent's request for increasing autonomy in two

ways: (1) they abruptly define rigid rules and re-create an earlier stage of dependency or (2) they establish premature independence. In the second scenario, the family supports only independence and ignores dependent needs. This may result in premature separation when the teenager is not really ready to be fully autonomous. The teenager may thus return home defeated. Parents need to shift from the parental role of "protector" to that of "preparer" for the challenges of adulthood.

2. **Refocus on midlife marital and career issues.** During this stage, parents are often struggling with what Erikson (1963) calls generativity, the need to be useful as a human being, partner, and mentor to another generation. The socially and sexually maturing teenager's frequent questioning and conflict about values, lifestyles, career plans, and so forth, can thrust the parents into an examination of their own marital and career issues. Depending on many factors, including cultural and gender expectations, this may be a period of positive growth or painful struggle for men and women.

3. **Beginning shift toward joint caring for older generation.** As parents are aging, so too are the grandparents. Parents (especially women) sometimes feel that they are besieged on both sides: teenagers are asking for more freedom and grandparents are asking for more support. With the trend of women having children later in life and seniors living longer, this double demand for attention and resources most likely will intensify.

Attachments

All family members continue to have their relationships within the family, or increasingly, the teenagers are more involved with their friends than with family members. The husband and wife need to reinvest in the marital relationship.

An example of an attachment pattern is illustrated in Figure 3–12. In the second diagram, the mother is overinvolved with the eldest son and has a negative relationship with the husband. The father tends to be minimally involved with all family members. There is conflict between the two sons.

> **Questions to Ask the Family.** What privileges do your teenagers have now that they did not have when they were younger? *Ask the adolescents:* How do you think your parents will handle it when your younger sister wants to date? Will it be different from when you wanted to date? On a scale of 1 to 10 (with 10 being the highest), how much confidence do your parents have in your ability to say no to drugs?

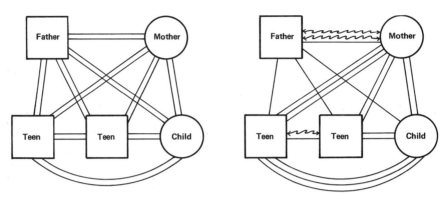

FIGURE 3–12. Sample attachments in stage 4.

Stage Five: Launching Children and Moving On

Many middle-class North Americans whose children have grown up assumed they would have an empty nest. However, these expectations are not being met. The United States Census Bureau reports that more young adults are living at home with their parents. In 1996, the proportion of 24-year-olds in the U.S. living in their parents' home was 53 percent. Among young adults age 25 to 34, the proportion rose from 9 percent in 1980 to 12 percent in 1996. Men are more likely to live "at home" than women and 93 percent of both the men and women have never married and do not have children of their own living with them in their parents' home (Saluta & Lugaila, 1998). Rising housing costs and beginning pay rates that have not gone up as fast as those of more experienced workers have been singled out as some causes of this trend. A different explanation is that young North Americans are having difficulty growing up and are unwilling to go out on their own and settle for less affluence than their parents.

Tasks

1. **Renegotiation of marital system as a dyad.** There is frequently a thrust to alter some of the basic tenets of the marital relationship. This is especially true if both partners are working and the children have left home. The couple bond can take on a more prominent position. The balance between dependency, independency, and interdependency has to be reexamined.

2. **Development of adult-to-adult relationships between grown children and their parents.** The family of origin must relinquish the pri-

mary roles of parent and child. They must adapt to the new roles of parent and adult child. This involves renegotiation of emotional and financial commitments. The key emotional process during this stage is for family members to deal with a multitude of exits from and entries into the family system.

3. **Realignment of relationships to include in-laws and grown children.** The parents adjust family ties and expectations to include their child's spouse or partner. The once-prevalent idea that the time after a grown child marries is a lonely, sad time, especially for women, has been replaced. Increases in marital satisfaction have frequently been noted.

4. **Dealing with disabilities and death of grandparents.** Many families regard the disability or death of an elderly parent as a natural occurrence. If, however, there is unfinished business between the couple and the elderly parents, there may be serious repercussions, not only for the children but also for the new third generation. The type of disability afflicting the seniors will determine the effects on the immediate family. For example, Pallett (1990) points out that care-givers who do not understand Alzheimer's dementia and its effects on cognitive function and behavior often attempt to deal with inappropriate or disruptive behavior in ineffective and counterproductive ways. Thus they inadvertently intensify their own stress.

Attachments

Each family member continues to have outside interests and establish new roles appropriate to this stage. Sample attachment patterns are illustrated in Figure 3–13. A problem may arise when both husband

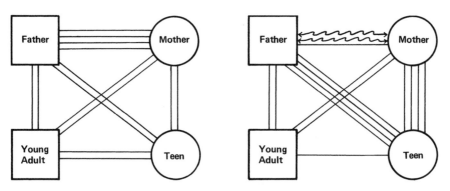

FIGURE 3–13. Sample attachments in stage 5.

and wife hold on to their last child. They may avoid conflict by allowing the eldest child to leave home and then focusing on the next child.

Questions to Ask the Family. How did your parents help you to leave home? What is the difference between how you left home and how your children are leaving home? Will your parents get along better, worse, or the same with each other once you have left home? Who, between your Mom and Dad, will miss the children the most? As you see your child moving on with a new relationship, what would you like your child to do differently than you did? If your parents are still alive, are there any issues you would like to discuss with them?

Stage Six: Families in Later Life

This stage begins with retirement and lasts until the death of both spouses. Potentially, it can last 20 to 25 years for many couples. The key emotional process in this stage is to accept the shift of generational roles.

Tasks

1. **Maintaining own or couple functioning and interest in the face of physiological decline: exploration of new familial and social role options.** Marital relationships continue to be important, and marital satisfaction contributes to both the morale and ongoing activity of both spouses. Bishop, Epstein, Baldwin, Miller, and Keitner (1988) found that the husband's morale is most strongly associated with health, socioeconomic status, income, and, to a lesser extent, family functioning. The wife's morale is most strongly associated with family functioning and, to a lesser extent, with health and socioeconomic status.

   As the older couple find themselves in new roles of grandparents and mother-in-law and father-in-law, they must adjust to their children's spouses and open space for the new grandchildren. Difficulty in making the status changes required can be reflected in an older family member refusing to relinquish some of his or her power: for example, refusing to turn over a company or making plans for succession in a family business. The shift in status between the senior family members and the middle-aged family members is a reciprocal one. Difficulties may occur in several ways. Older adults may give up and become totally dependent on the next generation, the next generation may not accept the seniors' diminishing powers and treat them as totally competent, or the next generation may see only the seniors' frailties and treat them as totally incompetent.

2. **Making room in the system for the wisdom and experience of the seniors.** The task of supporting the older generation without overfunctioning for them is particularly salient because people are living longer. The vast majority of adults over 65 do not live alone but rather with other family members, and less than 5 percent live in institutions. In the U.S. in 1996, 24 percent of people aged 65 to 74 years, excluding the institutionalized population, lived alone, and the percent increased to only 41 percent for those aged 75 and older (Saluto & Lugaila, 1998). It is not uncommon to have a 90-year-old parent being cared for by her 70-year-old daughter, with both of them living in close proximity to a 50-year-old son and grandson. The parents of the baby boomers are the current generation of "young-old." They are highly motivated to participate in self-help groups and are interested in improving their quality of life through counseling, traditional and alternative health activities, and education. Many have found "new" family connections through the use of e-mail. They do not live by the aging myths of the past. Rather, as consumers they expect and demand a good quality of life. Many grandparents continue to be involved in childrearing. In 1996 in the U.S., 6 percent of all children under 18 lived only with their grandparents. This was an increase from 3 percent in 1970 (Saluter & Lugaila, 1998).

3. **Dealing with loss of spouse, siblings, and other peers and preparation for death.** This is a time for life review and taking care of unfinished business with family as well as with business and social contacts. Many people find it helpful to discuss their life, review it, and enjoy the opportunity of passing this information along to succeeding generations.

Attachments

The couple reinvest and modify the marital relationship based on the level of functioning of both partners. In the U.S. in 1996, 63 percent of persons 65 to 74 were married and living with their spouses, and 41 percent of those age 75 and over lived with their spouses (Saluter & Lugaila, 1998). There is an appropriate interdependence with the next generation. This concept of interdependence is particularly important for nurses to understand in working with families with adult daughters and their parents. Middle-class older men and women seem equally likely to aid and support their children, especially daughters. Frequency of contact, however, tends to be higher with daughters than with sons. Thus, the possibility of strong intergenerational attachments between

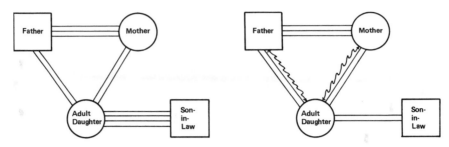

FIGURE 3–14. Sample attachments in stage 6.

a daughter and her parents exists. In the attachment pattern illustrated in Figure 3–14, the couple project their conflicts onto the extended family. This causes difficulty for the succeeding generations.

>**Questions to Ask the Family.** When you look back over your life, what aspects have you enjoyed the most? What has given you the most happiness? About what aspects do you feel the most regret? What would you hope that your children would do differently than you did? Similarly to what you did? As your health is declining, what plans have you and your son with schizophrenia made for alternate living arrangements for him?

THE DIVORCE AND POSTDIVORCE FAMILY LIFE CYCLE

Many changes in marital status and living arrangements are prevalent in North America today. Noteworthy is the high level of divorce. Saluter and Lugaila (1998) report that "the currently divorced population is the fastest growing marital status category" (p. 1). Divorced people represented 10 percent of adults age 18 and over in 1996 in the U.S., an increase from 3 percent in 1970. Whether the divorce rate will continue to climb, level off, or decline is a matter of speculation that can be backed up by various theories. There may be pressure for divorce to decline somewhat because of the possibility of unstable economic conditions and the AIDS epidemic. The proportion of children living with one parent has grown from 12 percent to 28 percent between 1970 and 1996 in the U.S. The majority (86 percent) live with their single-parent mother. An increasing proportion live with their father. In 1996, 14 percent lived with their father, up from 9 percent in 1970. The percentage of children living with one parent in 1996 varies: whites, 22 percent; Hispanics, 32 percent; blacks, 57 percent.

Families experiencing divorce are often under enormous pressure. Single-parent families must accomplish most of the same developmental tasks as two-parent families, but without all the resources. This places extra burdens on the remaining family members, who must compensate with increased effort to accomplish family tasks such as physical maintenance, social control, and tension management.

Quinn and Allen (1989) indicated from their study of 30 employed single parents that there were challenges in managing shortages of time, money, and energy. These parents voiced serious concerns about failure to meet perceived family and societal expectations for living "in a normal family" with two parents. "The women feel they must display behaviors which are contradictory to those they assumed they should exhibit if they were to remarry" (p. 390). They perceived ongoing pressure from family, friends, and church to marry again to give their children a "normal" family. The women reported being caught in a double bind, trying to demonstrate behaviors that might net them a new husband while trying to use seemingly opposing behaviors that allowed them to successfully manage their lives. We encourage nurses working with single-parent families to explore the parent's feelings about opposing expectations. This is a way of helping the women to plan their responses to various paradoxical situations.

It is also important for nurses to focus on the positive changes experienced by many separated women. Nelson's study (1994) found that recently "separated women used more growth-oriented coping, such as becoming more autonomous and furthering their education, and experienced more positive changes, such as, increased confidence and feelings of control, than did married women" (p. 158).

In our clinical supervision with nurses, we encourage focusing on the siblings, a subsystem that generally remains intact during the process of family reorganization. Schibuk (1989) reasons that sibling therapy can be effective, as children are the "unit of continuity" (p. 226). We also try to notice and support such cooperative postdivorce parenting environments as mutual parental support; teamwork; clear, flexible boundaries; high information exchange; constructive problem solving; and knowledgeable, experienced, involved, and authoritative parenting (Whiteside, 1998). Because many fathers are not used to taking care of their children without their wives orchestrating things, fathers often fade out of their children's lives. They want to avoid exwives and conflict and may feel uncomfortable if they have an unclear role of authority in their children's lives. Nurses can be extremely helpful in intervening in these situations and fostering mutually agreeable postdivorce arrangements for the benefit of the children.

Because divorce may occur at any stage of the family life cycle, it has a different impact on family functioning depending on its timing. The marital breakdown may be sudden or it may be long and drawn out. In either case, emotional work is required so that the family may deal with the shifts, gains, and losses in family membership. The phases involved in divorce and postdivorce are depicted in Table 3–2. Carter and McGoldrick (1999) found a clinical usefulness in the distinctions made between the three columns given in the tables. Column 1 lists the phase. Column 2 gives the prerequisite attitudes that will assist family members to make the transition and come through the developmental issues listed in column 3 en route to the next phase. We believe that clinical work directed at column 3 will not succeed if the family is having difficulty dealing with the issues in column 2.

Questions to Ask the Family. How do you explain to yourself the reasons for your divorce? Who initiated the idea of divorce? Who left whom? Who was most supportive of developing viable arrangements for *everyone* in the family? How was your spouse's willingness to continue a cooperative coparental relationship shown? How did you respond to this? As you changed your attachment to your spouse, what changes did you notice in your children? What would your in-laws say about how you have fostered your children's relationship with them? What would your children say? What methods have you found most successful in resolving conflicting issues with your ex-spouse? What advice would you give to other divorced parents on how to resolve conflictual issues with their ex-partners? How have your children helped you and your ex-spouse to maintain a supportive environment for them?

REMARRIED FAMILY LIFE CYCLE

The rise of remarriage and the stepfamily in North America in the recent decade has been striking. Between two-thirds and three-fourths of those who divorce eventually remarry. Glick (1989a) states that he sees "a preference for marriage in the observation that nine-tenths of young Americans are likely to marry; that close to one-half of the first marriages are likely to remain intact, despite the many options available to those involved; and that between two-thirds and three-fourths of those who divorce will eventually remarry" (p. 129). Glick (1989a) reports that an expected 72 percent of recently divorced women remarry. The level is higher (81 percent) for divorced women with no children, about the same (73 percent) for those with one or two children, and considerably lower (57 percent) for those with three or more children.

Glick (1989b) discusses the differences between a remarried family

TABLE 3–2.
STAGES OF DIVORCE FAMILY LIFE CYCLE

Phase	Emotional Process of Transition, Prerequisite Attitude	Developmental Issues
Divorce		
1. Deciding to divorce	Accepting inability to resolve marital tensions sufficiently to continue relationship	Accepting one's own part in the failure of the marriage
2. Planning the break-up of the system	Supporting viable arrangements for all parts of the system	1. Working cooperatively on problems of custody, visitation, and finances 2. Dealing with extended family about the divorce
3. Separation	1. Being willing to continue cooperative coparental relationship and joint financial support of children 2. Working on resolution of attachment to spouse	1. Mourning loss of nuclear family 2. Restructuring, marital and parent-child relationships and finances; adaptation to living apart 3. Realigning relationships with extended family; staying connected with spouse's extended family
4. Divorce	More work on emotional divorce: overcoming hurt, anger, guilt, and so forth	Retrieving hopes, dreams, and expectations from the marriage
Postdivorce		
1. Single-parent (custodial household or primary residence)	Being willing to maintain financial responsibilities, continue parental contact with ex-spouse, and support contact of children with ex-spouse and his or her family	1. Making flexible visitation arrangements with ex-spouse and his or her family 2. Rebuilding own financial resources 3. Rebuilding own social network
2. Single-parent (noncustodial)	Being willing to maintain parental contact with ex-spouse and support custodial parent's relationship with cihldren	1. Finding ways to continue effective parenting relationship with children 2. Maintaining financial responsibilities to ex-spouse and children 3. Rebuilding own social network

Source: Carter, B., & McGoldrick, M. (1999). The divorce cycle: A major variation in the American family life cycle. In B. Carter & M. McGoldrick (Eds.). *The expanded family life cycle: Individual, family and social perspectives* (3rd ed.). Boston: Allyn and Bacon, p 375. Copyright © 1999 by Allyn & Bacon. Reprinted by permission.

and a stepfamily with the latter being a "family remarried with a child under 18 years of age who is the biological child of one of the parents and was born before the remarriage occurred" (p. 24). In 1987, Glick estimates that there were 11 million remarried families and 4.3 million stepfamilies in the United States. He states that "21.3% of married couples/families are remarried families and 8.3% of all married couples/families are stepfamilies" (p. 25). In 1990 in the U.S., 21 percent of all married-couple households with children had a stepfather as compared to 1980, when it was about 15 percent. Berger (1998) reports that one in three Americans is a member of a stepfamily as a stepchild, stepparent, remarried parent, or stepgrandparent (p. 11).

Pill (1990) states that the redivorce rate for remarried couples is even higher than the divorce rate following first marriages. The high rate of redivorce within the first 5 years of remarriage suggests that these early years are a challenging period. Pill (1990) studied 29 nonclinical stepfamilies with custodial adolescent stepchildren and examined cohesion and adaptability. He found that they were in the process of revising their basic assumptions about family life and developing a stepfamily identity. The stepfamilies reported low to moderate levels of cohesion and moderate to high levels of adaptability, both of which were associated with stepfamily but not marital satisfaction. Stepfamily cohesion was lower than that of nuclear families, whereas adaptability was higher in the same life cycle stage.

The family emotional process at the transition to remarriage consists of struggling with fears about investment in new relationships: one's own fears, the new spouse's fears, and the fears of the children (of either or both spouses). It also consists of dealing with hostile or upset reactions of the children, the extended families, and ex-spouse. "Unlike biological families in which family membership is defined sanguinely, legally, and spatially and is characterized by explicit boundaries, the structure of a stepfamily is less clear" (Pasley, Rhoden, Visher, & Visher, 1996, p. 344). There is a need to address the ambiguity of the new family organization, including roles and relationships. Often there is an increased arousal of parental guilt and concerns about the children, and there may be a positive or negative rearousal of the old attachment to the ex-spouse (Carter & McGoldrick, 1999). In Table 3–3 Carter and McGoldrick have given a developmental outline for stepfamily formation.

Ahrons and Rodgers (1987) have advocated for models of healthy, well-functioning binuclear families. Having been angered by a predominant emphasis on pathology in the divorce literature, Ahrons began to study what she calls binuclear families. This term not only refers to joint-custody families or to families in which the relationship

TABLE 3–3.
REMARRIED FAMILY FORMATION: A DEVELOPMENT OUTLINE

Steps	Prerequisite Attitude	Developmental Issues
1. Entering the new relationship	Recovery from loss of first marriage (adequate "emotional divorce")	Recommitting to marriage and to forming a family with readiness to deal with the complexity and ambiguity
2. Conceptualizing and planning the new marriage and family	Accepting one's own fears and those of new spouse and children about remarriage and forming a stepfamily Accepting need for time and patience for adjustment to complexity and ambiguity of: 1. Multiple new roles 2. Boundaries: space, time, membership, authority 3. Affective issues: guilt, loyalty conflicts, desire for mutuality, unresolvable past hurts	1. Working on openness in the new relationships to avoid pseudomutuality 2. Planning for maintenance of cooperative financial and coparental relationships with ex-spouses 3. Planning to help children deal with fears, loyalty conflicts, and membership in two systems 4. Realigning relationships with extended family to include new spouse and children 5. Planning maintenance of connections for children with extended family of ex-spouse(s)
3. Remarriage and reconstruction of family	Final resolution of attachment to previous spouse and ideal of "intact" family Accepting a different model of family with permeable boundaries	1. Restructuring family boundaries to allow inclusion of new spouse-stepparent 2. Realignment of relationships and financial arrangements throughout subsystems to permit interweaving of several systems 3. Making room for relationships of all children with biological (noncustodial) parents, grandparents, and other extended family 4. Sharing memories and histories to enhance stepfamily integration

TABLE 3–4.
DIFFERENCES BETWEEN STEPFAMILIES AND NUCLEAR FAMILIES
AND THE THERAPEUTIC IMPLICATIONS

How Stepfamilies Differ from Nuclear Families	Therapeutic Implications
1. There are different structural characteristics.	1. Must evaluate the family using stepfamily norms. A nuclear family model is not valid.
2. There is little or no family loyalty.	2. Initially, seeing the family members together may be unproductive.
3. Before integration, the family reacts to transitional stresses.	3. The first focus needs to be on the transitional adjustment process, not on intrapsychic processes.
4. Society compares stepfamilies negatively to nuclear families.	4. There is a basic need for acceptance and validation as a worthwhile family unit.
5. There is a long integration period with predictable stages.	5. The stage of family development is very important in the assessment of whom to see in therapy.
6. There is not a breakdown of family homeostasis; equilibrium has never been established.	6. With normalization and education, stability can emerge from chaos and ignorance of the norms.
7. There is a complicated "supra family system."	7. The complications of the family need to be kept in mind during therapy. Drawing a genogram helps.
8. There have been many losses for all individuals.	8. Grief work may be necessary.
9. There are preexisting parent-child coalitions.	9. Developing a secure couple relationship is essential. Many times, "permission" is needed to do this.
10. A solid couple relationship does not signify good stepparent-stepchild relationships.	10. Steprelationships take special attention separate from the couple relationship.

TABLE 3–4. *(continued)*
**DIFFERENCES BETWEEN STEPFAMILIES AND NUCLEAR FAMILIES
AND THE THERAPEUTIC IMPLICATIONS**

How Stepfamilies Differ from Nuclear Families	Therapeutic Implications
11. There is a different balance of power.	11. Stepparents have very little authority in the family initially. Therefore, discipline issues need to be handled by the biological parent. Children have more power, which needs to be channeled positively.
12. There is less family control because there is an influential parent elsewhere or in memory.	12. Appropriate control can be fostered to lessen the anxiety engendered by helplessness
13. Children have more than two parenting figures.	13. There is a need to think in terms of a "parenting coalition," not a parenting couple.
14. There are ambiguous family boundaries with little agreement as to family history	14. These losses and stresses may require attention.
15. Initially there is no family history.	15. Members need to share their past histories and develop family rituals and ways of doing things.
16. The emotional climate is intense and unexpected.	16. Empathy with other family members can be encouraged by understanding the human needs that are not being met: to be loved and appreciated, to belong, and to have control over one's life.

Source: Visher, E. B., & Visher, J. S. (1996). *Therapy with stepfamilies.* pp 41–42. New York: Brunner/Mazel, with permission.

between ex-spouses is friendly, but indicates a different familial structure, without inferring anything about the nature or quality of the ex-spouses' relationship. Ahrons and Rodgers, who worked with 98 divorced couples over a 5-year period, produced some interesting relationship types, including "perfect pals," a small group of divorced spouses whose previous marriage had not overshadowed their long-standing friendship. The "cooperative colleagues" were a considerably larger and typical group found by Ahrons and Rodgers. Although not good friends, they worked well together on issues concerning their children. The third group were the "angry associates," and the fourth group were "fiery foes," who felt nothing but fury for their ex-spouses. Ahrons and Rodgers termed the fifth group "dissolved duos," who after the separation or divorce discontinued any contact with each other. Ahrons (1998) advocates for a normative process model of divorce rather than focusing on evidence of pathology or dysfunction. We agree with this stance.

We encourage nurses working with divorced and remarried families to bring to their patients or clients research knowledge of what works or does not work to foster continuing family relationships. Nurses should be cautioned, however, that there are seldom simple answers to complex problems. For example, Healy, Malley, and Stewart (1990) found that predictors such as child's age, gender, frequency and regularity of father-child visitation, father-child closeness, and the effect of parental legal conflict on the child's self-esteem were found to have different implications for different groups of 6- to 12-year-old children and for children in different situations. Their findings "suggest the futility of seeking simple answers to whether ongoing contact with fathers following divorce is beneficial or detrimental for children" (p. 531).

We also encourage nurses working with stepfamilies to increase their knowledge about stepfamily issues and respect the uniqueness of stepfamily life. The study conducted by Pasley, Rhoden, Visher, and Visher (1996) supports the idea that uninformed clinicians may unwittingly increase rather than decrease family tensions if they communicate to stepfamilies that they should be like biological families. In Table 3–4, Visher and Visher (1996) provide an outline of the differences between stepfamilies and nuclear families and the therapeutic implications.

> ***Questions to Ask the Family.*** What were the differences between you and your spouse in how you each successfully recovered from your first marriage? What most helped each of you deal with your own fears about remarriage? About forming a stepfamily? How did your spouse invite your children to adjust to him or her? What do your children think was the most useful thing you did in helping them deal with loyalty conflicts? What advice do you have for other stepfamilies on how to create a new family? What are you most proud of in how you have helped your stepfamily successfully make the transition from what they were before to what they are now?

COMPARISON OF PROFESSIONAL AND LOW-INCOME FAMILY LIFE CYCLE STAGES

The family life cycle of the poor frequently does not match the middle-class paradigm so often used to conceptualize their situations. Hines (1988) suggests that the family life cycle of the poor is actually three phases: the unattached young adult (perhaps younger than 12 years old) who is virtually unaccountable to any adults, families with children—a phase occupying most of the life span and including three- and four-generational households, and the final phase of the grandmother who continues to be involved in central childrearing in her senior years. In 1996 in the U.S., 6 percent of all children under 18 lived in their grandparents' household, an increase from 3 percent in 1950 (Saluter & Lugaila, 1998). We encourage nurses to consider the effects of ethnicity and religion, socioeconomic status, race, and environment on when and how a family makes its own transitions in its own life cycle.

Fulmer (1988) has suggested one comparison of the life cycle stages of professional and low-income families. His comparisons are outlined in Table 3–5. Although we do not believe in stereotypical life cycle stages or comparisons, we believe that the elements (education, timing, and pregnancy) suggested by Fulmer are worth considering. We encourage nurses to consider the great variability between various types of families as well as within types of families.

ADOPTIVE FAMILY LIFE CYCLE

In adoption, the family boundaries of all those involved are expanded. Reitz and Watson (1992) define adoption as:

> A means of providing some children with security and meeting their developmental needs by legally transferring ongoing parental responsibilities from their birth parents to their adoptive parents; recognizing that in so doing we have created a new kinship network that forever links those two families together through the child, who is shared by both. (p. 11)

We agree with this definition. As in marriage, the new legal status of the adoptive family does not automatically sever the psychological ties to the earlier family. Rather, the family boundaries are expanded and realigned. The data about how many children are adopted each year is sketchy because of multiple statistical systems. Fein (1998) found that in 1992 127,441 children were adopted in the U.S., a slight increase from 118,000 five years earlier. Approximately 42 percent of those adoptions involved stepparents and relatives. The biggest increase, ac-

TABLE 3–5.
COMPARISON OF FAMILY LIFE CYCLE STAGES

Age	Professional Families	Low-Income Families
12–17	1. Prevent pregnancy 2. Graduate from high school 3. Parents continue support while permitting child to achieve greater independence	1. First pregnancy 2. Attempt to graduate from high school 3. Parent attempts strict control before pregnancy. After pregnancy, relaxation of controls and continued support of new mother and infant
18–21	1. Prevent pregnancy 2. Leave parental household for college 3. Adapt to parent-child separation	1. Second pregnancy 2. No further education 3. Young mother acquires adult status in parental household
22–25	1. Prevent pregnancy 2. Develop professional identity in graduate school 3. Maintain separation from parental household, begin living in serious relationship	1. Third pregnancy 2. Marriage: leave parental household to establish stepfamily 3. Maintain connection with kinship network
26–30	1. Prevent pregnancy 2. Marriage: develop nuclear couple as separate from parents 3. Intense work involvement as career begins	1. Separate from husband 2. Mother becomes head of own household within kinship network
31–35	1. First pregnancy 2. Renew contact with parents as grandparents 3. Differentiate career and childrearing roles between husband and wife	1. First grandchild 2. Mother becomes grandmother and cares for daughter and infant

Source: Fulmer, R. (1988). Lower-income and professional families: A comparison of structure and life cycle process. In B. Carter & M. McGoldrick (Eds.), *The changing family life cycle: A framework for family therapy* (2nd ed.). Boston: Allyn & Bacon, p. 551. Copyright © 1988 by Allyn & Bacon. Reprinted by permission.

cording to Fein, has been children adopted from other countries. "Because they require visas, there are up to date statistics for these adoptions and since 1990, their numbers have nearly doubled from 7,093 to 13,620 in 1997" (Fein, 1998, p. 1). This has resulted in increased visibility for the adoption process and the issues involved for parents and children.

We believe that nurses should be aware of the trends and special circumstances in forming adoptive families. For example, most agencies offer adoption service along a continuum of openness. Silverstein and Demick (1994) outlined some potential benefits of open adoption for birth parents, including increased empathy for adoptive parents, reassurance that the child is safe and loved, and a reduction of shame and guilt. For adoptive parents, there is increased empathy for the birth parents, reduced stress imposed by secrecy and the unknown, and an embracing from the start of an affirmative acceptance of the child's cultural heritage. For the child, there is increased empathy for the adoptive parents, enriched connections with them, and reduced stress of disconnection. Simultaneously, for the child there is increased empathy for the birth parents and a reduction in fantasies about them, and with clear, consistent information, there is increased control in dealing with adoptive issues. We believe that these potential benefits are very significant, especially for families adopting babies from different cultures and races. There can also be divorced, single-parent, married, or remarried adoptive families. Reitz and Watson (1992) also have discussed adoptions within extended families as well as families with various forms of open dual parentage.

The adoption process, including the decision, application, and final adoption, can be a stressful as well as a joyful period for many couples. During the preschool developmental phase, the family must acknowledge the adoption as a fact of family life. The question of the permanency of the relationship sometimes arises from both the child and the parents. Hajal and Rosenberg (1991) have developed some hypotheses to explain the overrepresentation of adopted children (particularly those between 11 and 16) in the mental health outpatient system:

1. Genetic, hereditary factors
2. Deficiencies in prenatal and perinatal care
3. Adverse circumstances of adoption, including multiple disruptions in early life
4. Conditions in the adoptive home, including preexisting family problems
5. Temperamental differences between the adoptee and the adoptive parents or family

6. Fantasy system and communication regarding adoption, including parental attitudes about adoption
7. Difficulties establishing a firm sense of identity during adolescence
8. Greater age difference than usual between parents and adoptees

It should be noted that Cohen, Coyne, and Duvall (1996) found that problems with entitlement (the feeling of being entitled to be a parent to their child) were not specific to adoptive families but did differentiate between clinic and nonclinic control families regardless of whether the target child had been adopted. They point out that we must be mindful of assuming that adoptive families are unique on variables that have been examined only in adoptive populations.

We believe that it is important for nurses to recognize adoptive families' strengths and resources as they deal with challenging issues. During the adolescent stage of family development, a major task is to increase flexibility of family boundaries. In adoptive families, altercations may give rise to threats of desertion or rejection. During the young adult or launching phase, the young adult "adopts" the parents in a recontracting phase according to Hajal and Rosenberg (1991). As the adopted child proceeds to develop his or her own family of procreation, the integration of the adoptee's biological progeny can be a developmental challenge for everyone. Adoptive parents may be delighted with the psychological and social continuity. Simultaneously, they may mourn the loss of biological grandchildren and the pain of genealogical discontinuity. For the adoptee, reproduction includes both the thrill of a biological relationship and maybe some fears of the unknowns in their own genetic history.

In this CFAM developmental category, we have presented five sample types of family life cycles. Nursing has only begun to recognize the special characteristics of other family forms, such as gay male and lesbian couples. We encourage nurses to broaden their perspectives when interacting with various family forms. It is not clinically useful to consider what is *the* family form of the milennium. What we do know is that there is great variety: the poor and homeless family, the lesbian or gay male couple, the single parent, the adopted child with parent, the stepfamily, the divorced family, the separated family, the nuclear family, and the extended family. There may also be children living in households not headed by a parent.

■ ■ ■ FUNCTIONAL ASSESSMENT

The family functional assessment is concerned with details of how individuals *actually* behave in relation to one another. It is the here-

and-now aspect of a family's life that is observed and that the family presents. There are two basic aspects of family functioning: instrumental and expressive (Parsons & Bales, 1956). Each will be dealt with separately.

INSTRUMENTAL FUNCTIONING

The instrumental aspect of family functioning refers to the routine activities of daily living, such as eating, sleeping, preparing meals, giving injections, changing dressings, and so forth. For families with health problems, this is a particularly important area. The instrumental activities of daily life are generally more numerous and more frequent, and take on a greater significance because of a family member's illness. A quadriplegic, for example, requires assistance with almost every instrumental task. If a baby is attached to an apnea monitor, the parents almost always alter the manner in which they take care of instrumental tasks. For example, one parent will leave the apartment to do a load of wash only if the other parent is sufficiently awake to attend to the infant. If a senior family member is unable to distinguish what medication to take at a specific time, other family members often alter their daily routines to telephone or drop in on the senior.

EXPRESSIVE FUNCTIONING

The expressive aspect refers to nine categories:

1. Emotional communication
2. Verbal communication
3. Nonverbal communication
4. Circular communication
5. Problem solving
6. Roles
7. Influence and power
8. Beliefs
9. Alliances and coalitions

These nine subcategories are derived in part from the Family Categories Schema first developed by Epstein, Sigal, and Rakoff (1968) and later published by Epstein, Bishop, and Levin (1978). These categories were expanded by Tomm in 1977 and later published by Tomm and Sanders (1983). Earlier work (Westley & Epstein, 1969) had suggested that several of these categories distinguished emotionally healthy families from those that were experiencing more than the usual emotional distress. We have expanded on these works and now include nonverbal and circular communication, beliefs, and power (see Box 9–2).

Before discussing each subcategory, we would like to point out that most families have to deal with a combination of instrumental and expressive issues. For example, an older woman has a burn. The instrumental issues revolve around dressing changes and an exercise program. The expressive or affective issues might center on roles or problem solving. The family might be considering the following questions:

- Whose role is it to change Gram's dressing?
- Are women better "nurses" than men?
- Whose turn is it to call the physical therapist?
- Why is it that Milton never gets involved in Gram's care?
- How can we get Milton to drive Gram to see the doctor?

If a family is not coping well with instrumental issues, expressive issues almost always exist. However, a family can deal well with instrumental issues and still have expressive or emotional difficulties. It is therefore useful for the nurse and the family together to delineate the instrumental from the expressive issues. Both need to be explored when the nurse and family have a conversation about family functioning. Robinson (1998) points out the importance of nurses attending to what she calls "illness work" and "illness burden." Making arrangements for managing chronic or life-threatening illness does not just happen. The ordinary context of women shouldering the burden of homework is the one in which additional illness arrangements are made.

Although both past behaviors and future goals are taken into consideration in the functional assessment, the primary focus is on the here and now. It is helpful for both the nurse and family to identify a family's strengths and limitations in each of the following subcategories. We find it helpful to remember that the very conversation the nurse and family have about the family system shapes that system. People continually and actively reauthor their lives and stories (White & Epston, 1990). Our commitment to families is to show curiosity, delight, interest, and appreciation for their resiliency. Naturally, this does not mean that we condone family violence or abuse. Rather, it means that we recognize families are trying to make sense of their lives and stories. Our job is to witness this.

Patterns of interaction are the main thrust of the functional assessment category. Families are obviously composed of individuals, but the focus of a family assessment is less on the individual and more on the interaction *among* all of the individuals within the family. Thus, the family is viewed as a system of interacting members. In conducting this part of the family assessment, the nurse operates under the assumption that individuals are best understood within their immediate social context. The nurse conceives of the individual as defining and being defined by that context. The individual's relationships with family members and other meaningful members of the larger social environment are thus very important. If we do not attend to ideas and practices at play in the larger social context, we run the risk of focussing too narrowly on small, rather tight, recursive feedback loops (Freedman & Combs, 1996).

By interviewing family members together, the nurse can observe how they spontaneously interact with and influence each other. Furthermore, the nurse can ask questions about the impact family members have on one another and on the health problem. Reciprocally, the nurse can inquire about the impact of the health problem on the family. If the nurse thinks "interactionally" rather than "individually," each individual family member's behavior will not be seen in isolation but rather will be understood in context.

It is important for nurses to remember that, if they embrace a postmodern world view, they will not approach a family objectively to conduct an evaluation of them. Rather, the nurse and the family, in talking about the family's patterns of interacting, will bring forth a new story, rich in contextualized details. "Particular attention is paid to the ways that even the small and the ordinary—single words, single gestures, minor asides, trivial actions—can provide opportunities for generating new meanings" (Weingarten, 1998, p. 3). Unlike modernist nurses who define themselves as separate from the family with whom they are working, nurses with a postmodernist view assume that each participant in the family interview—wife, husband, partner, nurse—has an equal and often different contribution to the process. It is the nurse's task to help family members engage in conversations to make sense of their lives rather than to explain their behavior.

Emotional Communication

This subcategory refers to the range and types of emotions or feelings that are expressed, shown, or both. Families generally express a wide spectrum of feelings, from happiness to sadness to anger, whereas families with difficulties often have quite rigid patterns within a narrow range of emotional expression. For example, some families experiencing difficulties almost always argue and rarely show affection. In other families, parents may express anger but children may not, or the family may have no difficulty with women expressing tenderness but feel that men are not permitted to express it.

Questions to Ask the Family. Who in the family tends to start conversations about feelings? How can you tell when your Dad is feeling happy? Angry? Sad? How about your Mom? What effect does your anger have on your son? What does your Mom do when your Dad is angry? If your grandmother were to express sadness to your parents, how do you think your parents would react? When your brother Hiesem was killed in the accident, what helped your family the most to cope with grief?

Verbal Communication

This subcategory focuses primarily on the relationship expressed by the verbal content, and only secondarily on that expressed by the semantic content, of a communication. That is, the focus is on the meaning of the words in terms of the relationship.

Direct communication implies that the message is sent to the intended recipient. An elderly woman may be upset by what her husband is saying, but corrects her grandson's inconsequential fidgeting with the comment, "Stop doing that to me." This could represent a displaced message, whereas the same statement directed at her husband would be considered direct.

Clear versus masked is another way of looking at verbal communication. It refers to the lack of distortion in the message. A father's statement to his child, "Children who cry when they get needles are babies" may be masked criticism if the child is fighting back tears at the time of his injection. The old child management strategy of "say what you mean and mean what you say" is a good guideline for clear, direct communication.

Questions to Ask the Family. Who among your family members is the most clear and direct when communicating verbally? When you state clearly to your young adult son that he has to pay rent to you, what effect does that have on him? When your teenagers talk directly to each other about the use of condoms, what do you notice? If your adolescents were to talk more with you and your husband about safe sex, what do you think his reaction might be? What ways have you found for you and Manuel to have good, direct conversations?

Nonverbal Communication

This subcategory focuses on the various nonverbal and paraverbal messages that family members communicate. Nonverbal messages include body posture (slumped, fidgeting, open, closed), eye contact (intense, minimal), touch, gestures, facial movements (grimaces, stares, yawns), and so forth. The proximity or distance between family members is also an important nonverbal communication. Paraverbal communication includes tonality, guttural sounds, crying, stammering, and so forth. It is important to remember that nonverbal communication is highly influenced by culture. For example, Lewinsohn and Werner (1997) suggest that, in Taiwanese Chinese couples, indirect, nonverbal means of communicating and relating serve a positive function, but are viewed among Euro-Caucasian groups in the U.S. as an indicator of intrusiveness or overinvolvement.

Nurses should attend to the sequence of nonverbal messages as well as to their timing. For example, when an older man starts to talk about his terminal illness and his adult daughter turns her head and casts her tear-filled eyes toward the floor, the nurse can infer that the daughter is sad about her father's impending death. Her sequence of nonverbal behavior is congruent with sadness and the topic of conversation. It is not necessarily, however, the most supportive sequence for her father. Nonverbal communication is closely linked to emotional communication.

> ***Questions to Ask the Family.*** Who in your family shows the most distress when your father is drinking? How does Sheldon show it? What does your mother do when your father is drinking? When your sister Seema turns her head and stares out the window as your father is talking, what effect does it have on you? If your Dad were to stop talking at the same time as your Mom, what do you think she would feel like saying to him?

Circular Communication

This subcategory refers to the reciprocal communication between persons (Watzlawick, Beavin, & Jackson, 1967). There is a pattern to most relationship issues. For example, a common circular pattern occurs when the wife feels angry and criticizes her husband; the husband feels angry and avoids both the issues and her. The more he avoids, the angrier she becomes. The wife tends to see the problem only as her husband's, whereas the husband identifies the wife's criticism as the only problem. The circularity of this pattern is the most important aspect in understanding interaction in dyads. Each person influences the behavior of the other. More information about this is available in Chapter 2.

These circular communication patterns can also be adaptive. For example, an older parent feels competent and negotiates well with the landlord; the adult son feels proud and praises his parent. The more reinforcement the adult son gives, the more confident and self-assured the senior feels. This pattern is diagrammed in Figure 3–15.

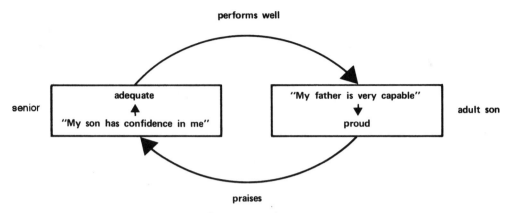

FIGURE 3–15. Adaptive circular pattern diagram.

Circular pattern diagrams (CPDs) concretize and simplify repetitive sequences noted in a relationship. A CPD may be applied to relationships between family members or between the nurse and the family. Since the nurse and the family also mutually influence each other, the nurse is encouraged to think interactionally about situations and offers the family an opportunity to think interactionally. This method of diagramming interaction patterns was first developed by Tomm (1980).

The simplest CPD includes two behaviors and two inferences of meaning. The inferences used are cognitive or affective or both. Inferences about cognition refer to ideas, concepts, or beliefs, whereas inferences about affect refer to emotional states. Affect or cognition, or both, propel the behavior. Figure 3–16 illustrates the relationship between these elements. "The inference is entered inside the enclosure and represents some internal process (what is going on inside each interactant). The connecting arrows represent information conveyed from each person to the other through behavior. The circular linkage implies an interaction pattern that is repetitive, stable, and self-regulatory" (Tomm, 1980, p. 8).

Although we use CPDs to foster circular thinking, we are mindful of their limitations. They can tempt us to look within families for collaborative causation of problems. This may distract from personal responsibility for unacceptable behavior such as violence. CPDs encourage a position of curiosity (Cecchin, 1987) rather than passion for particular values and a stand against others. Small, tight feedback loops may be highlighted and the "big picture" of the negative influence of particular values, institutions, and cultural practices may be

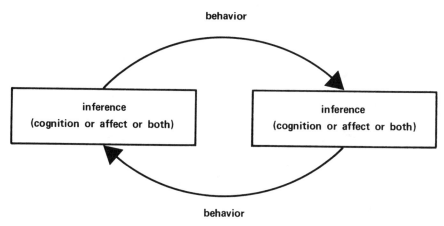

FIGURE 3–16. Basic elements of a CPD.

forgotten (Freedman & Combs,1996). Another limitation of CPDs is that they may encourage nurses to believe that they are outside the family system. As a participant observer in the larger system, the nurse is shown and hears about circular patterns reflecting family functioning. The interdependence of the nurse interviewer and family must be recognized. Both the nurse and family members cannot be decontextualized from their social and historical surroundings.

Several writers (Goldner, 1985; Ault-Rich', 1986), in what has come to be called the "feminist critique" of systems, have taken exception to the simplistic causation ideas advanced by a circular perspective. CPDs, by virtue of their neutral context, ignore power differentials and imply a discourse or relationship between equals. These writers criticize circularity for not being transparent about responsibility and minimizing power differentials in relationships. Of particular concern are such issues as incest, abuse, violence, intimidation, and battering. Despite these valid criticisms, we still find it useful in clinical work with families to subscribe to the notion of circularity but simultaneously hold to the idea of personal responsibility.

An example of a circular argument is illustrated in Figure 3–17. Each party blames and threatens the other.

A supportive relationship is illustrated in Figure 3–18. The husband trusts his wife and reveals his needs and fears. She is concerned and, in turn, sustains and supports him. This leads him to trust her more, and the relationship progresses.

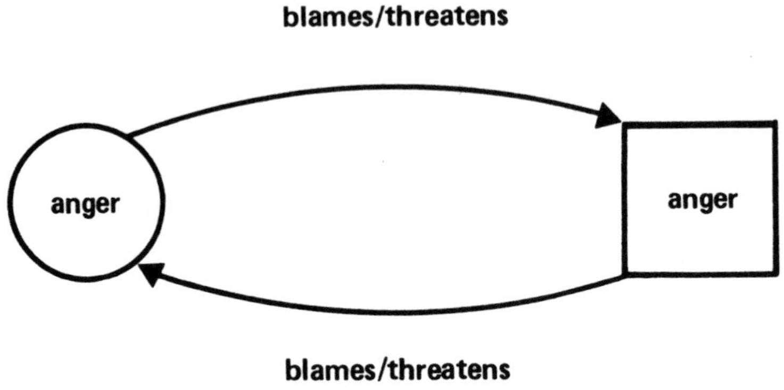

blames/threatens

anger   anger

blames/threatens

FIGURE 3–17. CPD of a circular argument.

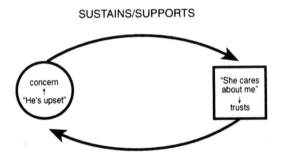

SUSTAINS/SUPPORTS

concern
↑
"He's upset"

"She cares
about me"
↓
trusts

EXPRESSES HIS NEEDS/FEARS

FIGURE 3–18. CPD of a supportive relationship.

Questions to Ask the Family

Nurse: You say your wife "always" criticizes you. (Nurse conceptualizes Figure 3–19). What do you do then? (Trying to fill in the husband's behavior in Figure 3–20.)

Husband: I don't like to discuss things. I avoid conflict. I leave. I go in the other room. What else can I do? She's always telling me what I did wrong.

Nurse: So she expresses her needs and you leave. How do you think that makes her feel? (Trying to fill in the inferred emotion in the wife's circle in Figure 3–21.)

Wife: I'll tell you. I get annoyed. I feel ignored, rejected.

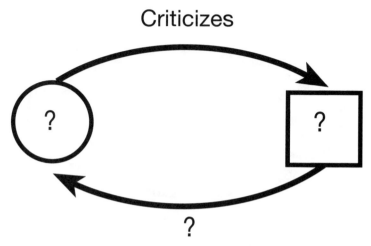

FIGURE 3–19. Beginning conceptualization of CPD.

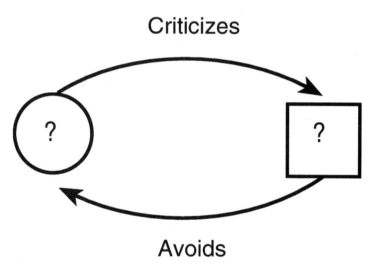

FIGURE 3–20. CPD illustrating husband and wife's behaviors.

Nurse: So you're annoyed when he leaves and ignores you. And then you become more critical. Is that right?

Wife: Well I don't really criticize, I just . . .

Husband: Yeah, you got it, nurse.

Nurse: So, when you try and express your concerns, how do you

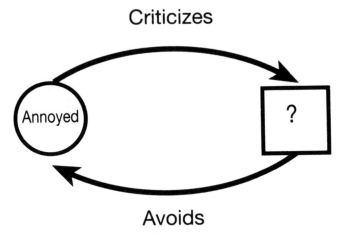

FIGURE 3–21. CPD illustrating wife's emotion.

	think it makes him feel? (Trying to fill in the inference in the square in Figure 3–21.)
Wife:	I don't know.
Nurse:	If he thinks you're lecturing, and he avoids the issues by leaving the room, what effect do you think your talking might be having on him?
Wife:	Well, I suppose he could be feeling frustrated. He sulks.
Nurse:	So the pattern seems to be that, no matter who starts it, the circle completes itself: Sometimes you're annoyed and you criticize. Your husband feels frustrated and ignores you. He sulks in the garage. Other times he avoids issues, and this arouses your frustration and criticism. (Explaining Figure 3–22.)
Wife:	It's a vicious circle.
Husband:	I don't want it to go on this way any more. We both get too upset.

Once the nurse has elicited a CPD, he or she should ask the family members to contextualize their discussion. One context might be that the wife is exhausted by her factory job and all the housework and childcare. The husband does not see why he should change his life because his wife has a stressful job and works long hours. They may engage in this particular negative circular interaction pattern every night while caring for their 3-year-old child with asthma.

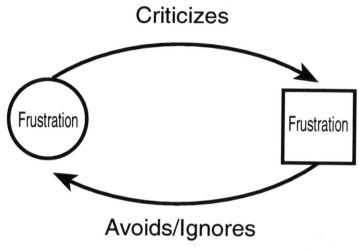

Criticizes

Frustration

Frustration

Avoids/Ignores

FIGURE 3–22. Nurse's conceptualization of this couple's communication pattern.

Problem Solving

This subcategory refers to the family's ability to solve its own problems effectively. Family problem solving is strongly influenced by the family's beliefs about its abilities and past successes. How much influence the family believes it has on the problem or illness is useful to know. Who identifies the problems is important. Is it characteristically someone from outside the family or from inside the family?

Once the problems are identified by someone, are they mainly instrumental (routine, day-to-day logistics) or are they emotional problems? Families sometimes get into difficulties when they identify an emotional problem as an instrumental one. For example, a mother who states that she cannot get her child who has phenylketonuria (PKU) to keep on the diet is really discussing an emotional issue rather than an instrumental one. She has difficulty influencing her child.

What are the family's solution patterns? Many close-knit extended families rely on relatives for assistance in time of need. Others tend to seek help from professionals. Knowing a family's usual solution style can give the nurse insight into why this family may seem to be "stuck" at this particular time with this particular issue. For example, older parents move to a retirement community. The wife breaks her hip. The husband is used to being self-reliant or, in a pinch, depending on his middle-aged daughter. The older couple know few people in their new community. The husband is reluctant to accept help from the visiting nurse. He states that he can manage all his wife's care despite the fact that he is losing weight and getting insufficient rest himself. The husband's solution pattern will be in conflict with that of the nurse.

Knowledge of whether or not a family evaluates the cost of its solutions can be helpful to the nurse. For example, a 68-year-old grandmother told Louise, the nurse, "I can't afford to let myself cry about the death of my son's infant. I have to go on for the sake of my other children." Louise was able to evaluate with the grandmother the cost of her solution pattern. Neither the grandmother nor the son discussed the infant's death with each other. The grandchildren's questions about "how come the baby didn't come home from the hospital?" were left unanswered. There was considerable tension, and the son was particularly overprotective with the 4-year-old boy (the only surviving male child). By gently exploring the cost of the solution (tension and overprotection), the nurse was able to suggest other solution patterns (e.g., shared grieving).

Questions to Ask the Family. Who first noticed the problem? Are you the one who usually notices such things? What most helped you to take the first step toward eliminating the violence pattern? What effect did it have when Toya also took steps to stop the cycle of violence in your family? How did the relationship between your son Jeremiah and your husband change when the violence stopped? If a violent episode were to occur again, how do you think you and your daughter would deal with it?

Roles

This subcategory refers to the established patterns of behavior for family members. A role is consistent behavior in a particular situation. Roles, however, are not static but rather are developed through an individual's interactions with others. Roles are thus influenced by others' sanctions and norms. McGoldrick (1988b) writes that the idea that women have a life cycle apart from their roles as wife and mother is a relatively recent one and still is not widely accepted in our culture. The expectation for women has been that they would take care of the needs of others, first men, then children, then the older generation.

Parks and Pilisuk (1991) examined the psychological cost of providing care for a parent with Alzheimer's disease and found that anxiety, depression, guilt, and resentment were evident. The fact that women dominated their sample of adult caregivers of a parent with Alzheimer's disease reflects an American pattern. The gender differences clearly profile women's more frequent, intensive, affective involvement with the caregiver role.

Women's roles have changed in recent years and are now less defined by the men in their lives. The birth rate has fallen below replacement levels, and many more women are concentrating on jobs and education. Nevertheless, women still make, on average, less than men do for the same job. Research has shown that a husband's income is negatively related to role sharing and the wife's education is positively related to role sharing (Ericksen, Yancey, & Ericksen, 1979).

Although role change is increasingly prevalent for both men and women in today's society, what is important for nurses to assess is how the family members cope with their roles. Is there role conflict or cooperation? Can the members cope with their roles? Are roles determined solely by age, rank order, or gender? Are there additional criteria such as social class and culture? Are the women in the family more involved with a wider network of people for whom they feel responsible? Do the men hear less than the women in the family about stress in their family network?

Formal roles are those for which the community has broadly agreed on a norm. Examples include the roles of mother, husband, and friend. Informal roles refer to the established patterns of behavior that are idiosyncratic to particular individuals in certain settings. Examples include the roles of "bad kid," "angel," and "class clown." These serve a specific function in a particular family. If Dad is the "softie," most likely Mom is the "heavy." If Giffy is the "good daughter," probably Kweisi is the "black sheep." The roles of "parentified child," "good child," and "symptomatic child" have been identified as having an impact in families in which there is adolescent drug abuse (Cleveland, 1981). Auxiliary roles of "child advocate," "analyst," "peacemaker," and "therapist" have also been described. It is helpful for the nurse to learn how family roles evolved, their impact on family functioning, and whether the family believes they need to be altered.

It is important for nurses to conceptualize the functional assessment category of roles in a family-oriented rather than an individual-oriented way.

> . . . the individual-oriented approach badly misrepresents the subject. For instance, to speak of the "role of the scapegoat" is to present the deviant as a person with fixed characteristics rather than a person involved in a process. "Scapegoating" technically applies to only one stage of a shifting scenario—the stage where the person is metaphorically cast out of the village. After all, the term originates from an ancient Hebrew ritual in which a goat was turned loose in the desert after the sins of the people had been symbolically laid on its head. The deviant can begin like a hero and go out like a villain, or vice versa. There is a positive-negative continuum on which he can be rated depending on which stage of the

deviation process we are looking at, which sequence the process follows, and the degree to which the social system is stressed.

At the time, the character of the deviant may vary in another direction, depending on the way his particular group does its typecasting. Which symptoms crop up in members of a group is itself a kind of typecasting. Thus the deviant may appear in many guises: the mascot, the clown, the sad sack, the erratic genius, the black sheep, the wise guy, the saint, the idiot, the fool, the imposter, the malingerer, the boaster, the villain, and so on. Literature and folklore abound with such figures. (Hoffman, 1981, p. 58)

Questions to Ask the Family. To whom do most of you go when you need someone to talk to? What effect does it have on Maxine when Ken helps with the baby's care? When Maxine and Ken collaborate instead of competing, who would be the first to notice? If Ken were to be more responsible for initiating contact with the relatives around Cherie's day-care arrangements, how do you think Maxine would feel?

Influence and Power

This subcategory refers to methods of affecting another's behavior. "Power is the ability of a person or group to regulate the criteria by which differing views of 'reality' are judged and resources apportioned" (Hartmann & Millea, 1996, p. 40). Gender issues are frequently intermingled with power issues. In a study conducted by Ball, Cowan, and Cowan (1995), husbands and wives were perceived to have a primary influence on different aspects of a discussion. "Women tended to raise issues and draw men out in the early phase of the discussion while men controlled the content and emotional depth of the later discussion phases and largely dominated the outcome" (p. 303). Shifts in power are preceded by changes in "reality," an expansion from a single perspective to a multiverse. Adopting a postmodern world view offers useful ideas about how power and "truth" are socially constructed, constituted through language, organized, and maintained in families and larger cultural contexts.

Weingarten (1998) discusses three views of power. Power can show up as overt acts of domination or coercion, an attribute of an individual behaving in the presence of observable conflict. Alternately, power can manifest itself in the suppression of conflicts and difference. A third view of power is having legitimacy of position to produce a consensus. It is the third view that is sometimes the most marginalizing of the disempowered. A nurse who is unaware of power differences among family members, in terms of roles, gender, economics, or social class can inadvertently encourage family members in positions of less power to accept goals that decrease their power and constrain their choices. Whether all family members contribute equally to problems and share responsibility for resolution is something that the nurse can pose for consideration (Dermer, Hemesath, & Russell, 1998). We believe that the most clinically useful stance to take with regard to the idea of power is to say "Power is. . . ." It can be used positively or negatively, overtly or covertly, to enhance or constrain options. There are power relations between the family members, the healthcare providers, and institutions.

Instrumental influence, power, or control refers to the use of objects or privileges as reinforcers (e.g., money, watching television, using the computer or telephone, candy, a vacation, and so forth). Psychological influence or power refers to the use of communication and feelings to influence behavior. Examples include directives, praise, criticism, threats, and guilt induction. Corporal control refers to actual body contact such as hugging, spanking, and so forth. It is important to note the positive and negative influences used in the family, especially with infants and seniors. Abuse of seniors by informal caregivers is not infrequent.

Lytton (1980) found that the "most important positive predictors of compliance (for 2-year-old boys) are mother's consistency of enforcement of rules, her encouragement of mature action, her use of psychological rewards (praise and approval), and her play with the child. The most important negative one is the amount of physical punishment by mother" (p. 182). This finding is not surprising; in our own clinical work we have found that the use of praise is positively related to success, whereas physical punishment and verbal, psychological punishment are constraining influences.

Questions to Ask the Family. Which of your parents is best at getting Nirmala to take her medication? When Delvecchio dominates the conversation, what effect does that have on Jamilett? What does your mother feel about how your stepfather disciplines your sister? If your stepfather were to be more positive with your sister Tiffany, how might his relationship with your mother change?

Beliefs

This subcategory refers to fundamental attitudes, premises, values, and assumptions held by individuals and families. Our beliefs are the blueprint from which we construct our lives and intermingle them with the lives of others. Families coevolve an ecology of beliefs that arise from interactional, social, and cultural contexts (Wright, Watson,

& Bell, 1996). Constraining beliefs decrease solution options to problems; facilitating beliefs increase solution options (Wright et al, 1996). However, any healing transaction involves at least three sets of beliefs: those of the ill patient, those of other family members, and those of the nurse (Watson & Lee, 1993; Wright & Nagy, 1993; Wright & Simpson, 1991; Wright & Watson, 1988; Wright, et al. 1996). Cousins (1979) offered the poignant idea that what we believe is the most powerful option of all.

Beliefs and behavior are intricately connected. Every action, every choice that families and individuals make evolves from their beliefs. Consequently, beliefs shape the way in which families adapt to chronic and life-threatening illness. For example, if a family believes that the best treatment for colon cancer is a nontraditional approach, it makes good sense if the family pursues acupuncture. Because our North American culture tends to use a paradigm of control about symptoms (it's good to be in control and bad to be out of control), it is very useful to explore family members' beliefs about control and mastery over their symptoms. The nurse may also focus on beliefs about etiology, diagnosis, healing and treatment, religion and spirituality, prognosis, the role of the family, and the role of the nurse (Wright et al., 1996).

Box 3–4 provides a list of areas for nurses to explore when assessing family beliefs about the health problem.

Questions to Ask the Family. How much control do you believe your family has over chronic pain? How much control does chronic pain have over your family? What do you believe the effect, if any, would be on chronic pain if you and your wife agreed on treatment? What do you believe has been the most useful thing health professionals have offered to help you cope with your suffering from fibromyalgia? What has been the least helpful?

Alliances and Coalitions

This subcategory focuses on the directionality, balance, and intensity of relationships between family members or between families and nurses. Although *complementary* and *symmetrical* are terms used to describe a two-person relationship (see Chap. 2), another term has been used to distinguish a three-person relationship. This term is *triangle.* The term was first coined by Murray Bowen (1978), a psychiatrist and family therapist, who explains:

> The two-person relationship is unstable in that it has a low tolerance for anxiety and it is easily disturbed by emotional forces

BOX 3–4. BELIEFS ABOUT THE HEALTH PROBLEM

A. Beliefs about:
1. Etiology
2. Treatment
3. Prognosis
4. Role of healthcare professionals
5. Role of the family
6. Mastery or control
7. Healing and treatment
8. Religion and spirituality
B. Influence of the family on the health problem
1. Resource utilization
a. Internal (to family)
b. External
2. Medication and treatment
C. Influence of the health problem on the family
1. Client response to the illness
2. Family members' responses to illness
3. Perceived difficulties and changes related to the health problem
D. Strenths related to the health problem at present
E. Concerns related to the health problem at present

Source: Adapted from Family Nursing Unit records, Faculty of Nursing, University of Calgary, Calgary, Alberta.

within the twosome and by relationship forces from outside the twosome. When anxiety increases, the emotional flow in a twosome intensifies and the relationship becomes uncomfortable. When the intensity reaches a certain level the twosome predictably and automatically involves a vulnerable third person in the emotional issue. The twosome might "reach out" and pull in the other person, the emotions might "overflow" to the third person, or the third person might be emotionally programmed to initiate the involvement. With involvement of the third person, the anxiety level decreases. It is as if the anxiety is diluted as it shifts from one to another of the three relationships in a triangle. The triangle is more stable and flexible than the twosome. It has a much higher tolerance of anxiety and is capable of handling a fair percentage of life stresses. (p. 400)

Most family relationships are organized around threesomes or triangles. Triangular alliances can be helpful or unhelpful. Johnson, Feldman, and Lubin (1995) found that in families of combat veterans experiencing post-traumatic stress disorder, the veteran can sometimes become triangulated with a dead buddy without the spouse's knowledge. Relationships are not unidirectional, even if one member of the triangle is an infant or an older person or has a handicap. The intensity of each relationship and the total amount of interaction is often fairly balanced. If one relationship becomes more intense, another one or two become less intense. Also, if one member of a threesome withdraws, the other two become closer. We believe that it is important for the nurse to note the degree of flexibility and fluidity within the family as they adjust to new arrivals, death, or illness.

As nurses assess this functional subcategory of alliances and coalitions, they will be aware of its interconnection with structural and developmental categories. The structural subcategory of boundaries is an important part of the alliance or coalition subcategory. The boundary defines who is part of the triangle and who is not. Of course, there are many triangles and many shifting alliances and coalitions within families. What is important for the nurse and family to note, therefore, is whether these are problematic or enriching.

We have observed that cross-generational coalitions sometimes coincide with symptomatic behavior. Hoffman (1981) has given an excellent example of a pattern of shifting cross-generational triadic processes. The pattern focuses around the inappropriate behavior of a youngster:

> Stage one: Mother coaxes, child refuses to obey, mother threatens to tell father (father-mother against child). Stage two: when father comes home, mother tells him how bad child has been, and father sends child to his room without supper. Mother sneaks up after father has left the table and brings child a little food on a plate (mother-child against father). Stage three: when child comes down later, father, trying to make up, offers to play a game with him that mother has expressly forbidden because it gets him too excited before bedtime (father-child against mother). Stage four: mother scolds father for this; the child, overexcited indeed, has a tantrum and is sent to bed; and the original triangle comes round again (mother-father against child). (p. 32)

In addition to noting the connection between the structural subcategory of boundaries and the functional subcategory of alliances and coalitions, nurses should be aware of the interconnection with the developmental subcategory of attachments. A family's attachments, or underlying emotional bonds that have an enduring or stable quality, are similar to alliances in that they are both unions. Attachments tend to differ from coalitions, however, in that the latter imply an alignment between two members with a third member being split off or opposed.

Questions to Ask the Family. When Demi and Tyson argue, who is most likely to get in the middle of the fight? If the children are playing very well together, who would mostly likely come along and *start* them fighting? Who would *stop* them from fighting? What impact has Don's brain tumor had on family members coming together or becoming further distanced?

■■■ CONCLUSIONS

The CFAM is a "map of the family" from the nurse's and the family's observer perspectives. The model provides a framework that can be drawn on as the nurse and the family discuss the issues. The nurse can use the three main categories (structural, developmental, and functional) to obtain a macro assessment of family strengths and problems. Depending on his or her confidence and competence level, the nurse may do a more micro assessment and explore in detail specific areas of family functioning. In either situation, the nurse needs to be able to draw together all relevant information into an integrated assessment. It is insufficient to focus on a family's difficulties with problem solving when the specific family structure is not known. Also, if the nurse focuses too much on previous developmental history, the nurse may be ignoring important current functioning issues. Naturally, past history cannot be ignored. It should be integrated, however, only insofar as it helps to explain current functioning.

Once a thorough family assessment has been completed, the nurse and the family may now determine whether intervention is needed or not. However, we wish to emphasize that the completion of a family assessment utilizing CFAM does not mean that the nurse or the family now has the "truth." Rather, the nurse and family have their own integrated assessment from their "observer perspectives."

■■■ REFERENCES

Ahrons, C.R. (1998). Divorce: An unscheduled family transition. In B. Carter & M. McGoldrick (Eds.). *The expanded family life cycle: Individual, family and social perspectives* (3rd ed.). Boston: Allyn and Bacon. pp. 381–398.

Ahrons, C., & Rodgers, R. H. (1987). *Divorced families: A multidisciplinary developmental view.* New York: W. W. Norton.

Anderson, D. A., & Worthen, D. (1997). Exploring a fourth dimension: Spirituality as a resource for the couple therapist. *Journal of Marital and Family Therapy, 23*(1), 3–12.

Anderson, H., & Goolishian, H. (1988). Human systems as linguistic systems: Preliminary and evolving ideas about the implications for clinical theory. *Family Process, 27,* 371–393.

Ashby, W. (1969). *Design for a brain.* London: Chapman & Hall, Science & Behavior Books.

Ault-Rich', M. (1986). A feminist critique of five schools of family therapy. *Family Therapy Collections, 16,* 1–15.

Ball, F. L.,Cowan, P., & Cowan, C. P. (1995). Who's got the power? Gender differences in partners' perceptions of influence during marital problem-solving discussions. *Family Process, 34*(3), 303–321.

Becvar, D.S. (1997). Soul healing and the family. In D. S. Becvar (Ed.). *The family, spirituality and social work.* Binghamton, New York: Haworth Press, pp 1–11.

Berenson, D. (1990). A systemic view of spirituality. *Journal of Strategic and Systemic Therapies, 9*(1), 59–70.

Berger, R. (1998). *Stepfamilies: A multidimensional perspective.* Binghamton, New York: Haworth Press.

Berliner, K., Jacob, D., & Schwartzberg, N. (1998). The single adult and the family life cycle. In B. Carter & M. McGoldrick (Eds.). *The expanded family life cycle: Individual, family and social perspectives* (3rd ed.). Boston: Allyn and Bacon, pp 362–372.

Bishop, D., Epstein, N., Baldwin, L., Miller, I., & Keitner, G. (1988). Older couples: The effect of health, retirement, and family functioning on morale. *Family Systems Medicine, 6*(2), 238–247.

Booth, A., Johnson, D. R., Branaman, A.,& Sica, A. (1995). Belief and behavior: Does religion matter in today's marriage? *Journal of Marriage and the Family, 57,* 661–671.

Boss, P. (1980). Normative family stress: Family boundary changes across the life-span. *Family Relationships, 29,* 445–450.

Bowen, M. (1978). *Family therapy in clinical practice.* Northvale, NJ: Jason Aronson.

Bowlby, J. (1977). The making and breaking of affectional bonds. *British Journal of Psychiatry, 130,* 201–210.

Burns, L. H. (1987). Infertility as boundary ambiguity: One theoretical perspective. *Family Process, 26*(3), 359–372.

Byng-Hall, J. (1995). Creating a secure family base: Some implications of attachment theory. *Family Process, 34*(1), 45–58.

Carter, B. (1999). Becoming parents: The family with young children. In B. Carter & M. McGoldrick (Eds.). *The expanded family life cycle: Individual, family and social perspectives* (3rd ed.). Boston: Allyn and Bacon, pp 249–273.

Carter, B., & McGoldrick, M. (Eds.) (1988). *The changing family life cycle: A framework for family therapy* (2nd ed.). New York: Gardner Press.

Carter, B., & McGoldrick, M. (1999). Overview: The expanded family life cycle: Individual, family and social perspectives. In B. Carter & M. McGoldrick (Eds.). *The expanded family life cycle: Individual, family and social perspective* (3rd ed.). Boston: Allyn and Bacon, pp 1–26.

Carter, B., & McGoldrick, M. (1998). The divorce cycle: A major variation in the American family life cycle. In B. Carter & M. McGoldrick (Eds). *The expanded family life cycle: Individual, family and social perspectives* (3rd ed.). Boston: Allyn and Bacon, pp 373–380.

Cheng-Ham, M. D. (1989). Family therapy with immigrant families: Constructing a bridge between different world views. *Journal of Strategic and Systemic Therapies, 8,* 1–2.

Cecchin, G. (1987). Hypothesizing, circularity and neutrality revisited: An invitation to curiosity. *Family Process, 26,* 405–413.

Cleveland, M. (1981). Families and adolescent drug abuse: Structural analysis of children's roles. *Family Process, 20,* 295–304.

Cohen, N. J., Coyne, J. C., & Duvall, J. D. (1996). Parents' sense of entitlement in adoptive and nonadoptive families. *Family Process, 35*(4), 441–456.

Cousins, N. (1979). *Anatomy of an illness as perceived by the patient.* New York: Bantam Books.

Dermer, SB., Hemesath, CW., & Russell, CS. (1998). A feminist critique of solution-focused therapy. *The American Journal of Family Therapy, 26,* 239–250.

Daneshpour, M. (1998). Muslim families and family therapy. *Journal of Marital and Family Therapy, 24*(3), 355–368.

Doherty, W. J., & Heinrich, R. (1996). Managing the ethics of managed healthcare: A systemic approach. *Families, Systems and Health, 14*(1), 17–28.

Duvall, E. (1977). *Marriage and family development* (5th ed.). Philadelphia: J. B. Lippincott.

Divorce rate drops. (1991, August). *Family Therapy News,* p. 16.

Epstein, N., Bishop, D., & Levin, S. (1978). The McMaster model of family functioning. *Journal of Marriage and Family Counseling, 4,* 19–31.

Epstein, N., Sigal, J., & Rakoff, V. (1968). *Family categories schema.* Unpublished manuscript, Jewish General Hospital, Department of Psychiatry, Montreal.

Ericksen, J., Yancey, W., & Ericksen, E. (1979). The division of family roles. *Journal of Marriage and the Family, 41,* 301–313.

Erickson, E. (1963). *Childhood and society* (2nd ed.). New York: W. W. Norton.

Falicov, C. J. (1988). Family sociology and family therapy contributions to the family development framework: A comparative analysis and thoughts on future trends. In C. J. Falivoc (Ed.), *Family transitions: Continuity and change over the life cycle.* New York: Guilford Press, pp 3–54.

Falicov, C. J. (1998). The cultural meaning of family triangles. In M. McGoldrick (Ed.) *Re-visioning family therapy: Race, culture and gender in clinical practice.* New York: Guilford Press, pp 37–49.

Fein, E. B. (1998,October 24). Secrecy and stigma no longer clouding adoptions. *The New York Times*, Section 1, p. 1.

Foot, D. K. (with Stoffman, D.) (1996). *Boom, bust & echo: How to profit from the coming demographic shift.* Toronto: Macfarlane, Walter & Ross.

Freedman, J., & Combs, G (1996). *Narrative therapy: The social construction of preferred realities.* New York: W.W. Norton & Co.

Fulmer, R. (1988). Lower-income and professional families: A comparison of structure and life cycle process. In B. Carter & M. McGoldrick (Eds.), *The changing family life cycle.* New York: Gardner Press, pp 545–578.

Giordano, J. (1988). Parents of the baby boomers: A new generation of young-old. *Family Relations, 37,* 411–414.

Glick, P. (1989b). Remarried families, stepfamilies, and stepchildren: A brief demographic profile. *Family Relations, 38,* 24–27.

Goldner, V. (1988). Generation and gender: Normative and covert hierarchies. *Family Process, 27,* 17–32.

Goldner, V. (1985). Feminism and family therapy. *Family Process, 24,* 31–47.

Green, R. J. (1996). Why ask? Why tell? Teaching and learning about lesbians and gays in family therapy. *Family Process, 35*(3), 389–400.

Green, R. J. (1998). Race and the field of family therapy. In M. Mc Goldrick (Ed.) *Re-visioning family therapy: Race, culture and gender in clinical practice.* New York: The Guilford Press, pp 93–110.

Green, R. J., & Werner, P. D. (1996). Intrusiveness and closeness–caregiving: Rethinking the concept of family "enmeshment." *Family Process, 35*(2), 115–136.

Hagestad, G. O. (1988). Demographic change and the life course: Some emerging trends in the family realm. *Family Relations, 37,* 405–410.

Hajal, F., & Rosenberg, E. (1991). The family life cycle in adoptive families. *American Journal of Orthopsychiatry, 61*(1), 78–85.

Halevey, J. (1998). A genogram with an attitude. *Journal of Marital and Family Therapy, 24*(2), 233–242.

Haley, J. (1977). Toward a theory of pathological systems. In P. Watzlawick & J. Weakland (Eds.), *The interactional view.* New York: W. W. Norton.

Hardy, K. V. (1990, September/October). Much more than techniques needed in treating minorities. *Family Therapy News.*

Hardy, K., & Laszloffy, T. (1995). The cultural genogram: Key to training culturally competent family therapists. *Journal of Marital and Family Therapy, 21*(3), 227–237.

Hartman, A. (1978). Diagrammatic assessment of family relationships. *Social Casework, 59,* 465–476.

Hartmann, B. R., & Millea, P. J. (1996). When belief systems collide: The rise and decline of the disease concept of alcoholism. *Journal of Systemic Therapies, 15*(2), 36–47.

Hawley, D. R., & DeHaan, L. (1996). Toward a definition of family resilience: Integrating life-span and family perspectives. *Family Process, 35*(3), 283–298.

Healy, J., Malley, J., & Stewart, A. (1990). Children and their fathers after parental separation. *American Journal of Orthopsychiatry, 60*(4), 531–543.

Hines, P. M. (1988). The family life cycle of poor black families. In B. Carter & M. McGoldrick (Eds.), *The changing family life cycle.* New York: Gardner Press, pp 513–544.

Hoffman, L. (1981). *Foundations of family therapy.* New York: Basic Books.

Imber-Black, E. (1991). The family—larger system perspective. *Family Systems Medicine, 9*(4), 371–396.

Johnson, D. R., Feldman, S., & Lubin, H. (1995). Critical interaction therapy: Couples therapy in combat-related post-traumatic stress disorder. *Family Process, 34*(4), 401–412.

Kliman, J. (1998). Social class as a relationship: Implications for family therapy. In M. Mc Goldrick (Ed.). *Re-visioning family therapy: Race, culture, and gender in clinical practice.* New York: The Guilford Press, pp 50–61.

Knudson-Martin,C., & Mahoney, A.R. (1996). Gender dilemmas and myth in the construction of marital bargains: Issues for marital therapy. *Family Process, 35,* 137–153.

Kuehl, B. (1995). The solution-oriented genogram: A collaborative approach. *Journal of Marital and Family Therapy, 21*(3), 239–250.

Laird, J. (1998). Theorizing culture: Narrative ideas and practice principles. In M. McGoldrick (Ed.) *Re-visioning family theapy: Race, culture and gender in clinical practice.* New York: The Guilford Press, pp 20–36.

Levac, A. M., Wright, L.M.,& Leahey, M. (1997). Children and families: Models for assessment and intervention. In J Fox (ed.). *Primary healthcare of children.* Baltimore, MD: Mosby, pp 3–13.

Lewinsohn, M. A., & Werner, P. D. (1997). Factors in Chinese marital process: Relationship to marital adjustment. *Family Process, 36*(1), 43–62.

Lewis, J. (1988a). The transition to parenthood: 1. The rating of prenatal marital competence. *Family Process, 27*(2), 149–166.

Lewis, J. (1988b). The transition to parenthood: 2. Stability and change in marital structure. *Family Process, 27*(3), 273–284.

Lewis, J., Owen, M. T., & Cox, M. (1988). The transition to parenthood: 3. Incorporation of the child into the family. *Family Process, 27*(4), 411–421.

Long, J. K. (1996). Working with lesbians, gays and bisexuals: Addressing heterosexism in supervision. *Family Process, 35*(3), 377–388.

Lytton, H. (1980). *Parent-child interaction: The socialization process observed in twin and singleton families.* New York: Plenum Press.

Maturana, H. R., & Varela, F.G. (1992). *The tree of knowledge: The biological roots of human understanding.* (Revised edition). Boston: Shambhala.

McGoldrick, M. (1982). Normal families: An ethnic perspective. In F. Walsh (Ed.), *Normal family processes.* New York: Guilford Press, pp. 399–424.

McGoldrick, M. (1988b). Women and the family life cycle. In B. Carter & M. McGoldrick (Eds.), *The changing family life cycle.* New York: Gardner Press, pp 29–68.

McGoldrick, M. (1991). Echoes from the past: Helping families mourn their losses. In F. Walsh & M. McGoldrick (Eds.), *Living beyond loss: Death in the family* New York: W. W. Norton, pp 50–78.

McGoldrick, M. (1998). Introduction: Revisioning family therapy through a cultural lens. In M. McGoldrick (Ed.) *Re-visioning family therapy: Race, culture, and gender.* New York: The Guilford Press, pp 3–19.

McGoldrick, M., Gerson, R., & Shellenberger, S. (1999). *Genograms: Assessment and Intervention* (2nd ed.). New York: W. W. Norton.

McGoldrick, M., & Gerson, R. (1988). Genograms and the family life cycle. In B. Carter & M. McGoldrick (Eds.), *The changing family life cycle: A framework for family therapy* (2nd ed.) Boston: Allyn & Bacon, pp 164–189.

Miller, J. J., & Gergen, K. (1998). Life on the line: The therapeutic potentials of computer mediated conversation. *Journal of Marital and Family Therapy, 24*(2), 189–202.

Minuchin, S. (1974). *Families and family therapy.* Cambridge, MA: Harvard University Press.

Nelson, G. (1994).Emotional well-being of separated and married women: Long term follow-up study. *American Journal of Orthopsychiatry, 64*(1),150–160.

Pallett, P. (1990). A conceptual framework for studying family caregiver burden in Alzheimer's type dementia. *Image, 22*(1), 52–58.

Parks, S. H., & Pilisuk, M. (1991). Caregiver burden: Gender and the psychological costs of caregiving. *American Journal of Orthopsychiatry, 61*(4), 50–509.

Parsons, T., & Bales, R. (1956). *Family: Socialization and interaction process.* London: Routledge & Kegan.

Pasley, K., Rhoden, L., Visher, E., & Visher, J. (1996). Successful stepfamily therapy: Clients' perspectives. *Journal of Marital and Family Therapy, 22*(3), 343–357.

Paterson, R.B. (1994). Learning from suffering. *Family Therapy News,* pp. 11–12.

Pill, C. (1990). Stepfamilies: Redefining the family. *Family Relations, 39,* 186–193.

Quinn, P., & Allen, K. (1989). Facing challenges and making compromises: How single mothers endure. *Family Relations, 38,* 390–395.

Reitz, M., & Watson, K. W. (1992). *Adoption and the family system.* New York: Guilford Press.

Radley, A., & Green, R. (1986). Bearing illness: Study of couples where the husband awaits coronary graft surgery. *Social Sciences and Medicine, 23,* 577–585.

Robinson, C. A. (1998) Women, families, chronic illness, and nursing interventions: From burden to balance. *Journal of Family Nursing, 4*(3), 271–290.

Ross, B., & Cobb, L. (1990). *Family nursing: A nursing process approach.* Redwood, CA: Addison-Wesley.

Saluter, A. F., & Lugaila, T. A. (1998). Marital status and living arrangements: March 1996. U.S. Dept. of Commerce, Census Bureau, Current Population Reports, Population Characteristics, P20–496, pp. 1–6.

Schibuk, M. (1989). Treating the sibling subsystem: An adjunct of divorce therapy. *American Journal of Orthopsychiatry, 59*(2), 226–237.

Schnittger, M., & Bird, G. (1990). Coping among dual-career men and women across the family life cycle. *Family Relations, 39*, 199–205.

Selvini, M., Boscolo, L., Cecchin, G., & Prata, G. (1989). Hypothesizing—circularity—neutrality: Three guidelines for the conduction of the session. *Family Process, 19*(1), 3–12.

Sheinberg, M., & Penn, P. (1991). Gender dilemmas, gender questions, and the gender mantra. *Journal of Marital and Family Therapy, 17*(1), 33–44.

Silverstein, D. R., & Demick, J. (1994). Toward an organizational-relational model of open adoption. *Family Process, 33*(2), 111–124.

Simon, R. (1988). Family life cycle issues in the therapy system. In B. Carter & M. McGoldrick (Eds.), *The changing family life cycle: A framework for family therapy* (2nd ed.). New York: Gardner Press, pp 107–118.

Siwolop, S. (1997). Conquering cancer, but depleting her savings. *The New York Times*, p. 4.

Stuart, M. (1991). An analysis of the concept of family. In A. Whall & J. Fawcett (Eds.), *Family theory development in nursing: State of the science and art.* Philadelphia: F. A. Davis, pp 31–42.

Suro, R. (1991). The new American family: Reality is wearing the pants. *The New York Times*, Section 4, p. 2.

Toman, W. (1976). *Family constellation: Its effects on personality and social behavior* (3rd ed.). New York: Springer.

Toman, W. (1988). Basics of family structure and sibling position. In M. D. Kahn & K. G. Lewis (Eds.), *Siblings in therapy: Life span and clinical issues.* New York: W. W. Norton, pp 46–65.

Tomm, K. (1977). *Tripartite family assessment.* Unpublished manuscript, University of Calgary, Alberta.

Tomm, K. (1980). Towards a cybernetic systems approach to family therapy at the University of Calgary. In D. Freeman (Ed.), *Perspectives on family therapy.* Vancouver: Butterworth, pp 3–18.

Tomm, K., & Sanders, G. (1983). Family assessment in a problem oriented record. In J. C. Hansen & B. F. Keeney (Eds.), *Diagnosis and assessment in family therapy* London: Aspen Systems, pp 101–122.

Tomm, W. (1994). Beyond "family models": Family as dialogical process in a cultural house of language. *Journal of Feminist Family Therapy, 6*(2),1–20.

Visher, E. B., & Visher, J.S. (1996). *Therapy with stepfamilies.* New York: Brunner/Mazel.

Waldegrave, C. (1990). Just therapy. *Dulwich Centre Newsletter, 1*, 5–46.

Walsh, F. (1996). The concept of family resilience: Crisis and challenge. *Family Process, 35*(3), 261–282.

Walsh, F. (1998). Beliefs, spirituality, and transcendence: Keys to family resilience. In M. McGoldrick (Ed.). *Re-visioning family therapy: Race, culture and gender in clinical practice.* New York: The Guilford Press, pp 62–77.

Walsh, F., & McGoldrick, M. (Eds.). (1991). *Living beyond loss: Death in the family.* New York: W. W. Norton.

Watson, W. L., & Lee, D. (1993). Is there life after suicide? The systemic belief approach for "survivors" of suicide. *Archives of Psychiatric Nursing, 7*(1), 37–43.

Watts-Jones, D. (1998). Toward an African American genogram. *Family Process, 36*(4), 375–384.

Watzlawick, P., Beavin, J., & Jackson, D. (1967). *Pragmatics of human communication.* New York: W. W. Norton.

Weaver, A. J., Koenig, H. G., &Larson, D. B. (1997). Marriage and family therapists and the clergy: A need for clinical collaboration, training and research. *Journal of Marital and Family Therapy, 23*(1), 13–25.

Weingarten, K. (1998). The small and the ordinary: The daily practice of a postmodern therapy. *Family Process, 37*(1), 3–16.

Westley, W., & Epstein, N. (1969). *The silent majority.* San Francisco: Jossey-Bass.

White, M. (1991). Deconstruction and therapy. *Dulwich Centre Newsletter, 3,* 21–40.

White, M. & Epston, D. (1990). *Narrative means to therapeutic ends.* New York: WW Norton Co.

Whiteside, M. F. (1998). The parental alliance following divorce: An overview. *Journal of Marital and Family Therapy, 24*(1), 3–24.

Wood, B. (1985) Proximity and hierarchy: Orthogonal dimensions of family interconnectedness. *Family Process, 24,* 487–507.

Wright, L.M. (in press). Spirituality, suffering and beliefs: the soul of healing with families. In F. Walsh (Ed.), *Spiritual Resources in Family Therapy.* New York: Guilford Press.

Wright, L. M., & Nagy, J. (1993). Death: The most troublesome family secret of all. In E. Imber-Black (Ed.), *Secrets in families and family therapy.* New York: W. W. Norton, pp 121–137.

Wright, L. M., & Simpson, P. (1991). A systemic belief approach to epileptic seizures: A case of being spellbound. *Contemporary Family Therapy: An International Journal, 13*(2), 165–180.

Wright, L. M., & Watson, W. L. (1988). Systemic family therapy and family development. In C. J. Falicov (Ed.), *Family transitions: Continuity and change over the life cycle.* New York: Guilford Press, pp 407–430.

Wright, L. M., Watson, W. L., & Bell, J. M. (1990). The family nursing unit: A unique integration of research, education and clinical practice. In J. M. Bell, W. L. Watson, & L. M. Wright (Eds.), *The cutting edge of family nursing.* Calgary, Alberta: Family Nursing Unit Publications, pp 95–109.

Wright, L. M., Watson, W. L., & Bell, J. M. (1996). *Beliefs: The heart of healing in families and illness.* New York: Basic Books.

CHAPTER 4

The Calgary Family
Intervention Model

The Calgary Family Intervention Model (CFIM) is a companion model to the Calgary Family Assessment Model (CFAM) (Chap. 3). Over the past 25 years, several family assessment models and family measurement instruments have been developed by nurses and others (Broome, Knafl, Pridham, & Feetham, 1998; Hanson, 1996; Mischke-Berkey, Warner, & Hanson, 1989). To our knowledge, the CFIM is the first family intervention model to emerge within nursing. No further intervention models have been developed since we first introduced our model in our second edition in 1994. However, there does seem to be much more recognition of the importance and effectiveness of family interventions in healthcare in the treatment of physical illness (Campbell & Patterson, 1995).

This chapter presents our definition and description of CFIM, examples of interventions at three domains of family functioning, and actual clinical examples using the CFIM. This chapter concludes with intervention ideas for common family situations that nurses encounter.

■■■ DEFINITION AND DESCRIPTION

After a comprehensive family assessment has been completed and family intervention is indicated, nurses need to consider how they should intervene to facilitate change. The CFIM is an organizing framework for conceptualizing the intersection between a particular domain of family functioning and the specific intervention offered by the nurse (Fig. 4–1). The CFIM visually portrays the "fit" between a domain of family functioning and a nursing intervention; that is, does the intervention effect change in the domain or not? The elements of the CFIM are interventions, domains of family functioning, and "fit" or effectiveness. The CFIM is focused on promoting, improving, and sustaining effective family functioning in three domains: cognitive, affective, and behavioral.

Interventions can be targeted to promote, improve, or sustain functioning at any or all of the three domains of family functioning, but a change in one domain will affect another domain. However, we believe that the most profound and sustaining change will be the one that occurs within the family's beliefs (cognition). In other words, as a family thinketh, so is it. One intervention could actually target cognitive, af-

157

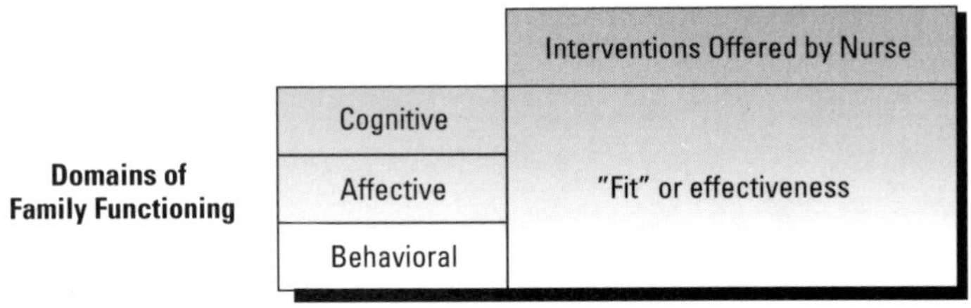

FIGURE 4–1. CFIM: Intersection of domains of family functioning and interventions.

fective, and behavioral domains of a family functioning simultaneously.

We believe that nurses can only *offer* interventions to the family. Whether the family opens space for an intervention depends on its genetic makeup and the family's history of interactions between family members (Maturana & Varela, 1992). The openness to particular interventions is also profoundly influenced by the relationship between the nurse and the family (Leahey & Harper-Jaques, 1996; Robinson, 1996; Robinson & Wright, 1995; Tapp, 1997; Thorne & Robinson, 1989) and the nurse's ability to invite the family to reflect about their health problems (Wright & Levac, 1992; Wright, Watson & Bell, 1996). Second-order cybernetics and the biology of cognition (Maturana & Varela, 1992) have influenced our ideas in this regard (see Chap. 2).

Intervening in a family system in a manner that will promote or facilitate change is the most challenging and exciting aspect of clinical work with families. The intervention process represents the core of clinical practice with families. It provides an appropriate context in which the family can make necessary changes. There are a myriad of interventions, but nurses need to tailor their interventions to each family and to the chosen domain of family functioning. Particular interventions will usually vary for each family, although there may be occasions when the same intervention is used for several families and for different problems. However, we wish to emphasize that each family is unique and that, although labeling particular interventions is of great importance in putting our practice into language, it does not represent a "cookbook" approach. The interventions we list are *examples* of interventions that could be used; they are not intended to be all-inclusive. We have given examples of interventions that we have found from our clinical practice and research to be very useful. The interventions that we cite are based on several important theoretical foundations: postmodernism, systems, cybernetics, communication, change theory, and biology of cognition (see Chap. 2).

In summary, the CFIM is not a list of nursing interventions or a list of family functions. Rather, it provides a means to conceptualize a fit between domains of family functioning and interventions offered by the nurse. The CFIM assists in determining the predominant domain of family functioning that needs changing and the most useful intervention that will effect change in that domain. Through therapeutic conversations, the family and nurse collaborate and co-evolve to discover the most useful fit (Tapp, 1997; Wright, Watson, & Bell, 1996). We use the qualitative term "fit" in a slightly different way than de Shazer (1988) did because we emphasize whether or not the interventions effect change in the presenting problem. Fit involves recognition of reciprocity between the nurse's ideas and opinions and the family's illness experience. Therefore, determining fit may involve some experimentation or trial and error. It also entails a belief by nurses that each family is unique and has particular strengths. In Chapter 7, we outline factors to enhance the likelihood that interventions will trigger change in the desired domain of family functioning.

▪▪▪ INTERVENTIVE QUESTIONS

One of the simplest but most powerful nursing interventions for families experiencing health problems is the use of interventive questions. Interventive questions are intended to actively effect change in any one or all three domains. Nurses conducting family interviews should remember, though, that knowledge of when, how, and to what purpose to pose questions is more important than simply choosing one type of question over another (Lipchik & de Shazer, 1986; Wright, Watson, & Bell, 1996).

LINEAR VERSUS CIRCULAR QUESTIONS

Interventive questions are usually of two types: linear and circular (Tomm, 1987; 1988). Linear questions are meant to inform the nurse, whereas circular questions are meant to effect change (Tomm, 1985; 1987; 1988). The important difference between these kinds of questions is their intent. Linear questions are investigative; they explore a family member's descriptions or perceptions of a problem. For example, when exploring family members' perceptions of their daughter's anorexia nervosa, the nurse could begin with linear questions: "When did you notice that your daughter had changed her eating habits?" "What do you think caused your daughter to stop eating as she normally would?" These linear questions, while informing the nurse of the history of the young woman's eating patterns, also help illuminate family perceptions or beliefs about eating patterns. Linear questions are frequently used to begin gathering information about families' problems, whereas circular questions reveal families' understanding of problems.

Circular questions are directed toward explanations of problems. For example, with the same family, the nurse could ask, "Who in the family is most worried about Cheyenne's anorexia?" "How does Mother show that she's the one worrying the most?" Circular questions help the nurse to discover valuable information because they seek out relationships between individuals, events, ideas, or beliefs.

The effect of these questions on families is quite distinct. Linear questions tend to be constraining, whereas circular questions are generative; the latter introduce new cognitive connections, paving the way for new or different family behaviors. The linear form of questioning implies that the nurse knows what is best for the family; it also implies that the nurse has become purposive and invested in a particular outcome. Linear questions are intended to correct behavior; circular questions are intended to facilitate behavioral change.

The primary distinction between circular and linear questions lies in the notion that information reveals differences in relationships (Bateson, 1979). With circular questions, a relationship or connection between individuals, events, ideas, or beliefs is always sought. With linear questions, the focus is on cause and effect. The idea of circular questions evolved from the concept of circularity and the method of circular interviewing developed by the originators of Milan Systemic Family Therapy (Fleuridas, Nelson, & Rosenthal, 1986; Selvini-Palazzoli, Boscolo, Cecchin, & Prata, 1980; Tomm, 1984; 1985; 1987) (see Chaps. 6 and 7).

Circularity involves the cycle of questions and answers between families and nurses that occurs during the interview process. The nurse's questions are based on information that the family gives in response to the questions the nurse asks, and thus the cycle continues (Watson, 1992). The family's responses to the questions provide information for the nurse and the family. Questions in and of themselves also provide new information and answers for the family. This is when the questions are considered interventions. Interventive questions may invite family members to see their problems in a new way and subsequently to see new solutions. Thus, as the family's answers provide information for the nurse, the nurse's questions may provide information for the family (Watson, 1992).

Tomm (1987) embellished the types of circular questions used by the Milan systemic family therapy team and identified, defined, and classified various circular questions. Loos and Bell (1990) creatively applied the use of circular questions to critical care nursing. Watson (1988a, 1988b, 1988c, 1989a, 1989b) and Wright, Watson, and Bell (1996) demonstrated the therapeutic aspect of circular questions with families experiencing chronic illness, life-threatening illness, and psychosocial problems. The circular questions identified by Tomm (1987) that we have found most useful in clinical practice with families are difference questions, behavioral effect questions, hypothetical or future-oriented questions, and triadic questions. We have expanded the use of circular questions by providing examples of questions that can be asked to intervene in the cognitive, affective and behavioral domains of family functioning. The types of questions, definitions, and examples are given in Table 4–1.

In summary, the four types of circular questions (i.e., difference, behavioral effect, hypothetical, and triadic) can be used to facilitate change in any one or all of the domains of family functioning. Figure 4–2 illustrates the intersection of various types of circular questions and the domains of family functioning. We wish to emphasize strongly that what is most critical is the effectiveness, usefulness, and fit of the question in influencing change rather than the specific question itself.

	Interventions Offered by Nurse: Circular Questions			
	Difference	Behavioral Effect	Hypothetical	Triadic
Cognitive				
Affective				
Behavioral				

Domains of Family Functioning

FIGURE 4–2. Intersection of circular questions and domains of family functioning.

TABLE 4–1.
CIRCULAR QUESTIONS TO CHANGE COGNITIVE, AFFECTIVE, AND BEHAVIORAL DOMAINS OF FAMILY FUNCTIONING

1. Type: Difference Question
Definition: Explores differences between people, relationships, time, ideas or beliefs.
Examples of intervening at three domains of family functioning:

Cognitive	Affective	Behavioral
• What's the best advice that you've had about managing your son's AIDS? What's the worst advice?	• Who in the family is most worried about how AIDS is transmitted?	• Who's the best in the family at getting your son to take his medication on time?
• What information would be most helpful to you about managing the effects of sexual abuse? Who in the family would benefit most with more information?	• Who is finding your disclosure of sexual abuse most difficult?	• When you first disclosed your sexual abuse, what was done by professionals that was most helpful?

2. Type: Behavioral Effect Question
Definition: Explores connections between the effect of one family member's behavior on another.
Examples of intervening at three domains of family functioning:

Cognitive	Affective	Behavioral
• How do you make sense of your husband not visiting your son in hospital?	• What do you feel when your son cries after his treatments?	• What do you do when your husband doesn't visit your son in hospital?
• What do you know about the effect of life-threatening illness on children?	• How does your mother show that she is afraid of dying?	• What could your father do to indicate to your mother that he understands her fears?

(continued)

TABLE 4–1. *(continued)*
CIRCULAR QUESTIONS TO CHANGE COGNITIVE, AFFECTIVE, AND BEHAVIORAL DOMAINS OF FAMILY FUNCTIONING

3. Type: Hypothetical/Future-Oriented Question
Definition: Explores family options and alternative actions or meanings in the future.
Examples of intervening at three domains of family functioning:

Cognitive	Affective	Behavioral
• What do you think will happen if these skin grafts continue to be so painful for your son? • If the worst occurs, how do you think your family will cope?	• If your son's skin grafts are not successful, what do you think his mood will be? Sad? Angry? Resigned? • If things do not go well with your grandmother's treatment, who will be most affected?	• How much longer will it be before your son will accept treatment for his contractures? • How long do you think your grandmother will have to remain in the hospital? If it's longer, what do you think your brothers and sisters will do?
• If you did decide to have your grandmother institutionalized, with whom would you discuss it?		

4. Type: Triadic Question
Definition: Question posed to a third person about the relationship between two other people.
Examples of intervening at three domains of family functioning:

Cognitive	Affective	Behavioral
• If your father were not drinking daily, what would your mother think about his going to the rehab center? • How does your father know that your sister needs support?	• What does your father do that encourages your mother to be less anxious about his condition? • When your father supports your sister, how does your mother feel?	• If your father were willing to talk with your mother about solutions to his addiction problem, what could he say? • What do you think your father needs to do to prepare for your sister's long treatment?

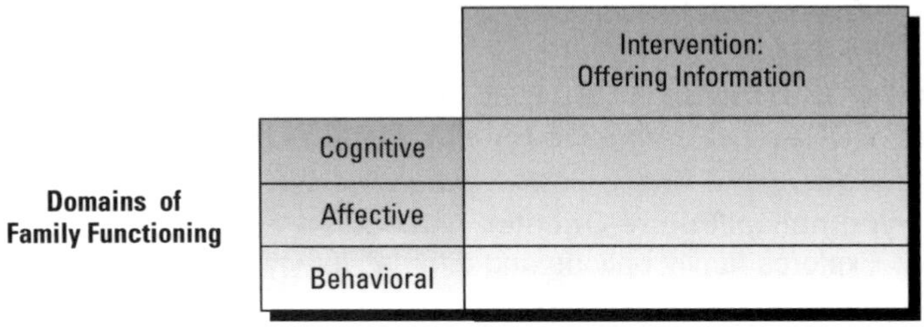

		Intervention: Offering Information
	Cognitive	
Domains of Family Functioning	Affective	
	Behavioral	

FIGURE 4–3. Intersection of intervention (offering information) and domains of family functioning.

OTHER EXAMPLES OF INTERVENTIONS

To illustrate the intersection of the three domains of family functioning (cognitive, affective, and behavioral) and various interventions, we have chosen several other examples of interventions in addition to circular questions. These examples are not meant to be an exhaustive list. Rather, they are interventions that we have found useful in our own clinical practice and research. The examples include:

- Commending family and individual strengths
- Offering information and opinions
- Validating or normalizing emotional responses
- Encouraging the telling of illness narratives
- Drawing forth family support
- Encouraging family members as caregivers
- Encouraging respite
- Devising rituals

These interventions can trigger change in any one or all of the domains of family functioning. For example, the nurse can use the intervention of offering information to promote change in cognitive, affective, or behavioral family functioning (Fig. 4–3).

We will now describe each intervention and offer a case example illustrating its application. We have chosen to cluster the sample interventions around a particular domain of family functioning. In doing this, we do not wish to imply that one intervention can be used to facilitate change in only one domain of family functioning. Nor do we imply that one intervention is a "cognitive intervention" and another an "affective intervention." Rather, these are examples of the fit between a specific problem or illness, a particular intervention, and a domain of family functioning.

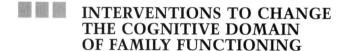

INTERVENTIONS TO CHANGE THE COGNITIVE DOMAIN OF FAMILY FUNCTIONING

Interventions directed at the cognitive domain of family functioning are usually those that offer new ideas, opinions, beliefs, information, or education on a particular health problem or risk. The treatment goal or desired outcome is to change the way in which a particular family perceives and believes regarding its health problems so that members can discover new solutions to these problems. We offer the following interventions as examples to change the cognitive domain of family functioning.

COMMENDING FAMILY AND INDIVIDUAL STRENGTHS

We routinely commend families in each session on the strengths observed during the interview. Commendations differ from compliments. de Shazer (1988) describes compliments as statements from the interviewer "about what the client has said that is useful, effective, good, or fun" with the purpose of promoting cooperation on the task at hand (p. 96). A commendation is an observation of patterns of behavior that occur across time (e.g., "Your family members are very loyal toward one another"), whereas a compliment is usually an observational comment of a one-time event (e.g., "You were very praising of your son today"). Families coping with chronic, life-threatening, or psychosocial problems frequently feel defeated, hopeless, or failing in their efforts to overcome their illnesses or live with them. Commonly, families coping with health problems have not been commended for their strengths or made aware of them (McElheran & Harper–Jaques, 1994). We choose to emphasize strengths rather than deficit, dysfunction, and deficiencies in family members. Wolin, O'Hanlon, and Hoffman (1995) have termed approaches that emphasize the latter "damage models."

The immediate and long-term positive reactions to such commendations indicate that they are effective therapeutic interventions. Robinson (1998) offered further credence to this belief in her study exploring the process and outcomes of nursing interventions with families having trouble with chronic illness. The families reported the clinical nursing team's "orientation to strengths, resources, and possibilities to be an extremely important facet of the process" (Robinson, 1998, p. 284). However, perhaps most surprising was that focusing on strengths was most significant and influential for the women in these families. Families who internalize commendations offered by nurses appear more receptive to other therapeutic interventions that may be offered.

In one family, an adopted son's behavioral and emotional problems had kept the family involved with healthcare professionals for 10 years. The nurse commended this family by telling them that she believed they were the best family for this boy because many other families would not have been as sensitive to his needs and probably would have given up years ago. Both parents became tearful and said that this was the first positive statement made to them as parents in many years.

By commending families' competence and strengths and offering them a new opinion of themselves, a context for change is created that allows families to then discover their own solutions to problems. Changing the view they have of themselves frequently enables families to view the health problem differently and thus move toward solutions that are more effective. Box 4–1 suggests helpful hints for offering interventions.

BOX 4–1. HELPFUL HINTS ABOUT OFFERING COMMENDATIONS:

- Be a "family strengths" detective and look for opportunities to commend families when strengths are discovered and uncovered.
- Ensure that sufficient evidence for the commendations is present; otherwise they may sound insincere and ingratiating.
- Use the family's language and integrate important family beliefs to strengthen the validity of the commendation.
- Offer commendations within the first 10 minutes of meeting with a family to enhance the practitioner-family relationship and to increase family receptivity to later ideas.
- Before you offer an opinion, routinely include commendations to families at the end of an interaction or meeting.

From Levac, A. M. C., Wright, L. M., & Leahey, M. (1997). Children and families: Models for assessment and intervention. In J. Fox (Ed.), *Primary health care of children*. St. Louis: Mosby, p. 13, reprinted by permission.

BOX 4–2. HELPFUL HINTS ABOUT OFFERING INFORMATION AND OPINIONS:

- Use language that is relevant, clear, and specific.
- Provide easy-to-read literature; write out key points on a small card.
- Inform families of community support groups and resources. Determine if they have been helpful to families who have used them and how.
- Build on family abilities by encouraging them to independently seek resources. Inquire about the family's reaction after seeking resources.
- Offer ideas, information, and reflections in a spirit of learning and wondering (e.g., "I wonder what would happen if you tried a slightly different approach to talking with Manisha about sex and birth control. Perhaps you might . . .").
- Do not be invested in the outcome. If the family does not apply the teaching materials, be curious about what did not fit for them rather than becoming judgmental and angry with the family.

From Levac, A. M. C., Wright, L. M., & Leahey, M. (1997). Children and families: Models for assessment and intervention. In J. Fox (Ed.), *Primary health care of children.* St. Louis: Mosby, p. 13, reprinted by permission.

OFFERING INFORMATION AND OPINIONS

The need for information from healthcare professionals is one of the most significant needs for families experiencing illness. The most pressing information desired by families is usually about developmental issues, health promotion, and illness management (Levac, Wright, & Leahey, 1997; Robinson, 1998). For example, helping parents to understand and help their children (Craft & Willadsen, 1992; Levac, Wright, & Leahey, 1997) is a common but important intervention for families. Nurses can teach families about normal physiological, emotional, and cognitive characteristics as well as identify developmental tasks or goals of children and adolescents that can be affected or altered during times of illness (Craft & Willadsen, 1992; Deatrick, 1998; Duhamel, 1987). One family found it very useful to have the nurse explain that siblings of children experiencing life-shortening illnesses often develop symptoms as a result of feelings of loneliness because parents are intently focused on their ill child. Box 4–2 suggests helpful hints about offering information.

Families with a hospitalized member have indicated that obtaining infromation is a high priority. Many families have expressed to us their frustration at their inability to obtain information or opinions readily from healthcare professionals. Nurses can offer to provide information about the impact of chronic or life-shortening illnesses on families. Nurses can empower *families* to obtain information about resources. We have learned that this latter approach is even more useful in some circumstances.

One clinical example concerns a family of two aging parents and their 34-year-old son who had severe multiple sclerosis. The parents were constant, devoted caretakers, but had not had any respite for several months. The nurse asked the son if he would be willing to challenge his belief about himself as being "helpless." The nurse asked him to take the leadership role in exploring possible resources for caregivers so that his parents might have a vacation. Because of his search, the son discovered that he was eligible for many financial benefits of which he had previously been unaware, including benefits to hire professional caregivers. Shortly afterward, the son arranged for 24-hour in-home nursing care while his parents took a vacation. His parents reported that they felt much less stressed and their son was much happier. He began making efforts to walk using parallel bars, which he had not done in several months.

In this case example, the nurse offered an opinion to empower the son to change his cognitive set. The intervention "fit" the cognitive domain and results took place in the affective and behavioral domains of family functioning.

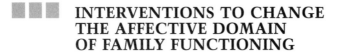 ## INTERVENTIONS TO CHANGE THE AFFECTIVE DOMAIN OF FAMILY FUNCTIONING

Interventions aimed at the affective domain of family functioning are designed to reduce or increase intense emotions that may be blocking families' problem-solving efforts. Following are examples of interventions that can change the affective domain of family functioning.

VALIDATING OR NORMALIZING EMOTIONAL RESPONSES

Validation of intense affect can alleviate feelings of isolation and loneliness and help family members to make the connection between a family member's illness and their emotional response. For example, after a diagnosis of a life-shortening illness, families frequently feel out of control or frightened for a period. It is important for nurses to validate these strong emotions and to reassure and offer hope to families that in time they will adjust and learn ways to cope.

ENCOURAGING THE TELLING OF ILLNESS NARRATIVES

Too often family members are encouraged to tell only the medical story or narrative of their illness rather than the story of their *experience* of their illness or illness narrative. However, when nurses encourage the telling of illness narratives by family members, not only are stories of sickness and suffering told but also stories of strength and tenacity (Wright, Watson, & Bell, 1996). Through therapeutic conversations, nurses can create a trusting environment for open expression of family members' fears, anger, and sadness about their illness experience (Tapp, 1997; Wright, et al., 1996). Having an opportunity to express the impact of the illness upon the family and the influence of the family on the illness from each family member's perspective gives validation to their experience. Listening to, witnessing, and documenting illness stories also has a profound impact on the nurse. Frank (1994; 1998) considers this an ethical practice. This approach is very different from limiting or constraining family stories to symptoms, medication, and physical treatments. By having a context provided for the sharing of the illness experience between family members, intense emotions are legitimized.

DRAWING FORTH FAMILY SUPPORT

Nurses can enhance family functioning in the affective domain by encouraging and assisting family members to listen to each other's concerns and feelings (Craft & Willadsen, 1992). This can be particularly useful if a family member is embracing some constraining beliefs when a loved one may be dying or has died (Moules, 1998). Through fostering opportunities for family members to express this painful experience, the nurse can enable the family to draw forth their own strengths and resources to support one another. Nurses can be the catalyst that facilitates communication between family members or between the family and other healthcare professionals. This type of family support can prevent families from becoming unduly burdened or defeated by an illness.

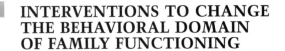

INTERVENTIONS TO CHANGE THE BEHAVIORAL DOMAIN OF FAMILY FUNCTIONING

Interventions directed at the behavioral domain help family members to interact and behave differently in relation to one another. This change is most often accomplished by inviting some or all family members to engage in specific behavioral tasks. Some tasks are given during a family meeting so that the nurse can observe the interaction; other tasks may be experimented with between sessions. Sometimes it is necessary to review with the family what the particular task and experiment is in order to check the family's understanding of what has been suggested.

We offer the following examples of interventions that could change the behavioral domain of family functioning.

ENCOURAGING FAMILY MEMBERS TO BE CAREGIVERS

Family members are often timid or afraid to become involved in the care of their ill family member unless they are supported by a nurse. Our experience has been that family members very much appreciate an opportunity to be *doing* something for their hospitalized family member as a way of feeling less helpless, anxious, and out of control. Of course, family caregivers are not immune to the well-known phenomena of caregiver burden. Health professionals must be alert to the risks involved in caregiving by family members and be willing to intervene when necessary.

ENCOURAGING RESPITE

It is often very difficult for a caretaking family to allow themselves adequate respite. Too frequently, family members feel guilty if they need or want to withdraw themselves from the caregiving role. Even the ill member must disengage himself or herself from time to time from the usual caregiving and accept another person's assistance. Each family's need for respite varies. The issues affecting respite requirements include the severity of the chronic illness, availability of family members to care for the ill person, and financial resources (Leahey & Wright, 1987). All of these issues must be considered before a nurse recommends a respite schedule. Caregiving, coping, and caring for one's own health need to be balanced. One example would be a family buying a less expensive prosthesis and using the extra money for a family vacation. Such "time-outs" or "times away" are essential for families facing excessive caretaking demands. Another example is a recommendation to a mother and father with a leukemic child to have grandparents babysit for a day while the couple spends time together.

DEVISING RITUALS

Families engage in many types of rituals: daily (e.g., bedtime reading), yearly (e.g., Thanksgiving dinner at Grandma's), and cultural (e.g., ethnic parades). Nurses can suggest therapeutic rituals that are not or have not been observed by the family. Roberts (1988) defines rituals as:

> Co-evolved symbolic acts that include not only the ceremonial aspects of the actual presentation of the ritual, but the process of preparing for it as well. It may or may not include words, but does have both open and closed parts which are 'held' together by a guiding metaphor. Repetition can be a part of rituals through the content, the form, or the occasion. There should be enough space in therapeutic rituals for the incorporation of multiple meanings by various family members and clinicians, as well as a variety of levels of participation. (p. 8)

In our clinical practice, we have observed that chronic illness and psychosocial problems frequently interrupt the usual rituals. Rituals are best introduced when there is an excessive level of confusion caused by the simultaneous presentation of incompatible injunctions. Rituals serve to provide clarity in a family system (Imber–Black, Roberts, & Whiting, 1988). For example, parents who cannot agree on parenting practices often end up giving conflicting messages to their families. This can result in chaos and confusion for their children. The introduction of an odd-day even-day ritual (Selvini–Palazzoli, Boscolo, Cecchin, & Prata, 1978) can often assist the family. The mother could be invited to experiment with being responsible for the children on Mondays, Wednesdays, and Fridays, and the father on Tuesdays, Thursdays, and Saturdays. On Sundays, they could behave spontaneously. On their "days off," parents could be asked to observe, without comment, their partner's parenting.

▖▖▖ CLINICAL CASE EXAMPLES

The following actual clinical case examples illustrate the use of the CFIM. Interventions were chosen to facilitate change in all three domains of family functioning.

CLINICAL CASE EXAMPLE 1

To illustrate a particular family intervention aimed at all three domains of family functioning (cognitive, affective, and behavioral) simultaneously, let us consider a parenting problem commonly presented to Community Health Nurses (CHN). This is the problem of young parents having difficulty putting their 3-year-old son to bed each night. Their efforts are always met with resistance from the son, then anger, then tears. In their efforts, the parents also become very frustrated and frequently end up angry with each other as well as with their son.

It is to be emphasized that it is not always necessary or even efficient to try to fit interventions to all *three* domains of family functioning simultaneously. Again, this depends on how well the family is engaged and the assessment of the nature of the problems.

With this particular problem of parents' chronic inability to have their 3-year-old son go to bed and stay there at a required time, the family intervention offered was information and opinions. This intervention is defined as the provision of assistance to parents to understand and help their young children (Craft & Willadsen, 1992). In describing this case example, we will also discuss particular executive skills the nurse can use to operationalize the intervention.

Parent–child system problem: Parents' chronic inability to have 3-year-old son go to bed and stay there at required time.

DOMAINS OF FAMILY FUNCTIONING	INTERVENTION: INFORMATION AND OPINIONS
Cognitive	Offer a parenting book for ideas on what bedtime means to children and how to put children to bed.

DOMAINS OF FAMILY FUNCTIONING	INTERVENTION: INFORMATION AND OPINIONS
Affective	Inform the parents that it is important to admit their frustrations to one another, especially if one spouse made an effort to put the child to bed but has not been successful. The other parent may give emotional support (e.g., "You tried real hard, dear; he's a handful").
Behavioral	Teach the parents that, when they put their son to bed, they should not respond to his efforts to gain attention (e.g., asking for a glass of water). Rather, be sure that these things have been attended to as part of his bedtime rituals. Warn parents that, before they can change their child's behavior of leaving his bed or continually calling them to his bedroom, his behavior will worsen for a few nights while he makes greater efforts to get his parents to respond. If the parents continue in a very matter-of-fact way to put him back in his room and tell him "no" to any further requests, his behavior will probably improve dramatically in a few nights.

CLINICAL CASE EXAMPLE 2

Next let us consider a clinical example illustrating the intervention of encouraging family members to be caregivers and caregiver support. Encouraging family members to be caregivers is inviting family members to be involved in the emotional and physical care of the patient. The problem illustrated in this case example was related to us by a nurse in a geriatric setting. Caregiver support is defined as a provision of the necessary information, advocacy, and support to facilitate primary patient care by people other than healthcare professionals (Craft & Willadsen, 1992). Again, the accompanying executive skills to operationalize the interventions are given.

Parent-Child System Problem: An elderly parent wants his or her adult children to visit more often; the adult children do not enjoy visiting because their elderly parent is always complaining.

DOMAINS OF FAMILY FUNCTIONING	INTERVENTIONS: ENCOURAGING FAMILY MEMBERS TO BE CAREGIVERS AND CAREGIVER SUPPORT
Cognitive and Behavioral	Teach adult children that their aging parent is having difficulty remembering their visits (short-term memory deficits), a common phenomenon of aging. Therefore it is not useful to remind their aging parent of when they visited last.
Affective	Empathize with the aging parent, saying that you understand that it must be lonely at times being a resident in a geriatric care center. The adult children would appreciate knowing that their parent is lonely so that they can respond appropriately. Therefore advise the elderly parent to avoid complaining to the children that they don't visit enough and, instead, tell them when they come that "Sometimes I feel lonely here. I'm really glad you came to visit me."

DOMAINS OF FAMILY FUNCTIONING	INTERVENTIONS: ENCOURAGING FAMILY MEMBERS TO BE CAREGIVERS AND CAREGIVER SUPPORT
Behavioral	Advise the adult children to stop giving excuses and explaining why they cannot come more often. Instead, obtain a guest book or calendar and write down each visit. Write down *who* visited and on *what* day, and perhaps any interesting news, so that the aging parent may read this between visits.

In each of the preceding examples, many other interventions and executive skills could have been suggested. We believe very strongly that there is no one "right" intervention, only "useful" or "effective" interventions. How useful or effective an intervention is can be evaluated only after it has been implemented. The element of time must be taken into account. With some interventions, the change or outcome may be noted immediately. However, changes (outcomes) are commonly not noticed for a long time. Most problems do not occur overnight, and therefore their resolution also requires a reasonable length of time. Change can be observed, as Bateson (1972a) states, as "difference which occurs across time" (p. 452).

CLINICAL CASE EXAMPLE 3

To appreciate that change is observed across time, we now offer two actual case examples of clinical work, from beginning to end, with the emphasis on the interventions that are used. A family was referred to one of our graduate nursing students with the presenting problems of enuresis and disciplinary problems at school in the eldest child, an 8-year-old boy. The family was composed of the father, age 28, self-employed; the stepmother, age 21, homemaker; and two sons, ages 8 and 6. The couple had been married for about 1 year. The family was seen (as a whole family and in various subsystems) for 6 sessions over 13 weeks from initial contact to termination. A thorough family assessment (using the CFAM model) revealed problems in the whole family system, in the parent-child subsystem, and at the individual level.

Whole Family System Problem: Adjustment to being a stepfamily.

All family members had to adjust to a new family structure. After being married only for a very short time, this stepmother found herself thrust into a parenting role when she and her husband became responsible for his two children, ages 6 and 4. The birth mother had deserted the children after living with them for 2 years in her home. The children had to adjust to a new set of parents, new surroundings, and no present contact with their biological mother.

Interventions. In the first session, the graduate student acknowledged that the problems the family was experiencing were a usual part of the adjustment of stepfamilies. The intervention of offering information and opinions was directed at the cognitive domain of family functioning. This new information seemed to relieve the parents a great deal. In addition, the student gave advice by encouraging the parents to allow the children to have contact with their biological mother when she again sought them out. Initially, the parents were hesitant about this suggestion, but later stated that they could see the importance of this for the children. The eldest child's problem of enuresis was conceptualized as a response to the adjustment to a stepfamily and the loss of his mother. This new opinion, also directed at the cognitive domain of family functioning, had a very positive effect on the family. The enuresis improved dramatically over the course of treatment.

Parent-Child Subsystem Problem: Maladaptive interactional pattern between stepmother and eldest son. (see circular pattern diagram below).

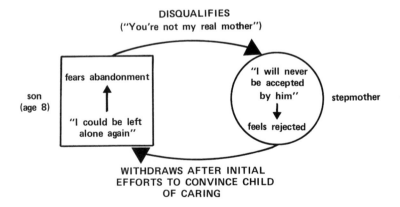

DISQUALIFIES
("You're not my real mother")

son
(age 8)

fears abandonment

"I could be left
alone again"

"I will never
be accepted
by him"

feels rejected

stepmother

WITHDRAWS AFTER INITIAL
EFFORTS TO CONVINCE CHILD
OF CARING

Because of the initial experience of the loss of their father (as a result of the biological parents' divorce) and then their literal abandonment by their biological mother, the children, particularly the eldest child, feared being abandoned again. Thus, the eldest child, hoping to be reassured that he would not be abandoned again, frequently reminded his young stepmother that she was not his real mother. Initially, the stepmother made efforts to reassure him, but eventually withdrew in frustration and felt rejected. This encouraged the child to maintain the maladaptive interactional pattern because he perceived this withdrawal as further evidence that he would be abandoned again. The vicious cycle was evident.

Interventions. The graduate nursing student encouraged the stepmother to stop withdrawing and to offer the child continual and sustained reassurance by stating, "I know I'm not your mother, but your father and I love and care for you and want to look after you. We will not leave you." This intervention of parent support and education was aimed at the behavioral, affective, and cognitive domains of family functioning. This behavioral task suggested to the stepmother proved quite successful. When the stepmother offered more reassurance to the boy, she reported that he stopped rejecting her. With decreased rejection, the stepmother was able to offer even more reassurance. Thus, a virtuous cycle began. The nursing student also offered commendations of family strengths (intervention directed at cognitive domain of family functioning) to the stepmother for her efforts to fulfill her role, saying that she was an exceptionally warm and caring young mother. The stepmother reported that she felt more relaxed in her parenting after this intervention.

Individual Problem: Eldest child's behavioral problems at school.

To assess this behavioral problem further, our graduate student met with the child's teacher at school and discussed the problem twice with the teacher by telephone. The stepmother was also present during the session at school.

Interventions. The main objective was to enhance the eldest child's self-esteem by focusing on his positive behavior. The teacher agreed to implement an intervention focused at the behavioral domain of family functioning: to acknowledge the child's positive behavior in front of his classmates to give him a different status than "class clown." It was also recommended to the stepmother that she minimize her contacts with the school and allow the teacher to assume more responsibility for the boy's behavior in class. Within a few weeks, the teacher reported a positive change in the child's behavior at school. The parents expressed great satisfaction over their child's improvement.

On termination with this family, the student recommended some readings on stepfamilies to the parents and informed them of a "self-help group" for stepfamilies. These two interventions of bibliotherapy and providing information on community resources were targeted at all three domains of family functioning: cognitive, affective, and behavioral.

CLINICAL CASE EXAMPLE 4

A family was referred to one of our undergraduate students while the student had a community-health field placement, with the presenting problem being the social isolation and frequent physical complaints of a 78-year-old widowed mother. This woman lived in a government-subsidized one-bedroom apartment. She had 6 adult children: 5 sons, ages 51, 48, 41, 37, and 35; a daughter, age 44; and 12 grandchildren. Five of the children were married, and all six lived in the same city as their mother. The family was seen as a whole and in various subsystems for 8 home visits over a period of 2 months.

After a thorough family assessment (using the CFAM model) and individual assessment, the following core problem was identified: Mother's lack of social contact beyond her immediate family.

Whole Family System Problem: It became apparent that this older woman was overly dependent on her adult children and therefore did not extend herself to be involved with her peers or in social activities appropriate to her age group. This resulted in frequent disagreements between the mother and the children over the frequency of visits with the mother. This was further exacerbated by the fact that the mother had no friends. After the death of her husband, about 10 years ago, she had lived intermittently with some of her children, but for the past 4 years had been living alone in her one-bedroom apartment. Presently the youngest son visits most often and does his mother's grocery shopping.

Interventions: The student's first significant intervention was to broaden the context in order to expand her view and understanding of this family member's problem. Thus, the student initially interviewed the mother alone, then with her youngest son (the adult child who visited most frequently). Then the student took on the ambitious task of arranging an interview with the mother and her six children. This was a most significant effort on the student's part to create a context for change. It had been agreed in the interview with the mother and her youngest son that the mother would contact the children. However, on follow-up by the student, it was learned that the mother had not called any of her children because she expected her youngest son to do it. This was further evidence of the mother's over-dependence on her children. Because the youngest son was anxious to have this meeting take place, he had taken on the task of inviting all of his siblings to an interview with his mother and the student.

At the family interview, all of the siblings were present and two of their spouses attended as well! Interestingly, the daughters-in-law were more vocal than their husbands and stated that they were very involved with their mother-in-law. In this large family interview, the issue of the mother's social isolation (apart from her family) was discussed. Through the process of circular questioning, the expectations of contact of both mother and children were assessed. Initially, the student encouraged the family to explore alternative solutions to their mother's lack of social activities and a peer group. This intervention aimed at the behavioral domain of family functioning was met by a statement that they had no ideas beyond what they had already tried. Therefore the student offered some more specific interventions that might open solutions to the problem of the mother's social isolation. This significant and most important interview revealed that this woman had always relied on her children for her main social interaction. She had never been a "joiner." In the past few years, she had even discontinued her attendance at church. Throughout her life, she had had few close friends.

The assessment also revealed that, collectively, the children had generally been supportive of their mother. Each week she had lunch with one or more of them. They included her in all special family occasions. However, the children always had to initiate contact. They were genuinely concerned about their mother's loneliness and lack of additional social contact, but had exhausted their ideas for changing the situation.

One of the first interventions the nursing student offered was directed at both the cognitive and behavioral domains of family functioning. The student offered information regarding community resources available to older people. Particularly, the student made the family aware of the Community Services Visitor Program. A decision was made that the mother would contact this program and the children would provide support. The mother also expressed interest in being involved in a choir again. The student offered to accompany her to a senior citizens' choir practice and introduce her to other participants.

The final major intervention discussed in that session was directed at the behavioral domain. The mother was asked if she would initiate contact with one of her children the next week. After the contact, the child would ask the mother to come for a visit as soon as possible. It has been our experience that the interest of family members in an older parent's activities does much to increase the parent's motivation. It is important to emphasize that the mother was involved in and receptive to these interventions.

The effect or outcome of these interventions was as follows:

1. The mother followed through on contacting the Community Services Visiting Program. The coordinator of the program contacted the mother and arranged for a regular visitor.
2. The student accompanied the mother to the senior citizens' choir. The older woman enjoyed the experience and two of the other women in the choir telephoned afterward!
3. The mother took the initiative to contact a couple of her children, and they, in turn, invited her for a family visit, which she accepted. The children reported that they enjoyed having their mother call them, and this appeared to increase their own desire to have more frequent contact with her.

In future interviews, the student encouraged the mother to reconnect with her church. The student also solicited the support of the children in this endeavor by requesting that they take an interest and inquire about their mother's church and choir activities when they called her.

Because this older mother was accustomed to a good deal of family support, it was not appropriate to totally remove that support. However, physical instrumental support (doing things for the mother) could be reduced without the mother feeling abandoned. Verbal (emotional) support for the mother's attempts at independence was most appropriate. When the mother began to increase her social contacts and activities, her nonspecific physical complaints decreased.

The student concluded treatment with this woman in a face-to-face interview. To involve the children in the termination process, the student sent a letter to each of them This letter, written by the student and her faculty supervisor, is printed verbatim below. It beautifully highlights the major interventions and again solicits further assistance from the children. In addition, the student very nicely included some of the family strengths in the letter. Hopefully, the change process in this particular family will continue to evolve long after this nursing student's termination of the therapeutic relationship with them.

Dear (real names omitted to preserve confidentiality)

I wish to thank you for your help and cooperation in my family assignment. I enjoyed meeting each of you and appreciated your individual input and assessment of your family. Your willingness to work together is certainly an excellent family strength.

I visited your mother on several occasions during my time with the Outreach Program. She continued to express her desire to be more socially independent. She has been able to make some increased community contact. She attended the choir and several of the choir ladies have called her to encourage her in continued participation. She met with the gentleman from the church and spoke with his wife. The Coordinator of the Visitor Program visited; she is arranging for a friend who will visit with your mother. Hopefully, they will develop some outside interests together. She has also been out to shop on her own on a few occasions.

I did contact Kerby Centre, as well as other seniors from Carter Place who go there, but was unable to find anyone going to the Wednesday lunch or any other suitable transportation. I have discussed this with your mother and she felt it might be something she could pursue on her own in the future.

Your mother expressed positive feelings about her attempts to be more socially active. However, she still looks to her children for her main support. At times, I found she needed more encouragement not to overly worry about her health to the point that she thinks she is unable to participate in any activities. I believe that each of you may help your mother by encouraging her in this area. I might suggest that if she says that she is unwell that she see her doctor. If there is no serious problem, gentle support for her independent activities might be helpful. This may be somewhat difficult at first, but if you are able to present a united front to your mother and support each other in a mutual approach to her being more socially active, she may be more able to accomplish this.

I am very impressed with the cohesiveness of your family and the continued concern and support you show toward your mother. Thank you very much again for letting me work with you.

Yours truly,
Leslie Henderson
Undergraduate Nursing Student
Faculty of Nursing, University of Calgary

This therapeutic letter sent by the student is in and of itself an intervention (Parry & Doan, 1994; White & Epston, 1990, Wright, Watson & Bell, 1996). In addition, several interventions were in the letter. They were aimed at all three domains of family functioning. Specifically, the student offered commendations and opinions directed at the cognitive domain of functioning. She invited the adult children to encourage their mother, which aimed at changes in the behavioral domain. By summarizing the clinical work with the family in the form of a therapeutic letter, the student intended to effect changes in both the affective and cognitive domains of family functioning. This very fine clinical work is an excellent example of effectively involving families in healthcare by the use of family assessment and intervention models with clear treatment goals by a student committed to improving family functioning and reducing suffering through the development of clinical skills.

▪▪▪ CONCLUSIONS

Interventions can be straightforward and simple or as innovative and dramatic as the nurse deems necessary for the health problem(s) presented. Ell and Northen (1990) convincingly support this statement with abundant research documentation that "interventions intended to promote health and prevent illness should be based on the assumption that individual health behaviors are strongly influenced by those around us, and that family general well-being can promote the physical health of its members" (p. 79). Any interventions should be directed toward the goals of treatment collaboratively generated by the nurse *and* the family. As nurses learn to actively engage and thoroughly assess the family, clearly identify problems, and set treatment goals, the conceptualizing, choosing, and implementing of specific interventions with each family becomes more rewarding and more effective. The ultimate goal, of course, is to aid family members in discovering new solutions to help reduce or alleviate emotional, physical, and spiritual suffering.

▪▪▪ REFERENCES

Bateson, G. (1972a). *Steps to an ecology of mind.* New York: Ballantine Books.

Broome, M. E., Knafl, K., Pridham, K., and Feetham, S. (Eds.) (1998). *Children and families in health and illness.* Thousand Oaks: Sage Publications.

Craft, M. J., & Willadsen, J. A. (1992). Interventions related to family. *Nursing Clinics of North America, 27*(2), 517–540.

Campbell, T. L., & Patterson, J. M. (1995). The effectiveness of family interventions in the treatment of physical illness. *Journal of Marital and Family Therapy, 21*(4), 545–583.

Deatrick, J. A. (1998). Integrative review of intervention research with children who have chronic conditions and their families. In M.E. Broome, K. Knafl, Pridham, K., and S. Feetham, (Eds.), *Children and Families in Health and Illness.* Thousand Oaks: Sage Publications.

de Shazer, S. (1988). Clues: *Investigating solutions in brief therapy.* New York: W. W. Norton.

Duhamel, F. (1987). Assessing families of adolescents with Crohn's disease. In L. M. Wright & M. Leahey (Eds.), *Families and chronic illness.* Springhouse, PA: Springhouse Corporation.

Ell, K. & Northen, H. (1990). *Families and health care.* New York: Aldine de Gruyter.

Fleuridas, C., Nelson, T., & Rosenthal, D. (1986). The evolution of circular questions: Training family therapists. *Journal of Marital and Family Therapy, 12*(2), 113–127.

Frank, A. W. (1994). Interrupted stories, interrupted lives. *Second Opinion, 20*(1), 11–18.

Frank, A. W. (1998). Just listening: Narrative and deep illness. *Families, Systems, and Health, 16*(3), 197–212.

Freedman, J., & Combs, G. (1996). *Narrative therapy: The social construction of preferred realities.* New York: W. W. Norton Co.

Hanson, S. M. H. (1996). Family assessment and intervention. In S.M.H. Hanson & Boyd, S. T. (Ed.), *Family health care nursing: Theory, practice, and research.* Philadelphia: F.A. Davis.

Hill, R. (1986). Life cycle stages for types of single-parent families: Of family development theory. *Family Relations, 35,* 19–29.

Imber-Black, E., Roberts, J., & Whiting, R. (Eds.). (1988). *Rituals in families and family therapy.* New York: W.W. Norton & Co.

Leahey, M., & Harper-Jaques, S. (1996). Family-nurse relationships: Core assumptions and clinical implications. *Journal of Family Nursing, 2*(2), 133-151.

Leahey, M., & Wright, L. M. (1987). Families and chronic illness: Assumptions, assessment, and intervention. In L.M. Wright & M. Leahey (Eds.), *Families and chronic illness.* Springhouse, PA: Springhouse Corp.

Levac, A. M. C., Wright, L. M., & Leahey, M. (1997). Children and families: Models for assessment and intervention. In J. Fox (Ed.), *Primary health care of children.* St. Louis: Mosby, pp. 3–13.

Lipchik, E., & deShazer, S. (1986). The purposeful interview. *Journal of Strategic and Systemic Therapies, 5,* 88–99.

Loos, F., & Bell, J. M. (1990). Circular questions: A family interviewing strategy. *Dimensions of Critical Care Nursing, 9*(1), 46–53.

Maturana, H., & Varela, F. (1992). *The tree of knowledge: The biological roots of human understanding.* Boston, MA: Shambhala Publications, Inc.

McElheran, N., & Harper-Jaques, S. (1994). Commendations: A resource intervention for clinical practice. *Clinical Nurse Specialist, 8*(1), 7–10.

Mischke-Berkey, K., Warner, P., & Hanson, S. (1989). Family health assessment and intervention. In P. J. Bomar (Ed.), *Nurses and family health promotion: concepts, assessment and intervention.* Baltimore: Williams and Wilkins.

Moules, N. J. (1998). Legitimizing grief: Challenging beliefs that constrain. *Journal of Family Nursing, 4*(2), 138–162.

Parry, A., & Doan, R. E. (1994). *Story re-visions: Narrative therapy in the postmodern world.* New York: Norton.

Roberts, J. (1988). Setting the frame: Definition, functions, and typology of rituals. In E. Imber-Black, J. Roberts, & R. Whiting (Eds.), *Rituals in families and family therapy*. New York: W. W. Norton & Co.

Robinson, C. A. (1998). Women, families, chronic illness, and nursing interventions: From burden to balance. *Journal of Family Nursing, 4*(3), 271–290.

Robinson C. A. (1996). Health care relationships revisited. *Journal of Family Nursing, 2*(2), 152-173.

Robinson, C. A., & Wright, L. M. (1995). Family nursing interventions: What families say makes a difference. *Journal of Family Nursing, 1*(2), 327-345.

Selvini-Palazzoli, M., Boscolo, L., Cecchin, G., & Prata, G. (1980). Hypothesizing circularity-neutrality: Three guidelines for the conductor of the session. *Family Process, 19*(3), 3–12.

Selvini-Palazzoli, M., Boscolo, L., Cecchin, G., & Prata, G. (1978). A ritualized prescription in family therapy: Odd days and even days. *Journal of Marriage and Family Counseling, 4*(3), 3–9.

Tapp, D. M. (1997). *Exploring therapeutic conversations between nurses and families experiencing ischemic heart disease*. Unpublished doctoral dissertation, University of Calgary, Alberta, Canada.

Thorne, S., & Robinson, C. A. (1989). Guarded alliance: Health-care relationships in chronic illness. *Image, 21*(3), 153-157.

Tomm, K. (1985). Circular interviewing: A multifaceted clinical tool. In Campbell, D., & Draper, R. (Eds.), *Applications of systemic family therapy: The Milan approach* (pp. 33–45). London: Grune & Stratton.

Tomm, K. (1987). Interventive interviewing—Part II. Reflexive questioning as a means to enable self–healing. *Family Process, 26,* 167–183.

Tomm, K. (1988). Interventive interviewing—Part III. Intending to ask lineal, circular, strategic, or reflexive questions? *Family Process, 27,* 1–15.

Tomm, K. (1984). One perspective on the Milan systemic approach: Part II. Description of session format, interviewing style and interventions. *Journal of Marital and Family Therapy, 10*(3), 253–271.

Watson, W. L. (Producer). (1989a). *Families and psychosocial problems* (videotape). Calgary, AB: University of Calgary.

Watson, W. L. (Producer). (1989b). *Family systems interventions* (videotape). Calgary, AB: University of Calgary.

Watson, W. L. (Producer). (1988a.) *A family with chronic illness: A "tough" family copes well* (videotape). Calgary, AB: University of Calgary.

Watson, W. L. (Producer). (1988b). *Aging families and Alzheimer's Disease* (videotape). Calgary, AB: University of Calgary.

Watson, W. L. (Producer). (1988c). *Fundamentals of family systems nursing* (videotape). Calgary, AB: University of Calgary.

Watson, W. L. & Nanchoff-Glatt, M. (1990). A family systems nursing approach to premenstrual syndrome. *Clinical nurse specialist, 4*(1), 3–9.

Wolin, S., O'Hanlon, B., & Hoffman, L. (1995, November). *Three strength-based therapies* [Audiotape]. A special symposium at the annual meeting of the American Association for Marriage and Family Therapy, Baltimore, MD.

White, M., & Epston, D. (1990). *Narrative means to therapeutic ends.* New York: Norton.

Wright, L. M., & Leahey, M. (1987). Families and life-threatening illness: Assumptions, assessment, and intervention. In M. Leahey & L. M. Wright (Eds.) *Families and Life-Threatening Illness.* Springhouse, PA: Springhouse Corporation.

Wright, L. M., & Levac, A.M. (1992). The non-existence of non-compliant families: The influence of Humberto Maturana. *Journal of Advanced Nursing, 17,* 913–917.

Wright, L. M, Watson, W. L, & Bell, J. M. (1996). *Beliefs: The heart of healing in families and illness.* New York: Basic Books.

CHAPTER 5

Family Nursing
Interviews:
Stages and Skills

When nurses have a clear conceptual framework for assessing and intervening with families, they can then begin to consider the various new competencies and skills needed for family interviews. The types of skills identified as necessary by various authors on family work reflect each author's particular theoretical orientation and unique preference as to how to approach and resolve problems. Therefore, the skills delineated in this chapter are based on our postmodernist world view. This includes, but is not limited to, the theoretical foundation of systems, cybernetic, communication, biology of cognition, and change theories that inform the CFAM and CFIM.

We favor a problem and solution-focused and time-effective approach. We emphasize that families possess the ability to solve their own problems, and that our task as nurses is to facilitate and help them to find their own solutions. We do not propose that we know what is "best" for families. We embrace the notion that there are multiple realities in and of "the world," that each family member and nurse sees a world that he or she brings forth through interacting with themselves and with others through language. We encourage an openness in ourselves, our students, and our families to the diversity of difference among us. However, to be involved in helping families change requires that nurses possess certain essential competencies and skills.

In the previous chapters we discussed the theoretical knowledge base that is necessary for beginning practice with families to competently assess and intervene with them. We also offered two practice models (the CFAM and CFIM) as frameworks to guide family data management, to conceptualize family dynamics, and to offer specific family interventions. This chapter focuses on the specific beginning-level skills necessary for family nursing interviews.

We concur with the Alberta Association of Registered Nurses (AARN, 1991) Nursing Practice Standards and Competencies for Nurses, which defines competencies as "the ability to demonstrate the requisite knowledge, skills and attitudes of nurses beginning to practice" (p. 2). The AARN (1991) specifically describes the importance of reciprocal or interactional knowledge of families by stating that one of the knowledge competencies required of nurses is that they "recognizes the influence of family structure and functioning on the patient/

client's health status and the influence of health status on family functioning" (p. 3).

In the past 20 years, the explosion of literature on family work suggests and implies a myriad of skills that can be used when working with families (Falicov, Constantine, & Breunlin, 1981; Flemons, Green, and Rambo, 1996; Liddle, 1991; Tomm & Wright, 1979; Watson, 1992). Some of these skills relate to the personal agency of the therapist (Blow & Piercy, 1997) whereas some focus on the therapist's external behavior. Simply stating general skills such as "the student must be able to label interactions accurately" says nothing about how that skill can be achieved. Figley and Nelson (1989) conducted a survey of educators and trainers of family therapists to identify the most important skills for beginners. The five most important skills identified were (1) basic interviewing skills, (2) establishing rapport, (3) giving credit for positive changes, (4) being able to distinguish content from process, and (5) setting reachable goals. Another very interesting finding of this study was that 31% of their top 100 generic skills referred to personal traits.

Through the use of specific learning objectives, the mystery of what a family interviewer actually does is removed. Thus, the learning objectives or skills become a tentative "map" for the interview. The skills described in this chapter emerge from our theoretical orientation and the application of the practice models CFAM and CFIM. These skills become the nurse behaviors that are unique to working with families. Of course, each nurse brings his or her own unique genetic and personality makeup and history of interactions, which personalize the application of these skills.

▌▌▌ STAGES OF FAMILY NURSING INTERVIEWS

Four major stages of family nursing interviews can be identified within the context of a therapeutic conversation between a nurse and a family. These are engagement, assessment, intervention, and termination. These stages tend to follow in a logical sequence during both the course of a given interview and the overall course of contact. For example, a nurse engages family members during each interview and terminates with them at the end of each interview, as well as at the beginning and end of the entire contact. Of course, there are times when a nurse may have to return to a previous stage. For example, interventions may be offered too quickly before a thorough assessment has been completed.

Engagement refers to the first stage, in which the nurse exercises skills that invite both himself or herself and the family to establish and maintain a therapeutic relationship. Our preferred stance or posture with families is to be collaborative and consultative (Leahey & Harper-Jaques, 1996). Selvini-Palazzoli, Boscolo, Cecchin, and Prata (1980) suggest that the interviewer should be allied with everyone and no one at the same time. They refer to this process as *neutrality*. It has also been called *curiosity* (Cecchin, 1987). When the nurse adopts a curious, interested stance, it impies greater equality and respect for the family's resiliency and resourcefulness. The nurse brings expertise to the relationship and the family members bring their own expertise. It is this synergy of combined expertise that can generate new outcomes to constraining situations. Factors that appear to inhibit engagement by the family interviewer are confrontation and interpretation too early in treatment. Further ideas and suggestions for the engagement stage are given in Chapters 6 and 7.

Assessment, the second stage, includes the substages of problem exploration and identification, plus delineation of a strengths and problem list. During this stage the nurse opens space for the family to tell their story. With some families, it may be an illness story, with others a story of loss and grief; with others it may be a story of uncertainty about the health of family members (e.g., a child's developmental delay or undiagnosed symptoms); and with still other families it may be stories of a desire to promote or maintain healthy lifestyles. We stress that the conversation between the nurse and the family is in and of itself part of the therapeutic discourse (Tapp, 1997). That is, if the nurse attends only to the signs and symptoms of disease, both nurse and family will find themselves in a discourse emphasizing pathology. Alternative discourses that would be equally unhelpful would emphasize "right answers" rather than an understanding of the family's frustrations, dilemmas, and yearnings (Freedman & Combs, 1996).

Beginning nurse interviewers generally lack a clear stepwise rationale to guide the collecting and processing of data during an interview. Thus, beginners often spend an inordinate amount of time collecting vast amounts of information. Frequently, this information is tangential to the presenting problem and is not usable. Alternatively, beginners sometimes rush into inappropriate treatment because they do not have a clear formulation of the presenting problem. It is better, however, for beginners to err on the side of taking longer than usual to complete the initial assessment than to rush to the intervention stage too prematurely. It needs to be noted that assessment in family work is an ongoing process. Thus, the strengths and problems list may change over time as the nurse's conceptual understanding of the family becomes more systemic. Ideas for conducting a time-effective 15-minute interview are given in Chapter 8. What areas to assess and how to integrate and document the information are available in Chapters 3 and 9, respectively.

The *intervention,* or third stage, is really the core of clinical work with families. It involves providing a context in which the family may make small or significant changes. There are numerous ways in which to intervene, and treatment plans should be co-constructed and tailored by the nurse and family for each family situation. The Calgary Family Intervention Model (Chap. 4) offers examples of specific interventions that can be used by nurses.

Termination, the last stage, refers to the process of ending the therapeutic relationship between the nurse and the family in a manner that allows the family not only to maintain but to continue constructive changes. Therapeutic termination encourages family members in their ability to solve problems in the future. Specific ideas for therapeutic termination are described in Chapter 10.

■ ■ ■ TYPES OF SKILLS

Within each stage of family interviewing there are three types of skills: perceptual, conceptual, and executive (Cleghorn & Levin, 1973). The identification and categorization of these three sets of skills by Cleghorn and Levin (1973) is considered a seminal contribution. These authors were the first to offer a systematic way to think about training family therapists and provided "a conceptual scaffolding" (Liddle, 1991, p. 640). Tomm and Wright (1979) used the perceptual, conceptual, and executive skills model as a guide for their comprehensive outline, which offered examples of therapist functions, competencies, and skills in each category over the course of family therapy. In our text, we have kept Wright's previous experience of identifying particular perceptual, conceptual, and executive skills across the four stages of family interviews. However, we have adapted the perceptual, conceptual, and executive skills to be congruent with nurses who are just beginning to practice with families.

The skills that we have identified fit within the context of our particular practice models, namely, the CFAM and CFIM. Perceptual and conceptual skills are paired because what is perceived is so intimately interrelated with what is thought. It is often difficult to separate the perceptual from the conceptual component. These perceptual and conceptual skills are then matched with executive skills.

Perceptual skills refer to the nurse's ability to make relevant observations. The nurse's own ethnicity, gender, sexual orientation, race, and class are but a few of the factors influencing his or her perceptions.

There is a major shift from the perceptual skills required in individual interviewing to those required in family interviewing. This shift can be explained in that the nurse is involved in observing multiple interactions and relationships simultaneously. The interaction among family members and the interaction between the nurse and the family are simultaneous.

Conceptual skills involve the ability to give meaning to observations. They also involve the ability to formulate one's observations of the family as a whole, as a system. We are always cognizant that the meanings derived from observations are not "the truth" but represent one nurse's effort to make sense of his or her observations.

We believe that the student entering the nursing field has intuitive *perceptual and conceptual skills* that have been learned in other roles in previous life experiences. The student however, is unaware of many of the skills. The nurse needs to develop an overt awareness of the perceptual process. The perceptual and conceptual skills are the basis of the executive skills.

Executive skills are the therapeutic interventions that the nurse actually carries out in an interview. These skills or therapeutic interventions elicit responses from family members and are the basis for the nurse's further observations and conceptualizations. As can be readily seen, the interview process is a circular phenomenon between the nurse and family. The process is highly influenced by the nurse's and the family's particular ethnicity, class, and race. Of course, the types of therapeutic interventions offered by the nurse are highly dependent on his or her clinical expertise and experience in working with families.

■ ■ ■ DEVELOPMENT OF FAMILY NURSING INTERVIEW SKILLS

In the education of nurses developing family nursing skills, emphasis should be placed first on the development of perceptual and conceptual skills. This can be accomplished by several methods. Lectures and readings are helpful. However, observation, role-playing, and videotapes of family interviews are a better way to increase perceptual and conceptual skill accuracy. When a nurse is unable to perform a specific executive skill, it is useful to find out whether the interviewer has developed a perceptual and conceptual base for that particular skill. This is the value of matching these skills in pairs.

Three surveys of nursing programs, one in Canada (Wright & Bell, 1989), one in the United States (Hanson & Heims, 1992), and one in Australia (St. John & Rolls, 1996) are an important beginning evaluation of our efforts as nurse educators to develop family interviewing skills. Both the Canadian and American studies found that family assessment is generally well taught at the baccalaureate level but that family intervention skills at both the undergraduate and graduate levels are sadly lacking. Of particular interest was the minimal provision of live supervised clinical practice with families, particularly at the graduate level (Wright & Bell, 1989). Case discussion and process recording were reported as the predominant method of supervision. To develop and achieve therapeutic competence in nursing practice with families, it is essential that live supervision be provided (Chesla, Gilliss & Leavitt, 1993; Tapp & Wright, 1996; Wright, 1994). The Australian study (St. John & Rolls, 1996) found that five strategies for teaching conceptual skills were useful for undergraduate students: presentation of exemplars from a range of clinical settings, role-playing, small group discussions, case studies, and family meetings.

It is especially encouraging to note the increase in the family nursing literature of descriptions and reports of how nurse educators are committed to enhancing the development of family nursing skills. Specific examples in the literature include teaching students to "think family" (Green, 1997), to appreciate family diversity (Friedman, 1997), to integrate family nursing within present conceptual models (De Montigny, Dumas, Bolduc, & Blais, 1997) and to practice family nursing skills in structured family nursing labs (Tapp, Moules, Bell, & Wright, 1997). These articles offer evidence for the continuing and deepening efforts to enhance and increase nursing students' competencies and skills in their care of families.

The specific skills for interviewing families are listed in logical sequence in Table 5–1. However, this does not mean that, during the course of an actual interview, the nurse must follow this outline rigidly. The nurse needs a "map of interviewing skills" that allows considerable flexibility in application. The family's cultural norms for giving and receiving information can provide a guide for the pacing of the meeting. We cannot emphasize enough the importance of the nurse and the family developing a collaborative working relationship during the interview.

▪▪▪ PERCEPTIONS OF SKILL ATTAINMENT

The competence of a nurse when working with a particular family will have a direct relationship to the success of treatment. The Family Nursing Unit, University of Calgary, has found it useful to conduct a follow-up evaluation of the perceptions of Master of Nursing (MN)

TABLE 5–1.
FAMILY INTERVIEWING SKILLS FOR NURSES

Stage 1: Engagement	
Perceptual/Conceptual Skills	**Executive Skills**
1. **Recognize that an individual family member is best understood in the context of the family.** That is, no individual exists in isolation.	1. **Invite all family members who are concerned/involved with the problem to attend the first interview.** For example, grandparents or other relatives or friends living outside of the home should also be invited to attend if they are involved with the problem.
2. **Appreciate that initial efforts to involve both spouses/parents enables, from the onset, a more holistic view of the family and increases engagement.** That is, fathers should definitely be involved for effective family work. Family therapy research (Gurman & Kniskern, 1981) indicates a much better outcome when fathers are present.	2. **Employ all efforts to initially involve both spouses/parents in initial sessions.**
3. **Recognize that providing a clear structure to the interview reduces anxiety and increases engagement.** That is, there is generally anxiety related to the uncertainty of being in a new setting and of not knowing how to behave in the situation. Structure is particularly important if the family is experiencing a crisis.	3. **Explain to family members the purpose, length, and structure of the interview and ask if they have any questions relating to the interview.** For example, "I thought we could spend about 15 minutes together discussing the issues that you are concerned about."

(continued)

TABLE 5–1. *(continued)*
FAMILY INTERVIEWING SKILLS FOR NURSES

Stage 1: Engagement *(continued)*

Perceptual/Conceptual Skills	Executive Skills
4. **Recognize that initially members are most comfortable talking about the structural aspects of the family.** That is, note nonverbal cues indicating level of comfort, such as taking coat off, adequate versus minimal time spent talking, and participating in versus ignoring conversation.	4. **Ask each family member to relate information with regard to name, age, work or school, years married, and so forth.** For example, introduce yourself directly by giving your name and either shaking hands or making some physical contact (e.g., touching a child's head).

Stage 2: Assessment

Perceptual/Conceptual Skills	Executive Skills
1. **Realize the importance of having a conceptual assessment map to understand family dynamics.** That is, a conceptual assessment map provides the nurse with several possible courses for focused exploration.	1. **Explore the components of the structural, developmental, and functional aspects of CFAM to assess strengths and problem areas.** All components of CFAM need not be explored if they are not relevant to the present issues.
2. **Realize the importance of beginning a family assessment by obtaining a detailed description and history of the presenting problem/concern/ issue.** The presenting problem usually serves as an entry point for the family to seek help. It is time-effective to be focused on addressing it.	2. **Ask each family member, including the children, to share his or her knowledge and understanding of the presenting problem.** For example, ask the father, "How do you see the problem?" or ask the whole family, "What is the main problem that each of you would like to see changed?"

(continued)

TABLE 5–1. *(continued)*
FAMILY INTERVIEWING SKILLS FOR NURSES

Stage 2: Assessment *(continued)*

Perceptual/Conceptual Skills	Executive Skills
3. **Realize that the presenting problem is often related to other problems in the family.** That is, a child's temper outbursts may be related to the family conflict (e.g., the child may be triangulated into the family conflict).	3. **Explore with the family if there are other problems/concerns connected to the presenting problem(s).** For example, "We've been talking for some time about the problem of Theo's refusal to take his Ritalin in the mornings. I'm wondering if there are any other problems the family is concerned about at present."
4. **Realize that eliciting differences generates more specific information for family assessment.** That is: (a) Clarification of differences between individuals is a significant source of information about *family functioning.* (b) Clarification of differences between relationships is a significant source of information about *family structure and alliances.* (c) Clarification of differences in family members or in relationships at various points in time is a significant source of information about *family development.*	4. **Inquire about differences between individuals, between relationships, and between various points in time.** For example: (a) To explore differences between individuals, ask the child: "What is expected of you before you go to bed at night?" and then ask, "Who is the best, Mother or Father, at getting you to do those things in the evening?" (b) To explore differences between relationships ask: "Do Father and Ingo fight more or less than Father and Hannah?" (c) To explore differences before or after important points in time ask: "Do you worry more, less, or the same about your husband's health since his heart attack?"

(continued)

TABLE 5–1. *(continued)*
FAMILY INTERVIEWING SKILLS FOR NURSES

Stage 2: Assessment *(continued)*

Perceptual/Conceptual Skills	Executive Skills
5. **Use the information obtained from the family assessment to begin formulating hypotheses in the form of a strengths/problems list.** That is, structural, developmental, and functional strengths/problems may be present at various systems levels. For example, whole family system problems: (a) Structural: adjusting to new family form of single-parent household. (b) Developmental: family in life cycle stage of children leaving home. (c) Functional: Family belief, "Father would be displeased with us for still crying about his death."	5. **Obtain verification of nurse's understanding of strengths/ problems by listing them to the family and eventually recording them. Offering the conclusions or summary of the nurse's assessment ideas enhances engagement and collaboration.** For example: "We've identified that being a new single parent and also having to cope with your children leaving home are your two major concerns. We've also discussed that your family is very well respected in the Latino community."
6. **Assess whether any of the identified problems are beyond the scope of the nurse's competence.** That is, it is appropriate to consider referral when medical symptoms have not been fully assessed or long-standing emotional or behavioral problems exist.	6. **Tell the family whether you will continue to work with them on problems. (If a decision is made to refer them to another professional, proceed to Stage 4A: Termination.)** For example, tell the family: "Now that I have a more complete understanding of your concerns, I think it necessary to have your son's headaches checked out medically. I would like to refer you to a pediatrician."

(continued)

TABLE 5–1. *(continued)*
FAMILY INTERVIEWING SKILLS FOR NURSES

Stage 2: Assessment *(continued)*

Perceptual/Conceptual Skills	Executive Skills
7. **Recognize that a more extensive inquiry into the most pressing problems is necessary before intervention plans can be implemented.** That is, initially families are usually most concerned with the presenting problem.	7. **Seek the family's opinion of which issue they perceive as most important and explore it in depth. If the family cannot agree, then discuss the lack of consensus.** For example, ask: "About which of the problems we have discussed today are you most concerned?"
8. **Recognize that the assessment is complete when sufficient information has been obtained to formulate a treatment plan.** That is, nurses sometimes rush into inappropriate treatment because they are without a clear understanding of the presenting problem or other significant related problems.	8. **State your integrated understanding of problem(s) to family and obtain their commitment to work on a specific problem.** For example, "Since everyone agrees that In Soo's bulimia is connected to the other addictions in the family, I would like to suggest that we focus on this problem for three interviews. Would you be willing?"

Stage 3: Intervention

Perceptual/Conceptual Skills	Executive Skills
1. **Recognize that families possess problem-solving abilities.** That is, a belief that families not only possess the capability to change but also can identify and implement solutions of how to change helps the nurse to avoid becoming overcontrolling or overresponsible.	1. **Encourage family members to explore possible solutions to problems.** For example, "Sanjeshna, you've mentioned that your mother is too critical of herself. Do you have any ideas of what she could do to feel better about herself as a mother coping with a chronic illness?"

(continued)

TABLE 5–1. *(continued)*
FAMILY INTERVIEWING SKILLS FOR NURSES

Stage 3: Intervention *(continued)*

Perceptual/Conceptual Skills	Executive Skills
2. **Recognize that interventions are focused on the cognitive, affective, and behavioral domains of functioning in families, as described in the CFIM.** That is, it is not always necessary or even efficient to target interventions at all *three* domains of functioning simultaneously.	2. **Plan interventions to target any one or all three of the domains of functioning described in the CFIM.** For example, (a) Cognitive: invite the family to think differently. (b) Affective: encourage different affective expression. (c) Behavioral: ask the family to perform new tasks either within or outside of the interview.
3. **Recognize that lack of information of an educational nature can inhibit the family's problem-solving abilities.** That is, often with additional information, families will be able to provide their own creative and unique solutions to problems.	3. **Provide information to the family that will enhance its knowledge and facilitate further problem solving.** For example, the nurse can ask the family if they would like to hear about some typical reactions of a 3-year-old to a new baby or about the aging process of an older adult with Alzheimer's disease. This type of intervention targets the family's cognitive domain of functioning.
4. **Recognize that persistent and intense emotions can often block the family's problem-solving abilities.** That is, families who predominantly experience emotions such as sadness or anger are often unable to deal with problems until the emotional constraint is removed.	4. **Validate family members' emotional responses, when appropriate.** For example, suppression of grief over the loss of a family member may only need confirmation of the normal grieving process to free family members to work through their bereavement. This type of intervention targets the family's affective domain of functioning.

(continued)

TABLE 5–1. *(continued)*
FAMILY INTERVIEWING SKILLS FOR NURSES

Stage 3: Intervention *(continued)*

Perceptual/Conceptual Skills	Executive Skills
5. **Recognize that suggesting specific tasks can often provide a new way for family members to behave in relation to one another that will improve problem-solving abilities.** That is, some tasks can serve to begin changes in the structure of the family or family rules.	5. **Assign tasks aimed at improving family functioning.** That is, suggest that the father and son spend one evening a week together in a common activity; suggest to the mother and father that one parent discipline the children on odd days and the other on even days. This type of intervention targets the family's behavioral domain of functioning.

Stage 4: Termination

Perceptual/Conceptual Skills	Executive Skills
A. If consultation or referral is necessary: 1. **Recognize that families appreciate additional professional resources when problems are quite complex.** That is, nurses cannot be expected to have expertise in all areas.	1. **Refer individuals and/or family members for consultation or ongoing treatment.** For example, "I feel that your family needs professional input beyond what I can offer for Guillermo's learning disability problems. Therefore, I would like to refer you to the learning center in the city. They have more expertise in dealing with these types of problems."

(continued)

TABLE 5–1. *(continued)*
FAMILY INTERVIEWING SKILLS FOR NURSES

Stage 4: Termination *(continued)*

Perceptual/Conceptual Skills	Executive Skills

B. If family interviewing with nurse continues:

Perceptual/Conceptual Skills	Executive Skills
1. **Recognize the importance of evaluating the family interviews at regular intervals.** That is, evaluating the progress of family interviews leads to more focused and purposeful time spent with the family.	1. **Obtain feedback from family members about the present status of their problems and initiate termination when the contracted problems have been resolved or sufficient progress has been made.** Families do not lead problem-free lives. Rather, what is important is their feeling of confidence to cope with life's stresses.
2. **Recognize when dependency on the nurse inadvertently may have been encouraged.** That is, many interviews over a prolonged period can foster excessive dependency.	2. **Mobilize other supports for the family if necessary, and begin to initiate termination by decreasing the frequency of sessions.** For example, nurses can inadvertently provide "paid friendship" with mothers in particular unless they mobilize other supports such as husband, friends, or relatives.
3. **Recognize family members' constructive efforts to solve problems.** It is the family's perception of progress that is more significant than the nurse's perception.	3. **Summarize positive efforts of family members to resolve problems whether or not the nurse believes significant improvement has occurred.**
4. **Recognize that backup support by professional resources is appreciated by individuals and families in times of stress.**	4. **End the family interviews with a face-to-face discussion when possible. Extend an invitation for further family interviews if appropriate, should problems recur or if the family desires consultation.**

students regarding their attainment of clinical skills. One year after graduation, each student receives a questionnaire about his or her perceptions of clinical skills. Wright, Watson, and Bell (1990) described the results in 1989. Since then, the number of graduates has increased to 105. The results to date suggest that family systems nursing skills can be acquired with supervision and maintained in clinical practice, regardless of the employment opportunities for direct clinical contact with families. The most surprising finding has been the graduates' reports of a dramatic conceptual shift from a linear perspective to a more systemic "world view." The concepts identified as having the most impact on graduates' thinking are circularity and systems theory concepts, understanding the individual in the context of the family, the use of circular questions as interventions, and the reciprocal influence of illness and family functioning. Wright, Watson, and Bell (1990) suggest that the family, as the system of focus, becomes a vehicle for learning systemic concepts and skills that the MN graduates are then able to extrapolate to apply to a variety of other settings and situations.

The application of family nursing knowledge in a variety of clinical settings has also been noted by St. John and Rolls (1996). They found in their study of 118 graduates of an undergraduate program that 57% of the graduates indicated that they gathered data on clients and their families' health in their nursing practice "routinely." They saw family nursing as an important component of their practice, especially in assessing and planning care.

▮▮▮ CONCLUSIONS

These family interviewing skills function as a guide for the nurse when working with a family. Thus, beginning family nurse interviewers, through the use of these skills, will be able to engage a family, assess, explore, and identify strengths and problems, and make a decision to intervene or to refer the family. The nurse is also able to recognize the importance of the termination phase of therapeutic family interviewing. These stages of a family interview, with their accompanying skills, are another useful blueprint for nurses working with families. We strongly encourage nurses to tailor the use of these skills to the family's unique context. The skills are not *applied* to families. Rather, the nurse and family converse together and bring forth old and new stories of suffering, problems, resiliencies, strengths, competence, and problem resolution. The ethnicity, culture, class, sexual orientation, and race of the nurse and family members will influence their collaboration.

▓▓▓ REFERENCES

Alberta Association of Registered Nurses (AARN). (1991). *Nursing practice standards.* Edmonton, Alberta: Alberta Association of Registered Nurses.

Blow, A., & Piercy, F. P. (1997). Teaching personal agency in family therapy training programs. *Journal of Systemic Therapies, 16,*(3), 274–283.

Cecchin, G. (1987). Hypothesizing, circularity, and neutrality revisited: An invitation to curiosity. *Family Process, 26*(4), 405–413.

Chesla, C. A., Gilliss, C. L., & Leavitt, M. B. (1993). Preparing specialists in family nursing: The benefits of live supervision. In S. L. Feetham, S. B. Meister, J. M. Bell, & C. L. Gillis, (Eds.), *The nursing of families: Theory/ research/education/practice* (pp. 163–176). Newbury Park, CA: Sage.

Cleghorn, J. M., & Levin, S. (1973). Training family therapists by setting learning objectives. *American Journal of Orthopsychiatry, 43,* 439–446.

De Montigny, F., Dumas, L., Bolduc, L., & Blais, S.(1997). Teaching family nursing based on conceptual models of nursing. *Journal of Family Nursing, 3*(3), 267–279.

Falicov, C. J., Constantine, J. A., & Breunlin, D. C. (1981). Teaching family therapy: A program based on training objectives. *Journal of Marriage and Family Therapy, 7,* 497–505.

Figley, C. R., & Nelson, T. S. (1989). Basic family therapy skills, 1: Conceptualization and initial findings. *Journal of Marital and Family Therapy, 15*(4), 349–366.

Flemons, D. G., Green, S. K., & Rambo, A. H. (1996). Evaluating therapists' practices in a post-modern world: A discussion and a scheme. *Family Process, 35*(1), 43–56.

Freedman, J., & Combs, G. (1996). *Narrative therapy: The social construction of preferred realities.* New York: W. W. Norton Co.

Green, C. P. (1997) Teaching students how to "think family." *Journal of Family Nursing, 3*(3), 230–246.

Friedman, M.(1997). Teaching about and for family diversity in nursing. *Journal of Family Nursing, 3(3),* 280–294.

Gurman, A. S., & Kniskern, D. P. (1981). Family therapy outcome research: Knowns and unknowns. In A. S. Gurman & D. P. Kniskern (Eds.), *Handbook of family therapy* (pp. 742–776). New York: Brunner/Mazel.

Hanson, S., & Heims, M. L. (1992). Family nursing curricula in U. S. schools of nursing. *Journal of Nursing Education, 31*(7), 303–308.

Kniskern, D. P., & Gurman, A. S. (1979). Research on training in marriage and family therapy: Status, issues, and directions. *Journal of Marriage and Family Therapy, 5,* 83–94.

Leahey, M., & Harper Jaques, S. (1996). Family-nurse relationships: Core assumptions and clinical implications. *Journal of Family Nursing, 2*(2), 133–151.

Liddle, H. A. (1991). Training and supervision in family therapy: A comprehensive and critical analysis. In A. S. Gurman & D. P. Kniskern (Eds.), *Handbook of family therapy* (pp. 638–697). New York: Brunner/Mazel.

Selvini-Palazzoli, M., Boscolo, L., Cecchin, G., & Prata, G. (1978). *Paradox and counterparadox.* Northvale, NJ: Jason Aronson.

Selvini-Palazzoli, M., Boscolo, L., Cecchin, G., & Prata, G. (1980). Hypothesizing, circularity and neutrality: Three guidelines for the conductor of the session. *Family Process, 19,* 3–12.

St. John, W. & Rolls, C. (1996). Teaching family nursing: Strategies and experiences. *Journal of Advanced Nursing, 23,* 91–96.

Tapp, D.M. (1997). *Exploring therapeutic conversations between nurses and families experiencing ischemic heart disease.* Unpublished doctoral dissertation. University of Calgary, Alberta, Canada.

Tapp, D. M., & Wright, L. M. (1996). Live supervision and family systems nursing: Postmodern influences and dilemmas. *Journal of Psychiatric and Mental Health Nursing, 3,* 225–233.

Tapp, D. M., Moules, N. J., Bell, J. M., & Wright, L. M. (1997). Family skills labs: Facilitating the development of family nursing skills in the undergraduate curriculum. *Journal of Family Nursing, 3(3),* 247–266.

Tomm, K., & Wright, L. M. (1979). Training in family therapy: Perceptual, conceptual, and executive skills. *Family Process, 18,* 227–280.

Watson, W. L. (1992). Family therapy. In G. M. Bulechek & J. C. McCloskey (Eds.), *Nursing interventions: Essential nursing treatments* (2nd ed.) (pp. 379–391). Philadelphia: W. B. Saunders.

Wright, L. M. (1994). Live supervision: Developing therapeutic competence in family systems nursing. *Journal of Nursing Education, 33(7),* 325–327.

Wright, L. M., & Bell, J. M. (1989). A survey of family nursing education in Canadian Universities. *Canadian Journal of Nursing Research, 21,* 59–74.

Wright, L. M., Watson, W. L., & Bell, J. M. (1990). The Family Nursing Unit: A unique integration of research, education and clinical practice. In J. M. Bell, W. L. Watson, & L. M. Wright (Eds.), *The cutting edge of family nursing* (pp. 95–109). Calgary, Alberta: Family Nursing Unit Publications.

How to Prepare for Family Interviews

Nurses who work in various types of settings often ask, "How do I prepare for family interviews?" For some nurses, there are chance family meetings. For others, interviews are a planned event and may be initiated by either the family or the nurse. For both the nurse and the family, the first interview is often filled with anxiety.

It is our belief that the less anxious the nurse is, the more he or she invites confidence in family members, thereby reducing their anxiety. The purpose of this chapter is to help reduce the nurse's anxiety by discussing how to plan for the first and subsequent interviews. How to develop hypotheses is also addressed. Concrete issues are then presented, such as how to decide about the interview setting, who will be present, and telephone contact with the family. Ideas are also offered for the nurse to reflect on the type of relationship to be co-constructed with a family.

■ ■ ■ HYPOTHESIZING

Before meeting the family for the first time, the nurse should develop an idea of the purpose of the interview and an understanding of the family's context. For example, if the nurse is going to conduct the interview to understand how the family is coping with a chronic or life-threatening illness, it will be conducted differently from an interview is trying to assess family violence, abuse, or some other specified problem. In the latter example, either the family or some other agency has already identified the problem. If the family were in crisis, for example, having just received news of an untimely death, the context for the interview would be different than if the family were not experiencing a crisis. Another purpose for an interview could be for the nurse to discover the family members' desires about how they would like to be involved in the patient's home care or hospitalization. Depending on the purpose of the interview, the types of questions asked and the flow of the therapeutic conversation may be quite different.

In our clinical supervision with nurses, we have encouraged them to generate hypotheses related to the purpose of the meeting before the interview. Several authors have defined hypotheses. In one of their earliest works, Selvini, Boscolo, Cecchin, and Prata (1980) refer to a hypothesis as a formulation based on information that the clinician processes regarding the family to be interviewed. They believe that a hypothesis establishes a starting point for tracking relational patterns. Fleuridas, Nelson, and Rosenthal (1986) define hypotheses as "suppositions, hunches, maps, explanations, or alternative explanations about the family and the 'problem' in its relational context" (p. 115). For them, the purpose of a hypothesis is to connect family behaviors with meaning and guide the interviewer's use of questions. A hypothesis provides order for the interviewing process. It introduces a systemic view of the family and generates new views of relationships, beliefs, and behaviors. Tomm (1987) considers a hypothesis to be a "conceptual posture." This is an "enduring constellation of cognitive operations that maintains a stable point of reference which supports a particular pattern of thoughts and actions and implicitly inhibits or precludes others" (p. 7). He advocates that the interviewer adopt a posture or stance of hypothesizing to deliberately focus his or her cognitive resources in order to generate explanations. Preferably, the hypothesis should be circular rather than linear to maximize the therapeutic potential. Breunlin, Schwartz, and Karrer (1990) have defined hypothesizing as "the selection of a set of ideas drawn from one or more meta frameworks which organizes and makes understandable specific feedback offered by the system" (p. 10).

The essence of all these definitions of hypothesis is similar. A hypothesis is a tentative proposition or hunch that provides a basis for further exploration. For example, we know from stress theories (McCubbin & Figley, 1984) and from our own personal and professional experiences that the time of diagnosis of an illness is generally stressful, and often symptoms temporarily become worse (Cousins, 1979). Using this as a hypothesis, the nurse can arrange a family interview to discuss the impact of the diagnosis on the family, the family's response to the illness, and the family's expectations of the nurse. In this way, the nurse can explore family patterns of adjusting to the diagnosis and also the family members' ideas of the types of relationships they would like to have with healthcare providers. The hypothesis provides general direction for the nurse interviewer in exploring with this particular family their unique adjustment to a diagnosis.

The value of curiosity and naïveté for the nurse working especially with immigrant and marginalized populations cannot be overestimated. Cultural naïveté and respectful curiosity can be as significant as or more significant than knowledge and skill (Dyche & Zayas, 1995).

Cathryn Ladoux, whose son suffered with Duchenne's muscular dystrophy, reminded us of the importance of cultural context to hypothesizing (Patterson, 1997). She states:

> When a child in our tribe acquires a disability or a chronic illness, we believe that this child is here to remind us that something is out of balance with the universe. We must pay attention to all this child will teach us, for in this way, we will be guided to discover what we need to know to move toward balance (p. 237).

It is important for us to point out how our thinking about hypotheses has changed as we work toward operating within a postmodernist paradigm and shift from a modernist point of view. Our attention has shifted from what *we* think about what patients and families are telling us to trying to grasp what *they* think about what they are telling us. Weingarten (1998) offers a useful exercise that she and Roth developed to help clinicians notice this postmodern shift to what she calls "radical listening" and attending to the other. For example, a family is describing a clinical or personal situation. One nurse listens and notices what the family is saying. This nurse asks herself: What am I thinking about what the family is saying? What hypotheses do I have about this family in their situation? How am I organizing the information I am taking in? Do I see patterns here? What are they? Another nurse listens to the family describing a personal situation. This nurse asks herself: What is the family saying? What do I think *they* think about what *they* are saying? Weingarten (1998) states that the second interviewer generates hypotheses having to do with what the family might be thinking, feeling, or meaning. The first nurse listens more to her own thinking and follows a modernist tradition. The second nurse is more attuned to the family and her thinking is more consistent with a collaborative, respectful appreciation of the family's world view. Her hypothesis includes a consideration of the influence of the family's spirituality, ethnicity, class, race, gender, and other such diverse factors on the conversation.

We are quite drawn to the ideas expressed by Griffith (1995b), who asks: "How is it possible to make cultural distinctions about work done in the culture where one was born and raised?" (p. 3). She encourages us to listen to the family's talk of suffering, make space for their words and voices, and enter into the family's meaning to work with them to alleviate suffering.

HOW TO GENERATE HYPOTHESES

Hypotheses can be formulated from many bases. They can be based on information about the family gathered during hospital admission, during visiting hours, or from the other staff. The information may consist of opinions, observations of behavior or interactive patterns, and other data. In considering this information, we encourage nurses to ask themselves what they think the other staff thinks about what they are saying. Hypotheses can also be based on the nurse's previous experience and knowledge. This experience and knowledge can be about families with what the nurse believes may be similar ethnic, racial, or religious backgrounds. The nurse may recall similar problems, symptoms, or situations and similar interactive patterns noticed with previous patients and families. He or she may generate a hypothesis based on knowledge about family development and life cycle stages or another conceptual framework that he or she finds most relevant. We encourage nurses to include in their hypotheses ideas about a family's strong spirit, generosity of heart, devotion to one another, deep caring, and commitment. These are enduring qualities that families can draw upon in times of stress.

In addition to formulating hypotheses based on information about the family or previous experience and knowledge, nurses may develop hypotheses based on whatever is salient or relevant to them about the health problem or risk that is encountered at this particular time. For example, if there has been a recent tragedy in the immediate community, the nurse may find such information relevant in generating a hypothesis about what might be most meaningful for this particular family at this point.

We believe that it is important for nurses to state (to themselves) their hypotheses explicitly and consciously before the interview. We do not concur with those who state that hypotheses are unnecessary. Our belief is that a nurse cannot *not* hypothesize or think about a family before the interview. It is important for nurses to explicate their hunches so that these thoughts may be refined and made transparent as nurse and family engage in the interview process. Pre-session hypothesizing is viewed as a way to start focusing on the family, churning up the gray matter, making connections, and generating questions. It is not preparing an agenda for the session that is imposed on the family regardless of what the family members desire and despite changes that may have occurred since the last session (Wright, Watson, & Bell, 1996).

The guidelines for designing hypotheses in Box 6–1 have been adapted from the work of Fleuridas and collaborators (1986). We encourage nurses to generate hypotheses that are useful. We do not be-

BOX 6–1. GUIDELINES FOR GENERATING HYPOTHESES

- Choose hypotheses that are useful.
- Generate the most helpful explanations of the family's behaviors for this particular time.
- Understand that there are no "right" or "true" explanations.
- Include all participants in the "problem-organizing system" to make the hypothesis as systemic as possible.
- Relate the hypothesis to the family's presenting concerns so the interview can proceed along the lines most relevant to the family.
- Make the hypothesis different from the family's to introduce new information into the system and avoid being entrapped with the family in solutions that are not working.
- Be as quick to discard unconfirmed or unhelpful hypotheses as you are to generate new ones.

Adapted with permission from Fleuridas, C., Nelson, T., & Rosenthal, D. (1986). The evolution of circular questions: Training family therapists. *Journal of Marital and Family Therapy*, *12*(2), 113–127. Reprinted from Vol. 12, No. 2 of the *Journal of Marital and Family Therapy* Copyright 1986. American Association for Marriage and Family Therapy. Reprinted with permission.

lieve that there is one "correct" or "right" hypothesis. Rather, the goal is to generate useful explanations that lead to desired outcomes. We agree with Freedman and Combs (1996) that stories are authored through conversations. The story that is co-constructed between the nurse and the family is uniquely personal. We cannot know which hypotheses will fit for a particular family or where people's stories will go. We can only attune ourselves one piece at a time to the story as it unfolds.

We encourage nurses to design hypotheses that are circular rather than linear. That is, a hypothesis that includes all the components of the system (e.g., the family *and* the nurse) is most likely to be more circular than one that includes *either* the nurse *or* the family. The hypothesis should be related to the family's concerns. This is important because, as stated previously, a hypothesis guides the interview. For example, if the nurse develops a hypothesis that is unrelated to the family's concerns, he or she will ask questions that are irrelevant to the reason why the family came to the interview.

The nurse who is attuned to the family's concerns will listen for openings, through questions and reflective discussion, of problem-saturated stories and "unique outcomes." These outcomes or "sparkling events" would not have been predicted in light of the problem-saturated story. Griffith (1995a) reminds us that it is clinicians' certainty that can oppress and constrain opportunities to hear the patient's and family's story as they experience it.

We also encourage nurses to design a hypothesis that is different from the family's explanation or hypothesis. For example, a family may have the explanation that Puichun is a "bad daughter" who is shirking her responsibility by not caring for her elderly mother in her own home. The nurse, on the other hand, may develop an alternate hypothesis that fits the same data. The nurse's hypothesis might be that Puichun is overwhelmed by having to take care of her two preschool children while maintaining a full-time job. Thus, she is stretched to the limit in also trying to take responsibility for her elderly parent. Furthermore, Puichun's elderly mother may be sensitive to her stress and thus may be reluctant to live with her.

Once hypotheses have been designed, the nurse can use them to guide the interview. The nurse can ask questions of each member and note the responses to questions, thus confirming, altering, or rejecting a hypothesis. It is the small and the ordinary that we try to pay attention to in our conversation with families. We agree with the notion put forth by Sadler and Hulgus (1989) that the "starting point for hypotheses is arbitrary and intuitive within the bounds of scientific context and therapeutic goals, but hypotheses are *validated* by evidence and either confirmed, disconfirmed or modified" (p. 265). Hypothesizing and interviewing constitute a reciprocal cycle and are interdependent. The nurse develops a hypothesis, asks questions, converses with the family about the "problem" and its influence on their lives, and gathers evidence that confirms or does not confirm the nurse's hypothesis. Box 6–2 illustrates questions that invite hypothesizing about the system and the problem (Watson, 1992). As new information is generated, the nurse modifies the previous hypothesis and evolves a more useful one. The goal of the interview is to bring forth the family's resources to deal with the presenting issue. More information about how to conduct family interviews is provided in Chapters 7 and 8.

Leahey and Wright (1987) have given an example illustrating how alternative hypotheses can be generated before the first family meeting.

> A nurse working in an extended-care facility noted that the family, especially the 9- and 10-year-old children, avoided visiting their 41-year-old mother who had Huntington's disease, and that the patient's symptoms worsened around visiting days. The children seemed depressed and withdrawn every time they came to the nursing unit on their monthly visits. During case conferences, the staff wondered whether there might be a connection between the

BOX 6–2. QUESTIONS THAT INVITE HYPOTHESIZING ABOUT THE SYSTEM AND THE PROBLEM

Who

Who is in the system? Who are the key players?

Who first noticed the problem?

Who is concerned about the problem?

Who is affected by the problem? (most, least)

Who is interested in keeping things the same? (most, least)

Who referred the system?

What

What is the problem at this time?

What is the meaning that the problem has for the system and for different members of the system?

What solutions have been attempted?

What question(s) do I feel obliged to ask?

To what question could this symptom or problem be an answer?

What beliefs perpetuate the problem?

What beliefs are perpetuated by the problem?

What problems perpetuate the beliefs?

What problems are perpetuated by the beliefs?

Why

Why is the system presenting at this time?

Why is this problem found in this system?

Where

Where has the information about this problem come from?

Where does the system see the problem originating?

Where does the system see the problem and the system going if there is no change or if there is change?

When

When did the problem begin?

When did the problem occur in relation to another phenomenon of the system?

When does the problem occur?

When does the problem not occur?

How

How might a change in the problem affect other parts of the system (i.e., key players, relationships, beliefs)?

How does a change in one part of the system affect another part of the system or the problem?

How does the symptom maintain the system?

How does the system maintain the symptom?

How will I know when my work with this system is over?

How might my work with this system constrain the system from finding its solution?

Adapted with permission from Watson, W. L. (1992). Family therapy. In G. M. Bulechek & J. C. McCloskey (Eds.), *Nursing interventions: Essential nursing treatments* (2nd ed., pp. 379–391). Philadelphia: W. B. Saunders.

family's avoidance and the patient's flailing and head banging. They generated several hypotheses to explain why the family might be avoiding the patient and why the patient's symptoms seem to exacerbate around the time of the family visits.

One hypothesis pertained to the children's belief that head banging and flailing were controllable. Perhaps the children felt that their mother was not trying to control herself so she would not have to return home to care for them. This made them angry and they avoided her. An alternate hypothesis concerned the children's conflicting loyalties toward their mother and the aunt who took care of them. Perhaps they felt that if they visited too often, their aunt might think they did not appreciate her care. Thus they spaced out their visits and seemed depressed and withdrawn. They demonstrated both loyalty to their aunt and affection for their mother.

Yet a third hypothesis involved the children's fears of developing Huntington's disease themselves. They avoided visiting and showed sadness because of their own expectations of contracting the disease (p. 60).

Having generated several hypotheses about the family and the problem in its relational context, the nurse arranged a meeting with the family. The purpose of the interview was to clarify how the family members wanted to be involved with the patient and how the staff could be most helpful to them. The nurse's hypotheses were relevant to the purpose of the interview. She did not know if the frequency of the family visits was a "problem" for either the children or the patient. Rather, the staff had identified the problem. Thus, the nurse chose to frame the purpose of the meeting as one in which the staff wanted to know how they could be most helpful to both the family and the patient during the patient's hospitalization. The patient and family were partners in care with the staff rather than the family being the object of care.

▌▌▌ INTERVIEW SETTINGS

A family interview can take place anywhere: in the home (in the kitchen, in the living room, or in the patient's bedroom); in an institution (at the bedside, in the nurse's office, or in an unused treatment room); or in the community (in an interviewing room, in schools, in an office, or on the street where a homeless family "reside").

Depending on the purpose of the clinical interview, some settings are more conducive to therapeutic conversation than others. Nurses and families, therefore, need to consider the advantages and disadvantages of various settings. They should be flexible in choosing a setting that is appropriate for the specific purpose of the interview.

HOME SETTING

Many nurses interview families in their home setting. There are some concrete advantages to interviewing in the home. Infants, children of all ages, and very old people are able to be present more easily. Chances are increased for meeting significant but perhaps elusive family members such as boarders, adolescents, or grandparents. Firsthand acquaintance with the physical environment is also possible. For example, sleeping arrangements and family photographs can be seen. The nurse can also experience the family's social environment. That is, rituals of eating or who answers the doorbell can be noted.

In addition to the concrete advantages to interviewing in the home, there are also other advantages. These are particularly important if the nurse is of a different social class or ethnic background than the family. Articulate middle-class parents may report in the office or school only the most exemplary family interactions. The nurse may thus have difficulty understanding how the apparent competence of the parents and the banality of the reported parent-child incidents are in such sharp contrast to the degree of behavioral upset manifested by the child. Lower-class families sometimes have difficulty bridging the gap and explaining their situation to middle-class nurses who are unfamiliar with their home milieu. For example, a nurse suggests that an older woman prepare her husband several small meals a day rather than one very large meal, which he is unable to consume. The nurse did not know (and the family members were too embarrassed to mention) that they shared cooking facilities with other people in their apartment building. A home interview can thus give the nurse a clearer direction for therapeutic suggestions.

Disadvantages of using the home setting for family interviews include the increased administrative and personal cost involved in traveling. There is also the increased possibility of disruptions to the interview and the increased skill that the nurse requires to structure the interview flexibly. Nurses should also be aware that a family's home is their sanctuary. If family members are asked in their own home to share intense and deep emotions, they are often left without a retreat. For example, if there is an issue of abuse, the nurse should anticipate that the family's affective disclosure would be quite intense. Perhaps they will need more physical and psychological space to deal with the issues than their home permits. On the other hand, if the purpose of the interview is to facilitate shared grieving following the loss of a family member, the home setting might be ideal.

The nurse can tell the family that he or she would like to have an interview in the home "to get a better feel for the situation." Explain that, in your experience, there are frequently interruptions to an interview in the home (e.g., telephone calls, neighbors dropping in, or Jasmine wanting to put on the television). Ask, "How should we handle this if it comes up?" In this way, you have already set the stage for work and for a specific purpose to the interview rather than for visiting. One way to handle social offerings, such as coffee or a cold drink, is to say, "Thanks, but maybe we could work first and then have coffee afterward." The work and social boundaries are thus clearly identified. This boundary might be useful for some nurses working with certain ethnic groups. Having such a boundary might be offensive with families from other ethnic groups or from rural areas.

OFFICE, HOSPITAL, OR OTHER WORK SETTING

The greatest advantage of using the work setting for the interview is that this is the nurse's base. Therefore, the nurse can capitalize on an opportunity and adapt the setting to the needs of the interview. There may be fewer telephone calls or visitor interruptions. Furthermore, the nurse has a greater opportunity to obtain consultation from a colleague when interviewing the family in the work setting.

Disadvantages of interviewing in the work setting focus around issues of context. A family can be intimidated by the professional trappings (e.g., large institution, plush furniture, and complicated equipment) and therefore display anxiety or reluctance to talk. Frank (1991), a sociology professor who experienced cancer, described the reluctance he and his wife had about sharing information in the hospital setting because of the lack of privacy:

> One incident can stand for all the deals I made during treatment. During my chemotherapy I had to spend three-day periods as an inpatient, receiving continuous drugs. In the three weeks or so between treatments I was examined weekly in the day-care part of the cancer center. Day care is a large room filled with easy chairs where patients sit while they are given briefer intravenous chemotherapy than mine. There are also beds, closely spaced with curtains between. Everyone can see everyone else and hear most of what is being said. Hospitals, however, depend on a myth of privacy. As soon as a curtain is pulled, that space is defined as private, and the patient is expected to answer all questions, no matter how intimate. The first time we went to day care, a young nurse interviewed Cathie (my wife) and me to assess our "psychosocial" needs. In the middle of this medical bus station she began asking some reasonable questions. Were we experiencing difficulties at work because of my illness? Were we having any problems with our families? Were we getting support from them? These questions

were precisely what a caregiver should ask. The problem was *where* they were being asked.

Our response to most of these questions was to lie. Without even looking at each other, we both understood that whatever problems we were having, we were not going to talk about them there. Why? To figure out our best deal, we had to assess the kind of support we thought we could get in that setting from that nurse. Nothing she did convinced us that what she could offer was equal to what we would risk by telling her the truth (p. 68).

Suggestions for how beginning interviewers can maximize privacy in hospital settings are given later in this chapter.

Another disadvantage of using the institution for interviewing can be the inadvertent fostering of the belief that pathology resides in the individual—for example, "Mom's the sick one. We're only coming to help Mom get over her depression." This attitude is particularly evident if the mother has been hospitalized on a psychiatric ward. This disadvantage can be handled by using the family's willingness to "help Mom." The interviewer can reframe or discuss the mother's hospitalization in a positive light. "Perhaps your mother's hospitalization has provided the family with an opportunity to all work together in a new way."

How to Use the Work Setting

Some places have elaborate interviewing rooms, but most nurses have to make do with the usual hospital or clinic setting. Therefore, they may have to negotiate with co-workers for space and privacy. We recommend that you choose a private place where you will not be interrupted. For example, an unused patient room or an office is often more quiet than a four-bed room with curtains, a visitor's lounge, or a waiting area. Remove any important equipment (e.g., machines or monitors). The discussion area should ideally be sparsely furnished with movable chairs and no big desks, couches, or examining tables. This allows family members to control their own space, move closer or farther away from someone, and not worry about children touching hospital equipment. A few quiet toys, such as rubber or cloth hand puppets or paper and crayons, are useful to have readily available in the room. Books and magazines should not be available during the interview because they give a mixed message to the family. The participants are expected to discuss issues. They should not expect to read during the interview.

Acquaint yourself with the physical layout of the room before the session. This will probably increase your feelings of comfort when first meeting the family.

At the beginning of the interview, if there are children, you can say to the parents, "I'd like you to handle the children in whatever way you usually do. That will give me a better idea of what you're coping with at home." If the baby starts to cry, observe who comforts the baby. If the noise level gets beyond your tolerance, notice what tolerance level the family has. Unless absolutely necessary, try to avoid giving behavioral directives during the first interview (e.g., "Watch out for that plant" or "Don't touch Dad's chest tube"). Valuable information can be lost by imposing your standards of behavior unless it is required for safety. At the same time, it is necessary to structure the interview to avoid chaos.

At the end of the session, you can assess the influence of the work setting. Ask the family if their members behaved differently than they usually do. For example, "Did the children behave better or worse to-day than they usually do?" "Were people more or less talkative than usual?"

▪▪▪ WHO WILL BE PRESENT

The decision as to who will be present for the first and subsequent interviews is an important one. It is generally determined mutually by the family members and the nurse. In our early days of working with families, we thought it imperative that *all* family members be present for family interviewing. However, we have changed our thinking about this. We believe that a nurse can develop hypotheses, assess, and intervene with a system regardless of who is in the interviewing room. The number of people in the room does not reflect the unit of treatment. Rather, what is more important is how the nurse conceptualizes human suffering and problems.

We have found the work of Anderson, Goolishian, and Winderman (1986) to be very helpful in thinking about human problems. The treatment system for human problems is a language system, with boundaries marked by a linguistically shared problem. These particular language systems or "problem-determined systems" may be an individual, a couple, a family, a unit group, an organization, or any combination of people that communicates around a shared, articulated problem. "In this *problem-determined systems view*, human systems defined by social constructs (e.g., families), do not cause or make problems; communicatively shared problems mark and define the system. Social-political constructions, such as family, are constructs relevant to a particular description of human experience; they are not necessary to the definition of a treatment system" (Anderson et al. 1986, p. 7).

find the id a of "problem-determined systems" very helpful in ou linical pra e. The appropriat escriptio for the system of tre ment is the problem-determined system rather than the individ l, the coupl the family, or the rger system. People are under the influence of problems; they are not the problem. This notion allows us to avoid becoming mired in the concept of "dysfunctional" family, work group, and so forth. We do not find it useful to use the term "dysfunctional family." People in active communication regarding a problem are the problem-determined system. We do not believe that problem-determined systems are fixed. Rather, they are fluid, always changing, and never stable. We agree with Anderson and Goolishian (1988) that, as the problem definition changes, so does the membership of people involved in describing a problem. The goal of interviewing is the dissolving of the problem.

"The role of the [nurse] is simply to engage in conversation with those who are relevant to the problem resolution in such a way that there is a co-evolved new reality, a new language system, and therefore a c sipation of he problem or share belief that a problem exists" (Anderson et al. 1986, p. 10). Through therapeutic conversation, the nurse creates a context wherein the participants in a problem-determined system no longer distinguish what they are thinking and talking about as a "problem." The nurse knows that change has occurred when the concerned membership of a problem-determined system can think and talk of their shared problems differently.

Although we believe in problem-determined systems, we also believe that nurses who are beginning to interview families will generally find it easiest to invite everyone living in the household to be present for the first interview. In this way, the nurse can more easily elicit information from members who most likely have a description of the problem. Haley (1987) points out that to begin family work "by interviewing one person is to begin with a handicap" (p. 10). We believe that this is generally a useful notion for nurses to consider. If the problem concerns a couple, we usually try to have both spouses together for the first meeting. Similarly, if it is a parenting issue, the father, mother, and child are all invited to the meeting.

The more people present, the more information it is possible to gather and the more viewpoints and descriptions of the influence of the problem can be considered. Family members at the first intervie y might include the young children, the grandparent "who never ha nuch to say and the nephew "v o just moved in for the weekend." Sometimes the most significant thing that the nurse is able to ac mplish in a f mily interview is ju to bring the whole family toge r in one s t at one time to cuss an mportant issue. We agree with Carr (1997), who suggests that it is very useful, when deciding who to invite to the first meeting, to consider the network of professional resources involved with the family as well as the family members themselves.

Nurses frequently question whether they should include psychotic family members or those who are mentally or cognitively handicapped in the initial interview. Generally, the answer is yes. It will provide the nurse with an opportunity to talk with the family about the impact of the psychosis or mental handicap on the family. In addition, it will show the nurse how the family and individual interact to deal with the presenting problem. A clinical example may help to illustrate this point. A family requested help for their 6-year-old daughter, who was "regressing, having imaginary friends, and refusing to play with peers or go to school." During the initial interview, the little girl walked over to the door and turned the doorknob. The nurse asked her not to leave the room. In response, the family members said that she was not leaving but rather "was letting the cat out the door." The nurse looked a bit startled because there was no cat in the room. The nurse then asked the other children how they knew that this was what the little girl was doing and proceeded to inquire if this was how they usually responded to the child's behavior. Had the "psychotic child" not been present, the nurse would have been unaware of the siblings' contribution to the presenting problem.

We agree with Anderson (1997) that deciding who should be present for the first meeting is an important indicator of the collaborative nurse-family relationship. A conversational partnership is encouraged. It is important for the nurse to be aware of who is in relevant conversation with whom about the problem outside the interview room. Given the increased use of e-mail and other telecommunication devices, it is useful for nurses to inquire not just about the family contacts in the immediate vicinity but also those "on line." We must respect family members' ideas about *what* is germane to the conversation and *who* should be involved in it. Anderson (1997) recommends that all decisions about who should be involved in meetings, when, and what is talked about are determined collaboratively conversation by conversation.

▪▪▪ FIRST CONTACT WITH THE FAMILY

The way in which the nurse makes the first contact with the family conveys an important message to the parents and the children. By inviting each person in the household to the family meeting, the nurse implicitly states that each is a significant family member. Each individual has a role to p y in u derstanding describing, and dealir with he problem.

The rationale for br nging in the whole family can be explained in several ways. If a baby is n the intensive care nursery, the nurse might use the following explanation. "When a baby is in the intensive care nursery, we often find that family members are concerned and often anxious as well. Bringing family members in together results in more information for the whole family on how best to help the baby." Another idea would be for the nurse to say, "In the past, we kept fathers and family members out of the delivery room and out of the hospital wards. We've recognized in recent years how important it is to have family members present for special events such as the birth of a baby. Now we recognize that it is even more important for family members to be present when there is some type of illness. Family members know and care about each other. Often they have a lot to offer each other."

With families experiencing a crisis, such as the diagnosis of a stage 4 glioblastoma brain tumor in a previously healthy 62-year-old father, nurses may want to focus on providing physical information relating to the patient. Nurses can also see if the family is interested in hearing about services for families coping with sudden-onset life-threatening illness. They may state that in times of crisis families often find comfort in meeting with health professionals so that they can gain accurate, up-to-date patient information. Nurses are aware from their knowledge of crisis theory that the time frame for intervention is limited because crises are self-limiting. Assertiveness and a calm demeanor are generally useful attitudes for nurses to take with a family overwhelmed by a crisis.

Sometimes spouses agree to come for an interview but object to either having the children present or taking the children out of school. One way to handle the latter problem is to have interviews before school, during the lunch hour, after school, or in the evening. If this is not possible because of the nurse's work schedule, the nurse may say, "I understand your concern about the children missing school. In my experience, though, children have a tremendous amount to contribute to a family interview. They generally feel quite relieved when they see that the family is dealing with an issue about which they may have been worrying. Schools also are usually quite agreeable to children missing an hour."

HOW TO SET UP AN APPOINTMENT

Generally, the first telephone contact sets the stage for subsequent interviews. Our advice is to pay careful attention to this contact, whether you call the family to set up an appointment or a family member calls you. Napier refers to the family member on the telephone as "the family's scout" (1976, p. 4). This scout is in pioneer country and will carry important information to the other family members about the nurse and the nurse's intentions.

The purpose of the initial telephone contact with the family is to set up an appointment for an interview, explain the rationale for involving family members, and determine with the family who will be present at the interview. Naturally, both nurse and family gather much useful information about each other over the telephone. Telephone contact is therefore part of the development of a collaborative working relationship, and the nurse should treat it as such. Following is a sample first telephone contact:

Mother: Hello.

Nurse: Mrs. Lopez, this is Louise Watkins. I'm the community health nurse in your neighborhood.

Mother: Yes.

Nurse: I understand that you have a new baby. It's our practice to come out and visit all families with new babies.

Mother: Oh, I didn't know that.

Nurse: Yes, we usually do a physical examination of the baby and discuss feeding or other concerns.

Mother: Oh, that seems like a good idea. The doctor didn't tell me much about feeding.

Nurse: Sure, we can get into that during our visit. I was just calling to set up a time that would be convenient for your family and for me. I would like to see the whole family because usually when a new baby arrives, the child has a great impact, not just on the mother but on the father and other children as well.

Mother: You can say that again! My 2-year-old usually seems to like his baby sister, but last night I saw him pinch her.

Nurse: Yes, these are the kind of things that we can discuss when the whole family and I get together. The meeting will probably take about an hour. I have some time available on Tuesday at 10 or on Thursday at 3. Which would be best for you, your husband, and the children?

Mother: Tuesday isn't good because my son is going to the doctor that day. Thursday would be better since my husband works shifts and gets off at 2:30.

Nurse: Would a 3:00 appointment give him enough time to get home, or should we make the appointment at 3:15?

Mother: Yes, 3:15 would be better.

Nurse: I look forward to seeing you and the whole family then.

Mother: Yes, me too.

Nurse: Goodbye.

Mother: 'Bye.

In the above selection, the nurse was clear, confident, focused, and accommodating. The nurse set forth the purpose of the interview and who she thought would be useful to be involved. She invited the family to a "meeting" by stating that this is the agency's usual practice. Whether the nurse refers to her collaborative time with a family as a "meeting" or an "interview" is arbitrary. But it's most important that the nurse use the most palatable language with families based on the context in which she encounters families. The nurse took charge by identifying and introducing herself without apologies and offered specific appointment times. Furthermore, the nurse also received much information that can be useful in the family meeting:

"The doctor didn't tell me much about feeding."

"I saw [the 2-year-old] pinch her."

"My son is going to the doctor . . ."

". . . my husband works shifts . . ."

It is not possible to provide written guidelines to cover all the various situations that nurses will encounter in trying to set up a family interview. Each family presents different challenges for the nurse; in addition, each nurse presents different challenges for families. Therefore, each interview must be approached with flexibility. A unique approach is always the rule in clinical practice. Each telephone contact demands a slightly different plan of action to invite family members to an interview or to elicit the family's permission for a home visit. We strongly encourage community health nurses especially to plan their telephone calls and appointments to maximize efficiency and the possibility of developing a collaborative partnership with the family.

▪ ▪ ▪ RESISTANCE AND NONCOMPLIANCE

Often in our clinical supervision with nurses, we have been asked how to deal with resistant or noncompliant families. When nurses ask this, they are generally referring to families whom they perceive as oppositional or not complying with ideas and advice that could promote, maintain, or restore health. The family is designated as "noncompliant" when they do not respond to particular nursing interventions; nurses interpret this behavior as unwillingness or a lack of readiness to change (Wright & Levac, 1992).

We do not use the terms *resistance* or *noncompliance* anymore, as we have not found them clinically useful. Resistance was initially used to describe a client's reluctance to uncover or recover from some anxiety-filled experience. The clinician's job was often to uncover this material, but when this area of the client's life was touched on, the client was seen to resist the interviewer's effort. Resistance is still generally seen as "located" in the client and is often described as something the client "does." This is a linear view that implies that problems with adherence to treatment regimens reside within individuals and families, not in the interactions or relationships between individuals (Anderson & Stewart, 1982; Wright & Levac, 1992). We disagree with this view because we see the idea of resistance as a *product* of client-interviewer interaction. We believe that resistance and noncompliance are not terms describing a unilateral phenomenon but rather an interactional phenomenon.

Rather than using *resistance* or *noncompliance*, we have found the multidirectional terms *cooperation* and *collaboration* to be very useful clinically. When nurses think of how they work collaboratively with families, they are less likely to impose their will on the family. They tend to open space for the family and to be more tentative and receptive to the family's point of view.

The theory behind the "death of resistance" (de Shazer, 1984) has emerged since the first edition of this book. There has been a dramatic increase in a solution-focused orientation to interviewing (Lipchik & de Shazer, 1986; de Shazer, 1991). With the emphasis on a solution comes an increasing emphasis on change, cooperation, and collaboration. Another orientation that we have embraced is the narrative approach developed by White and Epston (1990) and more recently advanced by Freedman and Combs (1996), Anderson (1997) and other postmodernists. These approaches provide far more positive direction for our work than the negative labels of resistance or noncompliance, which previously left us stymied in our clinical practice. They open us to reflect on conversation, language, and possibilities rather than pathologizing labels.

HOW TO DEAL WITH A HESITANT FAMILY

There are several possible reasons why one spouse may be hesitant to attend the family session. Each requires a different approach on the part of the nurse. Following are a few common situations that interviewers encounter.

1. "My husband would never come to a family interview. He thinks that my mother's stroke and how to handle it are my responsibility."

Ask what the wife thinks about her husband attending the interview. If she believes her mother's chronic illness is *her* responsibility and has very little to do with her husband, she will not be interested in inviting her husband to a family interview. You would need to engage in conversation with the wife to see if she wants to alter *her* cognitive set *before* you start talking to her about her husband.

2. "My husband wouldn't want to come to a family interview. Besides, I wouldn't know how to get him there."

If the wife would like her husband to attend but does not know how to invite him, you can explore with her why she feels her husband might be hesitant. There could be several reasons:

- He may view the problem as his wife's, not his own.
- The timing of the interview might be inconvenient.
- The thought of going to a hospital might be repugnant ("seeing all those sick people").
- He may be afraid of being blamed for not taking a more active role in his mother-in-law's care.

You can ask the wife if she thinks any of these feelings or thoughts might be stopping her husband from becoming involved. After she has speculated on the reasons for her husband's hesitance and her own desire for him to be present, you can discuss with her some alternate ways to engage him:

- She can discuss with her husband how *she needs his help* to deal with her mother's illness.
- She can find out convenient times for her husband to come to a half-hour interview.
- She can tell him exactly where the interview will be held, for example, not in the patient's room but rather in an office.
- She can tell him that *you are most hesitant* to see only parts of the family for an interview. That is, if you saw only the wife with her mother, there could be a danger that the husband would feel left out and perhaps blamed. If he were present, however, this could not happen. He could help you to understand more fully the relationship between his wife and her mother. She can let him know that he has a unique view of the family—a view that only he can provide. Most

husbands do not like to be left out of the original planning and decision making. Once they have a fuller understanding of the purpose of a family interview, they are often quite agreeable to attending.

When nurse-interviewers ask that the husband attend, although it may involve a little persuasion, and state that they need him to be there, they will have few problems with absent husbands. Conversely, nurses are likely to have difficulties in this area if they are timid or inconsistent in requesting the husband's presence.

Another idea for inviting an anxious or threatened family member to an interview is to suggest that the person be asked to be present as an observer, just to see what is happening. Also, the person can come whenever he or she is "in the mood" as a historian, an accuracy checker, or a consultant. If these suggestions are followed, it is important to ask the "observer" or "historian" to react at the *end* of the interview to what the family has discussed in the session. Gradually, as the family member continues to observe sessions, he or she often becomes more comfortable and is willing to participate *during* the interview. This may be a particularly useful way of engaging some adolescents. The idea of telling the member "not to talk" places no direct pressure on that member to participate. Silent members are often closely attuned to the process, and when a sensitive area is broached, they forget their defensive stance and join in the process. Other times, they may remain silent but hear the information.

HOW TO DEAL WITH FAMILY
NONENGAGEMENT AND REFERRAL SOURCES

If you have difficulty engaging the family on the telephone, you may need to contact the referral source. That is, physicians frequently tell a patient on discharge, "The nurse will be out to check up on you and see how you are doing." When you contact the patient, the patient may have forgotten what the physician said, or may be confused about the purpose of the visit, or simply may not be interested in being "checked up on." Sometimes in situations of suspected child abuse, the physician may contact the nurse and ask him or her to "drop in on the family just to see if there is any abuse." You may then find yourself in an awkward situation, trying to explain the purpose of your visit to a family who may be reluctant to have you come. One way to approach this is to say: "Doctor Fishkin asked me to set up a visit with your family to discuss things about raising children. Dr. Fishkin feels that most families who have infants and preschoolers as close together as yours sometimes find it helpful to talk to the nurse." You have clearly indicated that it is on Dr. Fishkin's request that you are calling and you have attempted to normalize the purpose of the interview. If, however, the family is still reluctant to have you visit, initiate contact with the physician and have the physician set the stage for future work with the family. You should not consider this inability to engage a family "your fault" or the fault of the family's resistance, but rather as a problem of inadequate preparation by the referral source.

Several other ideas have emerged over the past few years about dealing with referral sources. Colapinto (1988) advises interviewers to avoid focusing prematurely on family dynamics if the request for the interview comes from another agency or if the interview is compulsory. He suggests that treatment failure often ensues because of powerful conflict between the family and the referral source. We have also found this in our own clinical work. In such situations, we recommend that the nurse engage with the family and conceptualize their work together as collaboration to deal not with family issues per se but rather with dynamics between the family and the agency. In this way, the interviewer can join with the family around a problem such as "that school is always making trouble for us." Thus the focus of the nurse's work would not be on family dynamics but on work with the family to "get the school off their case."

Selvini (1985) also has talked about the problem of the sibling as the referring person. She advocates that special attention be paid to the influence of this person (generally a "most competent and prestigious family member") on the nurse-family contract. Gesuelle-Hart, Kaplan, and Kikoski (1990) have recommended that the interviewer identify and grapple with the expectations of the person referring the "problem family" for assessment. They suggest some useful questions to ask:

- Why is this referral being made to me at this time?
- What is the relationship between the referral source and my agency?
- Who is paying, for whom, for what?
- What are the expectations of the hierarchy within which I work?
- If the referral source is unhappy with the assessment, who will hear about it?
- If I am unhappy about the assessment process, who will hear about it? (p. 2)

In any situation in which there is nonengagement, it is important to realize that the reluctance is important information about the dynamics between the interviewer and the family. The hypothesized reason why a person is not present should be explored at the first interview. For example, we were once asked to consult with the family members of a 59-year-old woman who was terminally ill with cancer. The hospital staff nurse arranged the interview for a time convenient for the husband and adult daughter. Only the daughter and the mother, however, showed up for the interview. In exploring the reasons why the husband did not attend, we discovered that he was 73 years old and in poor health himself, a fact unknown to the hospital staff. In asking the adult daughter about the impact of her mother's illness, we also discovered information about the father's absence. The daughter wept openly about her mother's impending death. She then stated, "If you think I'm a basket case, you should see my father. He's in worse shape than I am." Thus, in this situation, the husband's absence from the interview provided important information about the family's emotional state. It is important for nurses to understand reluctance as a systems phenomenon rather than an individual issue. We hypothesized in this case not only that the father was reluctant to attend but that the adult daughter was trying to protect him.

■■■ REFLECTIONS ON THE NURSE-FAMILY RELATIONSHIP

Since the first edition of this book, there has been a steady increase in the attention paid to the "therapeutic conversation," meaning the therapist acting with, rather than on, patients. Bird (1993) has advocated self-reflection in relation to dominant societal ideas and practices, intimate relationships past and present, the client-therapist relationship, gender, sexual thoughts, and strong feelings. We believe that nurses cannot avoid their influence on families. We agree with Cecchin, Lane, and Ray (1994) that nurses and families inevitably influence each other, but not always with predictable results. We share their concern, not about influencing or not influencing, but about understanding the quality and nature of the relationship.

We believe that families and nurses each have their own healthcare system. Families provide diagnosis, advice, remedies, and support to their members in both sickness and health. They have constraining and facilitating beliefs (Wright, Watson, & Bell, 1996). Nurses also have their own constraining and facilitating beliefs, theories, and remedies that they share with families. Leahey and Harper-Jaques (1996) have outlined five assumptions relating to the family-nurse relationship and the clinical implications of each assumption. Emphasis is on *both* the nurse's *and* the family's contribution to establishing and maintaining the relationship. We believe that it is useful for a nurse to reflect on his or her potential contribution to the relationship *before* meeting with a family. It is also helpful for the nurse to reflect with the family about their working relationship at the end of their contract. More ideas on this topic are provided in Chapter 10.

The five assumptions related to the family-nurse relationship are as follows:

Assumption 1: The family-nurse relationship is characterized by reciprocity. The family and nurse are connected in a pattern that is quite distinct from the positivist-based idea of two separate components, either family or nurse. It is the "fit" between the family and the nurse that is important to foster a collaborative partnership. If the nurse wishes to foster a reciprocal relationship, he or she can reflect on the sample questions in Box 6–3.

Assumption 2: The family-nurse relationship is nonhierarchical. Each person's contribution is sought, acknowledged, and valued. Conversation is a co-construction of ideas and mutual discoveries. Both the nurse and the family are aware, however, that they are bound by moral, legal, and ethical norms. Box 6–4 contains some sample questions that nurses can ask themselves and the family about hierarchy.

Assumption 3: Nurses and families each have specialized expertise in maintaining health and managing health problems. Families who live with chronic conditions develop expertise in managing symptoms, adapting their environments, and adjusting their lifestyles. When they

---

BOX 6–3. QUESTIONS ABOUT RECIPROCITY

For the nurse's self-reflection:
  To what extent did I:
• Elicit the patient's and family members' expectations, hopes, questions, and ideas?
• Consider the patient's and family members' expectations, knowledge, experience, and desires when planning nursing care?
• Communicate information, ideas, and recommendations to patients and families on a regular basis?
• Involve the patient and family to their satisfaction in making decisions for the overall treatment plan?
To ask the family when evaluating care:
  To what extent do you feel that:
• I heard your opinions and ideas?
• I was available and approachable to answer your questions?
• I showed interest in your ideas and experience with illness?

From Leahey, M., & Harper-Jaques, S. (1996). Family-nurse relationships: Core assumptions and clinical implications. *Journal of Family Nursing, 2*(2), pp. 133–151, copyright © 1996 by M. Leahey and S. Harper-Jaques. Reprinted by permission of Sage Publications, Inc.

BOX 6–4. QUESTIONS ABOUT HIERARCHY

For the nurse's self-reflection:
- To what extent am I imposing my beliefs on the family? Allowing the family to impose their beliefs upon me?
- How well do the expectations between the family and myself match?
- When there is a mismatch, whose opinion usually predominates?
- How frequently are decisions about the patient's healthcare made mutually by the patient, family, and myself?

To ask the family when evaluating care:
- Overall, what percentage of time were decisions about your health-care made in a mutual way between you and me?
- To what extent did I help you feel more in control of your health?

From Leahey, M., & Harper-Jaques, S. (1996). Family-nurse relationships: Core assumptions and clinical implications. *Journal of Family Nursing, 2*(2), pp. 133–151, copyright © 1996 by M. Leahey and S. Harper-Jaques. Reprinted by permission of Sage Publications, Inc.

meet with the nurse, they bring a wealth of information and personal expertise to the encounter. Nurses, through their education and experience, also bring expertise to the relationship with the family. Nurses can think about their own and the family's expertise as they prepare to meet with a family to discuss managing a particular health problem. Box 6–5 provides sample questions that the nurse can consider.

Assumption 4: Nurses and families each bring strengths and resources to the family-nurse relationship. Nurses who use a resource-identification lens will strive to draw forth the family's cultural, ethnic, spiritual, and other beliefs that have been helpful in dealing with the health problem. Nurses also have their own life experience, clinical intuition, and educational background available to bring to the relationship. Box 6–6 offers sample questions that nurses could ask themselves about how they would like the relationship with the family to be focused on strengths.

Assumption 5: Feedback processes can occur simultaneously at several different relationship levels. Nurses have often focused on family dynamics and interactional patterns within family systems. More recently, they have begun to address family-nurse relationships and reflect on their own patterns with families. Rarely do nurses address the interactive patterns that can simultaneously occur at different relational levels. Box 6–7 offers sample questions that the nurse can consider about the family-nurse relationship.

BOX 6–5. QUESTIONS ABOUT EXPERTISE

For the nurse's self reflection:
- What do I know about the family's ideas and plans for care during this course of treatment?
- What can I learn from this family about their experiences in living with this health problem?
- What knowledge and expertise do I have to offer this family?
- How does this family demonstrate its trust in my expertise?
- Who in the family has the most expertise in getting grandpa to take his medications?

To ask the family:
- What are the things that you or other family members do to help you to relieve the pain?
- What ways have you found most useful to invite your father to take care of his own personal needs?

BOX 6–6. QUESTIONS ABOUT STRENGTHS

For the nurse's self-reflection:
- Do my actions and comments acknowledge the strengths and abilities of this family?
- What interventions can I use to further enhance this family's strengths?
- How am I inviting this family to trust my knowledge and skill in helping them with this health problem?
- What are the strengths that I bring to this relationship?

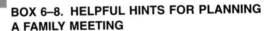

BOX 6–7. QUESTIONS ABOUT THE FAMILY-NURSE RELATIONSHIP

For the nurse's self-reflection:
To what extent did my relationship with the patient and family help to:
- Increase their knowledge? Insight? Coping?
- Improve or enhance their emotional well-being?
- Improve the patient's physical health?
- Build stronger relationships between the patient and family members?

To ask the family when evaluating care:
To what extent did our meetings together:
- Meet your needs?
- Contribute to your having an increased sense of confidence in living with your illness?

From Leahey, M., & Harper-Jaques, S. (1996). Family-nurse relationships: Core assumptions and clinical implications. *Journal of Family Nursing, 2*(2), pp. 133–151, copyright © 1996 by M. Leahey and S. Harper-Jaques. Reprinted by permission of Sage Publications, Inc.

BOX 6–8. HELPFUL HINTS FOR PLANNING A FAMILY MEETING

Before initiating a family meeting, the nurse needs to:
- Ascertain the purpose and benefit of a family meeting from the family's perspective.
- Explain why a family meeting may be beneficial to the family.
- Determine who in the family agrees that a problem exists and who might be willing to come to a family meeting.
- Mutually determine with the family when and where a meeting could take place (home, office, school).
- Begin to formulate hypotheses (hunches about connections between the family system and the particular problem).
- Read literature about working with families experiencing similar health problems to better understand the issues and concerns of that specific population.
- Prepare linear and circular questions that will draw forth relevant data about family structure, development, and function. (See the discussions of CFAM in Chap. 3 and CFIM in Chap. 4 for examples of questions).

Adapted with permission from Levac, A. C., Wright, L. M., & Leahey, M. (1997). Children and families: Models for assessment and intervention. In J. Fox (Ed.), *Primary health care of children.* St. Louis: Mosby, p. 4.

■■■ **CONCLUSIONS**

In preparing for family interviews, it is important for nurses first to remind themselves of the purpose of the meeting and then to generate hypotheses related to this purpose. Box 6–8 outlines areas for nurses to consider in preparing for family interviews. Decisions about the interview setting and who will be present flow from ideas about who has a description of the problem and who is a customer for change. These ideas are the result of a collaborative partnership between the nurse and the family.

■■■ **REFERENCES**

Anderson, H. (1997). *Conversation, language, and possibilities: A postmodern approach to therapy.* New York: Harper Collins Publishers, Inc.

Anderson, H., & Goolishian, H. (1988). Human systems as linguistic systems: Preliminary and evolving ideas about the implications for clinical theory. *Family Process, 27*(4), 371–394.

Anderson, H., & Goolishian, H., & Winderman, L. (1986). Beyond family therapy. *Journal of Strategic and Systemic Therapies, 5*(4), 1–13.

Anderson, C., & Stewart, S. (1983). *Mastering resistance.* New York: Guilford Press.

Bird, J. (1993). Coming out of the closet: Illuminating the therapeutic relationship. *Journal of Feminist Family Therapy, 5*(2), 47–64.

Breunlin, D., Schwartz, R., & Karrer, B. (1990). The "metaframeworks" perspective in action. *Family Therapy Case Studies, 5*(2), 9–30.

Carr, A.. (1997). Positive practice in family therapy. *Journal of Marital and Family Therapy, 23*,(3), 271–293.

Cecchin, G., Lane, G., & Ray, W. (1994). Influence, effect, and emerging systems. *Journal of Systemic Therapies, 13*(4), 13–21.

Colapinto, J. (1988). Avoiding a common pitfall in compulsory school referrals. *Journal of Marital and Family Therapy, 14*(1), 89–96.

Cousins, N. (1979). *Anatomy of an illness as perceived by the patient.* New York: Bantam Books.

de Shazer, S. (1984). The death of resistance. *Family Process, 23*(1), 11–16.

de Shazer, S. (1991). *Putting difference to work.* New York: W. W. Norton.

Dyche, L., & Zayas, L. H. (1995). The value of curiosity and naivete for the cross-cultural therapist. *Family Process, 34*(4), 389–399.

Fleuridas, C., Nelson, T., & Rosenthal, D. (1986). The evolution of circular questions: Training family therapists. *Journal of Marital and Family Therapy, 12*(2), 113–127.

Frank, A. (1991). *At the will of the body: Reflections on illness.* Boston: Houghton Mifflin.

Freedman, J., & Combs, G. (1996). *Narrative therapy: The social construction of preferred realities.* New York: W. W. Norton & Co.

Gesuelle-Hart, S., Kaplan, L., & Kikoski, C. (1990). Assessing the family in context. *Journal of Strategic and Systemic Therapies, 9*(3), 1–13.

Griffith, M. E. (1995a). Opening therapy to conversations with a personal God. *Journal of Feminist Family Therapy, 7*(1/2), 123–139).

Griffith, M. E. (1995b). Stories of the South, stories of suffering, stories of God. *Family Systems Medicine,13*(1), 3–9.

Haley, J. (1987). *Problem-solving therapy.* San Francisco: Jossey-Bass.

Leahey, M., & Harper-Jaques, S. (1996). Family-nurse relationships: Core assumptions and clinical implications. *Journal of Family Nursing, 2*(2), 133–151.

Leahey, M., & Wright, L. M. (1987). Families and chronic illness: Assumptions, assessment and intervention. In L. M. Wright & M. Leahey (Eds.), *Families and chronic illness* (pp. 55–76). Springhouse, PA: Springhouse.

Levac, A. C. , Wright, L. M., & Leahey, M. (1997). Children and families: Models for assessment and intervention. In J. Fox (Ed.) *Primary health care of children.* St. Louis: Mosby, pp. 3–13.

Lipchik, E., & de Shazer, S. (1986). The purposeful interview. *Journal of Strategic and Systemic Therapies, 5*(1), 88–99.

McCubbin, H., & Figley, C. (Eds). (1984). *Stress and the family: Vol. 2. Coping with catastrophic stress.* New York: Brunner/Mazel.

Napier, A. (1976). Beginning struggles with families. *Journal of Marriage and Family Counseling, 2,* 3–12.

Patterson, J. M.(1997). Meeting the needs of Native American families and their children with chronic health conditions. *Families, Systems and Health, 15*(3), 237–241.

Sadler, J., & Hulgus, Y. (1989). Hypothesizing and evidence-gathering: The nexus of understanding. *Family Process, 28*(3), 255–268.

Selvini, M. (1985). The problem of the sibling as the referring person. *Journal of Marital and Family Therapy, 11*(1), 21–34.

Selvini, M., Boscolo L., Cecchin, G., & Prata, G. (1980). Hypothesizing—circularity—neutrality: Three guidelines for the conductor of the session. *Family Process, 19*(1), 3–12.

Tomm, K. (1987). Interventive interviewing: 1. Strategizing as a fourth guideline for the therapist. *Family Process, 26*(1), 3–14.

Watson, W. L. (1992). Family therapy. In G. M. Bulechek & J. C. McCloskey (Eds.), *Nursing interventions: Essential nursing treatments* (2nd ed.) (pp. 379–391). Philadelphia: W. B. Saunders.

Weingarten, K. (1998). The small and the ordinary: The daily practice of a postmodern narrative therapy. *Family Process, 37*(1), 3–16.

White, M., & Epston, D. (1990). *Narrative means to therapeutic ends.* New York: W.W. Norton.

Wright, L. M., & Levac, A. M. (1992). The non-existence of non-compliant families: The influence of Humberto Maturana. *Journal of Advanced Nursing, 17,* 913–917.

Wright, L. M., Watson, W. L., & Bell, J. M. (1996). *The heart of healing in families and illness.* New York: Basic Books.

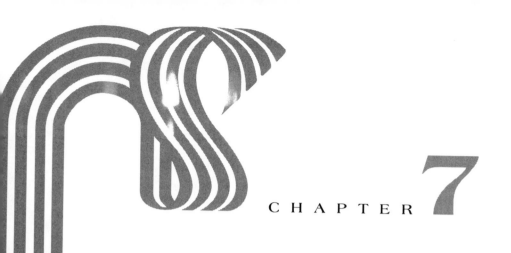

CHAPTER **7**

How to Conduct Family Interviews

Once the nurse and a family have decided to meet for an interview, the nurse can consider how to conduct the meeting. Just as there are stages in the whole interviewing process, there are also stages in initial interviews. An awareness of these stages provides the nurse with a general interview structure and can help to allay the nurse's anxiety.

In this chapter, we present guidelines for each stage of an initial interview. After this, we address the stages involved in the entire interviewing process.

▪▪▪ GUIDELINES FOR FAMILY INTERVIEWS

The following stages generally occur in initial interviews:

1. *Engagement stage,* in which the family is greeted and made comfortable.
2. *Assessment stage*
   a. **Problem identification,** in which the nurse explores the family's presenting concerns
   b. **Relationship between family interactions and health problem,** in which the nurse explores the family's typical responses to the health problem
   c. **Attempted solutions,** in which the family and nurse talk with each other about solutions and their effect on the presenting issues
   d. **Goal exploration,** in which the nurse draws together the information and the family specifies what goals, changes, or outcomes they are seeking
3. *Intervention stage,* in which the nurse and family collaborate on areas for change
4. *Termination stage,* in which the nurse and family end the interview

ENGAGEMENT STAGE

During the engagement, or first stage of the interview, the nurse and family begin to establish a therapeutic relationship. Engagement has

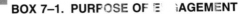

BOX 7–1. PURPOSE OF ENGAGEMENT

- To promote a positive nurse-family relationship by developing an atmosphere of comfort, mutual trust, and cooperation between the practitioner and the family
- To recognize that the family members bring strengths and resources to this relationship that may have previously gone unnoticed by healthcare professionals
- To prevent potential practitioner-family misunderstandings or problems later on in the therapeutic relationship

Adapted from Levac, A. C., Wright, L. M., & Leahey, M. (1997). Children and families: Models for assessment and intervention. In J. Fox (Ed.), *Primary health care of children*. St. Louis: Mosby (p. 4). Reprinted by permission.

several purposes. These are outlined in Box 7–1. The goal in this stage is for the family members and the nurse to develop a mutual alliance. In the beginning, the nurse is often perceived as a stranger, unknown and potentially helpful or not helpful. Because family members do not know what to expect from the nurse, he or she must establish a relationship with the members by demonstrating understanding, competence, and caring.

We encourage nurses to consider the type of relationship that they would like to establish with families over the course of time. Thorne and Robinson (1989) have described various stages of the evolution of relationships between families experiencing chronic illness and their healthcare professionals: "naïve trust," "disenchantment," and "guarded alliance." They propose that naïve trust among the chronically ill, their families, and healthcare providers is inevitably shattered in the face of unmet expectations and conflicting perspectives. Anxiety, frustration, and confusion often result in disenchantment. Trust can then be reconstructed on a more guarded basis so that the chronically ill patient, the family, and the nurse can continue to engage in healthcare activities. Thorne and Robinson (1989) state that this reconstructed trust is highly selective and is based on revised expectations of the roles of both patient and provider. They suggest that there are four relationship types in guarded alliance: "hero worship," "resignation," "consumerism," and "team playing." In hero worship and team playing, the trust dimension is high, whereas in resignation and consumerism, it is low. Both team playing and consumerism value competence highly, whereas hero worship and resignation put a low

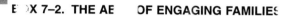

BOX 7–2. THE ABC OF ENGAGING FAMILIES

A	B	C
Assume an active, confident approach.	Begin by providing structure for the meeting (time frame, orientation to the context).	Create a context of mutual trust.
Ask purposeful questions that draw forth family assessment data.	Behave in a curious manner and take an equal interest in all family members.	Clarify expectations about your role with the family.
Acknowledge the importance of all family members perceived as significant, whether present or not.	Build on family strengths by offering commendations to the family.	Collaborate in decision making, health promotion, and health management.
Address all who are present, including small children.	Bring relevant resources to the meeting (list of agencies, phone numbers, pamphlets).	Cultivate a context of racial and ethnic sensitivity.

Adapted from Levac, A. C., Wright, L. M., & Leahey, M. (1997). Children and families: Models for assessment and intervention. In J. Fox (Ed.). *Primary health care of children.* St. Louis: Mosby, p. 5, with permission.

value on competence. Important ABC's for the engagement of families with children are provided in Box 7–2.

Reciprocal trust is a very critical dimension to consider during the engagement phase of family interviewing. The nurse helps the patient and family to feel more confident in their own competence in managing illness. To develop a high degree of trust in the nurse, the patient and family are encouraged to explicitly state their expectations for healthcare. The nurse provides the opportunity for family members to express their desires. If the patient and family are to have a high degree of trust in their own competence, their own resources must be acknowledged by family members and healthcare providers. We agree with Griffith (1995) that there is no completely open conversational space. We have found her ideas helpful in continuing to move from a stance of certainty to wonder. She outlines four "certainties" that constrain opportunities to hear the family's story as they experience it. Although she applies these to religion, we have used them in our teaching and continually try to apply them when talking with families experiencing chronic or life-threatening illness.

1. **Constraint:** I know what God is like for you because I know your religious denomination.
2. **Constraint:** I know what God is like for you because I know what your language about God means.
3. **Constraint:** I know what God is like for you because your image of God is a reflection of your early attachment figures.
4. **Constraint:** I know what God is like and you need to know God as I do.

One way of reminding ourselves not to fall into the trap of certainty and expertness on the family's situation has been to develop a strong sense of curiosity. When initiating engagement, we assume a position of neutrality or curiosity. Cecchin (1987) draws connections between neutrality or curiosity and hypothesizing. He maintains that curiosity is a delight in the invention and discovery of multiple patterns. "Curiosity helps us to continue looking for different descriptions and explanations, even when we cannot immediately imagine the possibility of another one . . . hypothesizing is connected to curiosity. Hypothesizing has more to do with technique. Curiosity is a stance, whereas hypothesizing is what we do to try to maintain this stance" (p. 411). We believe that curiosity nurtures circularity and is useful in the development of hypotheses. We have found hypothesizing, circularity, and curiosity to be extremely important components of our clinical work. We agree with Cecchin (1987), who states that "circular questioning can be understood as a method by which a clinician creates curiosity within the family system and therapy system" (p. 412). We have found that, by using hypothesizing, circularity, and curiosity, we have become more open to families and they, in turn, have developed more reciprocal trust in us. The family perceives the nurse as curious when he or she does not take sides with any one member or subgroup. Nurses who are curious are seen as aligned with everyone and no one in particular at the same time. They are seen as nonjudgmental and accepting of everyone.

Wright, Watson, and Bell (1996) pose a reflective question when they ask, "Are clinicians to remain neutral and non-hierarchical when confronted with illegal or dangerous behaviors?" (p. 103). They answer this important question by stating that each family functions in the way that members desire and in a way that they determine most effective. However, being part of a larger system, clinicians are bound by moral, legal, cultural, and societal norms that require them to act in accordance with those norms in regard to illegal or dangerous behavior. Cecchin (1987) assented that in these situations "clinicians may need to take different position—one which is distinct from a non-hierarchical, collaborative stance. Confronted by illegal behavior, a clinician may have to abandon a curious, therapeutic manner and become a social controller" (p. 409) to conform to the moral or legal rules and their consequences.

To enhance engagement, the nurse must provide structure, be active and empathic, and involve all members of the family. To provide structure, the nurse might say something such as, "We'll meet now for about 10 minutes so that I can get a better sense of your expectations and any concerns you have about hospitalization. We can then talk about what I might be able to help you with. How does that sound to you?" By stating the structure at the beginning of the eeting, the nurse reduces the family's anxiety about how long they will meet and also gives some direction for the conversation.

One way in which the nurse can be active during the engagement phase of the interview is to find out who is present. Many times we have found that "extra" family members attend interviews in the hospital. Leahey, Stout, and Myrah (1991) found an attendance rate of 94 percent of families invited to meetings on an inpatient mental health unit in a Canadian community hospital. These data held constant over a 7-year period. Often we find that family members of whom the nurse was unaware show up for the family meeting. For example, extended family members or ex-spouses have been invited by other family members or the patient, who believes it is important for them be present. Another way that nurses have found useful to start an interview is to work with the family in constructing a genogram or ecomap (see Chap. 3). Families generally find constructing a genogram an easy way to involve themselves in giving the nurse relevant information.

At the start of the interview, the nurse should ask questions of each member. We recommend that nurses initially attempt to spend an equal amount of time with each family member. We suggest that the nurse ask the same question or a similar one of each member to gather each person's ideas about a particular topic. It is important to note that, when we ask questions, we believe (in agreement with Freedman and Combs [1996]) that families are not retrieving particular experiences. Rather, in the conversation with us, the family members "put a spin on the experiences they call up; they suggest beginnings and endings for these experiences; they highlight portions of experience while diminishing or excluding others" (p. 117).

Examples of questions used to foster a collaborative working relationship and engagement have been offered by Levac, Wright, and Leahey (1997). These provide an implicit message to family members that the practitioner cares about them. They also open space for the family to exert more power in the conversation, voice concerns, and clarify the working arrangement. These examples are:

- What was most useful or not useful in your past working relationships with health professionals like me?
- On a scale of 1 to 10 (with 1 being very low and 10 being very high), how well do you think I understand your situation?
- If you were to become frustrated about our work together, would you be open to having a conversation with me about your concerns?
- In what ways was our discussion useful to each of you?

If the engagement between the nurse and family does not proceed well or if a fit cannot be established, we recommend that the nurse take a metaposition and critically reflect on the relationship. Jaber, Trilling, and Kelso (1997) have observed that three unspoken, implicit rules tend to operate in "stuck" family-healthcare provider relationships:

1. The healthcare provider is the expert.
2. The healthcare provider is the agent of change.
3. The healthcare provider's interpretation of the symptoms is sufficient to design a successful management plan.

These authors suggest revising these rules in the following ways:

1. Both the healthcare provider and patient are experts. The patient is expert in the illness story and (usually but not always) the healthcare provider in the physiology of the disease process.
2. The healthcare provider will try to facilitate change, but the ultimate agent of change is the patient.
3. To construct a workable management plan, the patient's and the healthcare provider's interpretation of the symptoms must both be acknowledged.

The engagement stage may also be thought of as the phase of the interview for creating a context for change that constitutes the central and enduring foundations of the therapeutic process (Wright, Watson, & Bell, 1996). Wright et al. (1996) suggest that all obstacles for change need to be removed during this stage so that a full and meaningful family assessment may be made. Examples of obstacles to change include a family member who does not want to be present or attends the meeting under duress, previous negative experiences with healthcare professionals, and unrealistic or unknown expectations of the referring person about treatment.

ASSESSMENT STAGE

During the assessment stage, the nurse and family explore four areas: problem identification, relationships between family interaction and the health problem, attempted solutions, and goals.

Problem Identification: Exploration and Definition

During this phase of the family interview, the nurse asks the family about its main concerns, complaints, or problems. That is, what is the problem that each family member would most like to see changed? After the exploration of each family member's perception of the most pressing concern, we have found it useful to ask the "one question" suggested by Wright (1989). That is, "If you could have only one question answered in our work together, what would that one question be?" This is a particularly effective way to elicit the family's deepest concerns at the beginning of the clinical work. It provides a focus for the conversation and generates new information shared among family members and between the nurse and the family. For example, the husband of a 44-year-old woman with a new diagnosis of multiple myeloma asked, "How can I support my wife and children better during this time?" The teenage daughter asked, "How can I learn more about my mother's illness?" The patient asked, "How long do I have to live?" The young adult son asked, "Should I avoid having my friends come over to the house so as to keep it more quiet for my mother when she returns home?" It is evident from the four questions asked by the family members that they each had a different expectation for the interview and for their relationship with the nurse.

Fleuridas, Nelson, and Rosenthal (1986) recommend that the family's definition of the concern be elicited by focusing on the three time frames of present, past, and future. Within each time frame, the nurse can ask questions pertaining to areas of difference, areas of agreement and disagreement, and explanations as to the meaning of the concern. It is important to emphasize that an effective interview does not depend on the use of any one type of question but rather on the knowledge of when, how, and to what purpose questions are used with particular family members at particular points in time. We have found the results from the study conducted by Dozier, Hicks, Cornille, and Peterson (1998) useful in deciding which types of questions to use. These authors found that circular and reflexive questions contribute most to early therapeutic alliance In Chapter 4 we provided information on various types of questions.

Leahey and Wright (1987) give examples of how to elicit the family's concerns by asking circular questions focusing on the present, past, and future:

Present. The nurse should ask each family member, including the children, to share their knowledge and understanding of the present situation. For example, the community health nurse working with a diabetic family could ask such questions as:

- What is the family's main concern *now* about Mahathir's diabetes?
- How is this concern a problem for the family *now* as compared to before?
- Who agrees with you that this is a problem?
- What is your explanation for this?

Past. In exploring the past, the nurse can again ask questions pertaining to:

- *Differences:* (How was Mahathir's behavior before his diabetes was diagnosed?)
- *Agreement or disagreement:* (Who agrees with Dad that this was the main concern when the family lived in Seattle?)
- *Explanation or meaning:* (What do you think was the significance of Mahathir's decision to stop injecting his own insulin?)

Future. During the initial interview with a new family, the nurse must learn about the family's own hypotheses or beliefs about the problems. In asking the family to explain the present situation, the nurse should attempt to identify previously unrecognized connections. This might be done by asking such questions as:

- If Tololwa suddenly developed renal disease, how would things be different from the way they are now?
- Does Tololwa agree with you?
- If this were to happen, how would you explain the change in Mahathir's relationship with Mom?

If the nurse finds that children or adolescents are reluctant to identify concerns in the family, he or she may need to ask the children alternative questions. Children may hesitate to disagree with their parents' description of the situation. A nurse can ask a child what he or she would like to see different in the family or how he or she would know if the problems went away. For example, one 8-year-old repeatedly stated that there were no difficulties surrounding his brother's diabetes and his mother's intense involvement with the sick child. However, when the nurse asked a future-oriented question about what differences he would notice in the family if his brother did not have diabetes, the 8-year-old said that he and his mother could go to basketball games after school. At the time of the interview, the mother had stated she was hesitant to leave the house after the boys returned from school for fear that her oldest son, Raja, would have an insulin reaction.

Other ideas for involving children in interviews have also been presented. Benson, Schindler-Zimmerman, and Martin (1991) suggested modifications of circular questions to be used with young children. These modifications, based on Piagetian theory, take into account the cognitive developmental limitations of children. For example, they suggest that relationship differences can be explored by providing props such as scarves, hats, and glasses for the children. This role-playing technique using props enables children and adults to display their perceptions. Another idea would be to give the child an ordered array of pictures ranging from a frowning face to a smiling face. The nurse could then ask, "Which one of these is most like how you and your brothers got along this week?" (p. 367).

In exploring the presenting concern, the nurse should obtain a clear and specific definition of the situation. Box 7–3 lists some factors for the nurse to consider when defining the problem. We try to remember, in our conversations with families, that each family expresses its pain and suffering in a unique way. Al-Krenawi (1998) points out that Bedouin-Arab patients routinely express their personal or family problems in proverbs. For example, a co-wife of a husband engaged in polygamy described how her husband's multiple marriages affected her deeply by saying, "My eye is blind and my hand is short." She meant that she felt unable to do anything (p. 73). Another example of how a presenting problem can be described is offered by Fraser (1998), who cites African-American couples' frequent use of metaphors to describe issues. One metaphor used by a couple experiencing major disagreement and conflict was "a glass wall between us, we can see each other, but we never seem to touch" (p. 142). The nurse can identify conflict among family members about the problem definition if this arises. When differences exist, the nurse clarifies the issues further to help define the problem for which the family is seeking change.

The nurse can also ask questions of each member about his or her own explanation for the situation now. Rolland (1998) stresses that exploring family beliefs in first meetings and at times of crisis is particularly important. The family members are joining with the nurse and

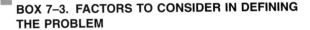

BOX 7–3. FACTORS TO CONSIDER IN DEFINING THE PROBLEM

1. Presenting Problem
   - Specify
2. Problem Identification
   - Who in the family was the first to identify the problem? And then who?
   - When was the problem identified?
   - What were the concurrent life events or stressors at time of identification of problem?
   - Who else (family members, friends) agrees that it is a problem? Who disagrees?
   - How does the family understand that this problem developed (beliefs)?
3. Problem Evolution
   - What behaviors became problematic?
   - Pattern of development
   - Frequency of problem emergence
   - Time intervals of quiescence
   - Factors aggravating
   - Factors alleviating
   - Who in the family is most and least concerned?

Adapted from Family Nursing Unit records, Faculty of Nursing, University of Calgary.

entrusting the nurse with their well-being. If they feel that their beliefs or explanations about the illness are not acknowledged, they may quickly feel marginalized. The nurse can ask, for example, their explanation or theory as to why this problem exists at this point in time. Furman and Ahola (1988) have given a number of useful suggestions for exploring a family's causal explanations for its own and other people's behavior. They suggest that the simplest way to do this is to ask direct, explanation-seeking questions such as, "What do you think is the reason for your son's psychosis?"

Another idea is to ask the clients to use their imagination to discuss an explanation. The interviewer can also offer a variety of alternative explanations or "gossip in the presence" by asking triadic questions such as, "What do you, Jordan, think is Ashley's explanation for your mother's depression?" In exploring the family's preexisting explanations, it is essential that the interviewer be curious and avoid agreeing or disagreeing with the explanation. Furman and Ahola (1988) suggest that there are several advantages to exploring the family's causal explanations, including improving cooperation between the interviewer and the family, developing systemic empathy with all family members versus selective empathy with one or two, detaching oneself from explanations provided by other professionals, recognizing and avoiding coalitions, loosening firmly held explanations, diluting negative explanations, and developing an ability to speculate with the clients about the effects of believing in one explanation or the other.

The problem-defining process or "co-evolving the definition" is a critical aspect of family work. Cecchin (1987) warns clinicians to accept neither their own nor the client's definition too quickly, and Maturana and Varela (1992) caution clinicians to adopt a attitude of permanent vigilance against the temptation of certainty. By remaining curious, a clinician has a greater chance of escaping the sin of certainty, or the sin of being too invested in one's own opinion.

Relationship between Family Interaction and the Health Problem

Once the main problems have been identified, the nurse asks questions about the relationship of family interaction to the health problem. Box 7–4 lists some factors to consider in exploring family interaction related to the presenting problem. The nurse conceptualizes the information that he or she has already gathered from the family in light of the meaning it has for the family and the hypotheses generated before the interview. The nurse then begins to develop additional questions that focus on *interactional* behaviors dealing with the three time frames of present, past, and future. Within each time frame, the nurse once again explores differences, agreements and disagreements, and ex-

---

BOX 7–4. FACTORS TO CONSIDER IN EXPLORING FAMILY INTERACTION RELATED TO THE PROBLEM

- Current manifestations of the problem.
- Typical responses of family members and others to the problem.
- Other current associated problems or concerns.
- How does the problem influence family functioning?
- How do family members understand that they have not been successful in conquering this problem (beliefs)?

Adapted from Family Nursing Unit records, Faculty of Nursing, University of Calgary.

planations or meanings. It is important to emphasize that the purpose of asking these questions is not merely to gather data. Rather, the nurse and the family are co-authoring a new story to replace a problem-saturated description (White & Epston, 1990). That is, by asking circular questions, the nurse generates new ideas and explanations for himself or herself *and* the family to consider.

Present. In exploring the present situation, the nurse could ask, "Who does what, when? Then what happens? Who is the first to notice that something has been done?" The nurse steers away from asking about traits tha t are supposedly intrinsic to a person, for example, being "shy." Rather, the nurse might ask, "When does he *act* shy?" or "To whom does he *show* shyness?" Then, "What does Jennifer do when Carley shows shyness?" The nurse can inquire about differences between individuals: "Who is better at getting grandmother to make her meals, Shanghi or Puichun?" The nurse can also inquire about differences between relationships: "Do your ex-husband and Danielle fight more or less than your ex-husband and Nadiya?" In working with families with chronic or life-threatening illness, the nurse should explore differences before or after important events or milestones. For example, the nurse could inquire: "Do you worry more, less, or the same about your wife's health since her emergency surgery?"

In addition to exploring areas of difference, the nurse can inquire about areas of agreement or disagreement: "Who agrees with you that Brandon is the most forgetful of giving your mother eyedrops three times a day? Who disagrees with you?" The nurse should explore the family's explanation for the sequence of interaction: "How do you understand Brandon's tendency to be most forgetful about the eyedrops? Are there ever times when he does remember? What seems to be different about the times when he remembers?"

Past. In exploring the past, the nurse uses similar types of questions to explore:

Differences: "How was it different? How does that differ from now?"

Agreement or disagreement: "Who agrees with Len that Dad was more involved in Lori Ann's exercise program?"

Explanation or meaning: "What does it mean to you that, after all this time, things between your wife and her mother have not changed?"

In addition to exploring how the family saw the problem in the past, we have found it extremely useful to explore how they have seen changes in the problem. Weiner-Davis, De Shazer, and Gingerich (1987) have found that change in the problem situation frequently occurs before the first meeting with the interviewer. Families can often recall and describe such changes if prompted. It is important to note that often the family must be prompted to emerge from their problem-saturated view of the situation. For example, a man may tell the nurse at the community mental health center that his male partner drinks very heavily and has always done this "until recently." If the nurse is attuned to inquiring about pretreatment changes, he or she will ask questions about the differences that the man has noticed recently. For example, the nurse might inquire, "Is his recent behavior the kind of change you would like to continue to have happen?" The idea of noticing exceptions to problems is one that we have used frequently in our clinical work, and we are indebted to de Shazer (1982, 1991) and White (1991) for emphasizing it.

Future. By focusing on the future and how the family would like things to be, the nurse instills hope for more adaptive interaction regarding the presenting concern. He or she also co-constructs a reality between family members and herself for a "problem-dissolved system" (Anderson & Goolishian, 1988). The nurse can ask questions pertaining to:

Differences: "How would it be different if your grandfather didn't side with your mother against your father in managing Paola's Crohn's disease?"

Agreement or disagreement: "Do you think your mother would agree that, if your grandfather stayed out of the discussions, things would be better?"

Explanation or meaning: "Dad, if your wife stopped phoning her father for advice about Paola's Crohn's disease, what would that mean to you?"

During this part of the interview, the nurse attempts to gain a systemic view of the situation and a description of the cycle of repeated interactions. These interactions may be between family members or between family members and the nurse. We stress that it is not important for the nurse to understand or agree with the problem but rather to be curious. The nurse should be able to describe the sequence of the development of the problem over time and the current contextual problem interaction, as well as the times when the problem does not show itself.

Attempted Solutions to Solving Problems

During this next phase of the assessment, the nurse explores the family's attempted solutions to the problem. Box 7–5 lists some factors to consider when exploring the family's attempted solutions. The process can begin with general questions related to the problem. For example, "How have you tried to obtain information from physicians and nurses

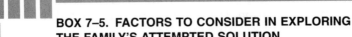

BOX 7–5. FACTORS TO CONSIDER IN EXPLORING THE FAMILY'S ATTEMPTED SOLUTION

- How has the family tried to resolve the problem?
- Who tried?
- With whom?
- What results?
- What were the events precipitating the search for professional help?
- Who is most in favor of agency help? Most opposed?
- What was the sequence of events resulting in actual contact with the agency?

Adapted from Family Nursing Unit records, Faculty of Nursing, University of Calgary.

about Eli's condition in previous hospitalizations?" More specific questions should then be used to identify the least and most effective solutions for achieving what the family desires. The nurse can ask when these solutions were used. For example, "What was least helpful in trying to get information from the nurses? What was most effective?" The nurse can ask if any successful elements in the solutions are still being used, and, if not, why not. Similar types of sequences of interaction questions that focus on difference, agreement or disagreement, and explanation or meaning can be used to explore the family's attempted solutions to the presenting concerns.

White (1991) has discussed the idea of attempted solutions as "unique outcomes." These are experiences that contradict the client's dominant or problem-saturated story. Unique outcomes provide a window to what might be considered to be the alternative territories of a person's life. "For an event to comprise a unique outcome, it must be qualified as such by the persons to whose life the event relates" (p. 30). It must be judged important and significant and represent a preferred outcome and an appealing development to which people are attracted as a new possibility. He recommends "re-authoring," in which the interviewer can ask a variety of questions to facilitate the process of preferring unique outcomes. For example, White (1991) suggests the following questions:

- How did you get yourself ready to take this step?
- What preparations led up to it?
- Just before taking this step, did you nearly turn back?

- If so, how did you stop yourself from doing so?
- Looking back from this vantage point, what did you notice yourself doing that might have contributed to this achievement?
- What developments have occurred in other areas of your life that may relate to this?
- How do you think these developments prepare the way for you to take these steps? (p. 30)

White also discusses the value of what he calls "experience of experience questions." Such questions "invite persons to reach back into their stock of lived experience and to express certain aspects that have been forgotten or neglected with the passage of time" (p. 32). They "recruit the imagination of persons in ways that are constitutive of alternative experiences of themselves" (p. 32). Examples include:

"If I had been a spectator to your life when you were a younger person, what do you think I might have witnessed you doing then that might help me to understand how you were able to achieve what you have recently achieved?"

"What do you think this tells me about what you have wanted for your life, and about what you have been trying for in your life?"

"How do you think that knowing this has affected my view of you as a person?"

"Exactly what actions would you be committing yourself to if you were to more fully embrace this knowledge of who you are?"

"If you were to side more strongly with this other view of who you are, and of what your life has been about, what difference would this make to your life on a day to day basis?" (p. 32)

In our work with families, we have frequently been told that no solutions have been attempted or that "nothing has worked." We find it useful to draw on the concept of resilience in these situations. Hawley and DeHaan (1996) have defined it: "Family resilience describes the path a family follows as it adapts and prospers in the face of stress, both in the present and over time. Resilient families respond positively to these conditions in unique ways, depending on the context, developmental level, the interactive combination of risk and protective factors, and the family's shared outlook" (p. 293) In talking with families about their resilience, we use terms such as endurance, withstanding, adaptation, coping, and survival and try to draw forth other qualities surfacing in the face of hardship or adversity. We talk about the ability to "bounce back" or make up for losses. We agree with Walsh (1996) that "resilience is forged *through* adversity not *despite* it" (p. 271). Bouncing back is not the same as "breezing through" a crisis. Walsh (1996) points out that resilience involves multiple recursive processes over time. It is this layering and recursiveness that we inquire about when we ask families about their coping and attempted solutions.

In working with families dealing with life-threatening or chronic illness, the nurse should be aware of additional "helping agencies" involved in healthcare delivery. We have found it important to ask such questions as "Have any other agencies attempted to help you with this problem? What has been the most useful advice that you have received? Did you follow this advice? What has been the least helpful advice?" Leahey and Slive (1983) point out the usefulness of exploring the differing ideas espoused by the helping systems. If there is unclear leadership or a confused hierarchy within the helping systems, the family can be placed in a conflictual situation that is similar to that of a child whose parents continually disagree. Confusion among helping agencies can exacerbate the family's concerns. In this way, the attempted solution (assistance by helping agencies) can become an entirely new problem for both the family and other agencies. It is important for the nurse to be aware of whether this situation exists before attempting to intervene.

Goal Exploration

At some point during the interview, the nurse and family establish what goals or outcomes the family expects as a result of change. Box 7–6 lists some factors for nurses to consider when exploring goals. We believe that families are seeking practical results when they come to a healthcare provider; families are pragmatists. They are "in pain" or "suffering" and their desire is to get rid of a problem. The problem may be between themselves as family members or between the family and the nurse (e.g., the family desires practical information about the acceptable level of physical activity after a myocardial infarction [MI]

BOX 7–6. FACTORS TO CONSIDER WHEN EXPLORING GOALS

- What general changes does the family believe would improve the problem?
- What specific changes?
- What are the expectations of how the agency may facilitate change in the problem?

Adapted from Family Nursing Unit records, Faculty of Nursing, University of Calgary.

and the nurse has not provided such concrete information). Family members may expect a large change, such as "My brother Sheldon will be able to walk without the aid of a cane" or a small but significant change, such as "We will be able to leave our handicapped daughter with a babysitter for 1 hour a week."

In many cases, a small change is sufficient. We believe that a small change in a person's behavior can have profound and far-reaching effects on the behavior of all persons involved. Experienced nurses are aware that small changes lead to further progress. de Shazer (1991) indicates that workable goals tend to have the following general characteristics. They are:

1. Small rather than large
2. Salient to clients
3. Described in specific, concrete behavioral terms
4. Achievable within the practical contexts of clients' lives
5. Perceived by the clients as involving their "hard work"
6. Described as the "start of" and not the "end of" something
7. Treated as involving new behavior(s) rather than the absence or cessation of existing behavior(s) (p. 112)

Goals describe what will be present or what will be happening when the complaint or concern is absent. We believe that unidimensional behavioral goal statements, such as "I will be eating less," are not as desirable as multidimensional, interactional, and situational goal statements that describe the "who, what, when, where, and how" of the solution. Such a multidimensional goal statement might be, "I will be eating a small, balanced meal in the evening at the dinner table with my husband, and we will not be watching television but rather talking to each other."

There are many ways in which the nurse can clarify the family's goals with such future or hypothetical questions as, "What would your parents do differently if they did not stay at home every evening with Frazer?" The nurse can explore future or hypothetical areas of difference ("How would your parents' relationship be different if your dad allowed your uncle to take care of Frazer one evening a week?"); areas of agreement or disagreement ("Do you think your Dad would agree that your parents would probably have little to talk about if they went out one evening a week?"); and explanation or meaning ("Tell me more about why you believe your parents would have a lot to talk about when they went out that one evening a week. What would that mean to you?").

Hewson (1991) has elaborated an interesting idea of combining past and future questions. She terms these "past prediction questions." For example, "if you were to tell me next week (or month or year) that you had done X, what could I find in your past history that would have allowed me to predict that you would have done X?" (p. 10). "The questions capitalize on the 'possibility to probability' phenomena at the same time as inviting a richer account of the history of the new/old story" (p. 10).

We have found it particularly useful in our clinical work to ask the "miracle question" (de Shazer, 1988) to elicit the family's goals. de Shazer (1991) describes the question in this way:

> Suppose that one night there is a miracle and while you are sleeping the problem . . . is solved: How would you know? What would be different?
>   What will you notice different the next morning that will tell you there has been a miracle? What will your spouse notice? (p. 113)

The miracle question elicits interactional information. The person is asked to imagine someone else's ideas as well as his or her own. The framework of the miracle question (and others of this type) allows family members to bypass their causal explanations. They do not have to imagine how they will get rid of the problem, but rather can focus on results. de Shazer (1991) states that "this then allows them to bring more of their previous non-problem experiences into the conversation; thus, the goals developed from the miracle question are not limited to just getting rid of the ~~problem/complaint~~.* Clients frequently are able to construct answers to this 'miracle question' quite concretely and specifically. 'Easy, I'll be able to say "no" to cocaine.' 'She'll see me smile more and go to work with more enthusiasm'" (p. 113).

Nurses working with families having a member with a chronic or life-threatening illness often find family members quite vague about the changes they expect. For example, "We would like Jordan to feel good about himself even though he has had a colostomy." Experienced clinical nurses know that "feeling good about oneself" is very difficult to describe or measure. We recommend that the nurse should ask the family to describe the smallest concrete change that Jordan could make to show that he "feels good about himself." By asking for this degree of specificity about desired change early in the nurse-family relationship, we believe it is more likely that the family and nurse can accomplish the desired change.

When discussing goals, we have found the work of Prochaska, DiClemente, and Norcross (1992) quite useful. They describe various

---

*To emphasize the elimination of the problem, de Shazer often strikes out the word problem *or* complaint.

stages an individual can go through on a continuum toward effecting self-change. In precontemplation, the first stage, the individual is not yet considering change. The second stage, contemplation, emerges where there is an increased recognition of the negative consequences of the behavior. Preparation for action, the third stage, denotes motivation and a realization that change is essential. Action, the fourth stage, includes an effort to modify behavior. The fifth stage, maintenance, entails retaining changes implemented in the action stage. We do not reify these stages nor consider them absolute progressions. Rather, we use them as talking points with family members, recognizing that each member may be at a different stage of readiness. We listen for openings to new stories, ask for openings, and check to make sure that the opening represents a preferred experience for the family.

▪▪▪ GUIDELINES FOR THE REMAINING INTERVIEWING PROCESS

Once the nurse has completed the initial interviews or assessment, he or she can consider the entire interviewing process. The stages of the interviewing process generally include:

1. Engagement
2. Assessment
3. Intervention
4. Termination

PLANNING

After an initial assessment is completed, a beginning nurse interviewer frequently worries about whether or not to intervene with a family. The following questions often arise: Am I the appropriate person to offer intervention? Do I have sufficient skills? Or, perhaps, should another professional, such as a social worker, psychologist, or family therapist, be called in?

Does every family that is assessed need further intervention? This is not to say that interventions begin only at the intervention stage. Rather, they are part of the total interview process from engagement to closure. For example, just by asking the family to come together for an interview, the nurse has intervened. Each time the nurse asks a circular question, he or she influences the family, generates new information, and intervenes.

For nurses, the decision to offer interventions, refer the family to others, or discharge them is a complex one. Several factors need to be examined before making the choice: the level of the family's functioning, the level of the nurse's competence, and the work context.

Level of the Family's Functioning

The nurse should recognize the complexity of the case. Christophersen (1979) advocates that treatment begin if the referring problem has been detected early and clearly defined procedures for management have been published. Most nurses would agree with this position but would find it very idealistic. Community health nurses and mental health nurses, in particular, often work with families who are not referred early. Some of these families who present have an unusual number of physical and emotional problems and are frequently involved in one crisis after another. These families offer specific challenges to the clinician.

Our recommendation is that nurses carefully assess the family's level of functioning and its desire to work on specific issues, such as management of hemiplegia after a stroke, impact of cystic fibrosis on the family, negotiation of services for elderly family members, or caring for a child with special needs. If the family is at all amenable to working on such an issue, it is incumbent on the nurse to either offer intervention or help them to get appropriate assistance by referring them to others. Guidelines for the referral process are given in Chapter 10.

Grace and Camilleri (1981) discuss the ethical issues involved in who should be treated. They point out that "with the popularizing of psychiatry, a surface inspection would seem to indicate that everyone is in need of psychotherapy in one form or another" (p. 565). The childless couple, the family with young infants, the family with adolescents, the single-parent family, and the aging family are all considered to be candidates for psychotherapeutic aid. Many people lead psychologically constricted and difficult lives, but should they be "treated"? This is a troublesome question for helping professionals.

Our recommendation is that nurses ethically weigh two opposing positions when they make the decision to intervene with, refer, or discharge a family. One position states that if a person is potentially dangerous to self or others, that person should receive intervention. On an individual level, a suicidal patient is such an example. On a larger system level, a family in which there is physical, sexual, or emotional abuse or violence is an example. An opposing position has been voiced by Szasz (1973). He asserts that the individual should decide whether to be treated or hospitalized. A person's self-responsibility is vehemently defended. Szasz's position on individual rights can be extrapolated to cover a family's rights. Today, many families that previously were considered deviant are seen to be functioning adaptively, such as sole-parent adoptive families or gay, lesbian, or bisexual couples. It is our hope that nurses will ethically and wisely consider the family's level of functioning. This is a necessary step before deciding to offer further treatment. In Chapter 10, we present some ideas that we have used when we have decided not to offer additional treatment to families.

Another ethical consideration for nurses to weigh is the balance between judgment about families and respect for their cultural, religious, and ethnic self-determination. To avoid ethnocentrism and paternalism, nurses have embraced certain politically correct ideas with enthusiasm. Kikuchi (1996) states that "as cultural relativism has become firmly entrenched within nursing, it has become the fashion not to question the tenability of . . . injunctions for nursing practice" (p.159). We advocate that nurses engage in critical thinking about responsible practice, safeguard human dignity, and not blindly follow injunctions to be politically correct. We have found it useful in our clinical work with families to be open and direct with them in discussing ethical dilemmas involving them.

The Nurse's Level of Competence

Nurses should consider their personal and professional capacity when choosing to work with a family. If the nurse has experienced a recent death of a family member, he or she may not be able to facilitate grieving in family members. Likewise, a nurse with strong views that people with psychosomatic illnesses are hypochondriacs would be best advised not to attempt work with such families. We do not subscribe to the view that a nurse has to have personally dealt with a situation (e.g., raised teenagers) to be of help to a family. Most noteworthy in a nurse is clinical competence. We do believe, however, that the nurse should attempt to be well informed and not just offer advice that might or might not be helpful. On a professional level, the nurse needs to evaluate his or her competence. Am I at the beginning or the advanced level of family interviewing skill? Can I obtain supervision to aid in dealing with complex families? Each nurse should examine these questions and the answers before making a decision about intervening with families.

Work Context

Sometimes considerable controversy is raised about the issue of who is competent to treat clients. This controversy involves issues of definition and professionalism. How a "family problem" and a "medical problem" are defined in a particular work setting can fuel the controversy. If a nurse (working with a patient who has had a stroke) invites the relatives to come for a class, is the nurse treating a family or a medical problem? We take the approach that the definition of the problem is less important than the solution. That is, if the whole family is involved, the definition of the problem is a question of semantics.

The issue of professional territoriality is a very thorny one with no pat answers. Sometimes the patient sees the psychologist for psychodiagnostic testing and the social worker to deal with the family and outside agencies. The role of the nurse with the family in this situation can become controversial. If the nurse does a family assessment and decides to intervene with the family, is the nurse usurping the social worker's position? Or, perhaps, is the nurse usurping the physician's position by making the decision to intervene? We view as progress in mutidisciplinary cooperation the name change for the journal *Families, Systems and Health.* The journal used to be called *Family Systems Medicine.* Also constricting has been the use of the term "medical family therapy" (McDaniel, Hepworth & Doherty, 1992). This type of language, particularly the use of the word "medical," can inadvertently exclude or diminish nursing's involvement with families (Bell, Wright, & Watson, 1992).

We support the generic core competencies outlined by McDaniel and Campbell (1996) for all professionals involved in delivering collaborative healthcare. These are listed in Box 7–7. There are no simple answers to complex professional and territorial issues. We urge nurses to work cooperatively to ensure the best family care possible. In general, we believe the best person to intervene in a situation is the one with the most ready access to the system level in which the problems manifest themselves. However, we believe that, in the past, nurses have been too quick to turn over family care to other professionals. Nurses are now reclaiming their important role in providing family-centered care.

The advent of managed care has required all nurses and healthcare providers to examine and adapt their practices to account for the provision of timely, efficient, and cost-effective services. Managed care, health insurance reform, and other complex issues have changed the face of nursing practice. The coming together of the consumer movement and health economics has huge implications for practice in the 21st century. Nurses have to do more than just heal their patients. Day after day, they must also attend to the socioeconomic and political context of healthcare as well as to the survival of their careers. We believe that it is vital for nurses to find ways to thrive professionally and for families to receive optimal care. Strategies to address bureaucratic

BOX 7–7. GENERIC CORE COMPETENCIES FOR ALL PROFESSIONALS TRAINING IN COLLABORATION

1. Bring in the patient and family members as full partners in health-care.
2. Maintain attention to collaborative values.
   - Focus primarily on capacities as opposed to deficits.
   - Promote universal access to healthcare.
   - Empower, educate, and learn from families.
   - Value interdependency.
   - Collaborate to improve the health of communities through social change.
3. Become accountable for the use of resources.
   - Track statistics and outcomes.
4. Discuss, monitor, and deal with issues of shared power among professionals and between professionals, patient, and families.
   - Create space for everyone to have a place in the discourse.
   - Examine the relationship between power and helping professions and between competition and collaboration.
   - Develop case-specific leadership, dependent on the needs of the patient and the context.
   - Learn to be both a leader and a follower.
   - Develop the ability to talk about differences.
   - Help trainees deal with the realities of hierarchy in much of today's healthcare system.
5. Examine issues of culture, race, class, and disabilities in health-care.
   - Make services culturally responsive.
   - Develop ways to accept and support differences.
   - Examine cultural countertransference.
6. Learn to enhance others' competencies.
7. Learn to contract regarding how and how much to communicate with other professionals about patients.
8. Attend to issues of spirituality.
9. Teach each professional and each individual to know, accept, and embrace their limits.
10. Attend to the development of the self of the healthcare professional.

disentitlement of cultural, ethnic, racial, and other minority groups must be put forth. Models for access to healthcare for economically disadvantaged families need further refinement and implementation. Freedman and Combs (1996) and other Narrative therapists have put forth ideas emphasizing accountability structures and practices as a way of recognizing the centrality of structured power differences in our society. We believe that, as nurses work with diverse families and are increasingly transparent in this work, they will find ways to positively influence their employment contexts.

INTERVENTION STAGE

Once the nurse has decided to intervene with the family, we recommend that he or she review CFIM (see Chap. 4). This will stimulate ideas about change, and the nurse can then design interventions to work with the family addressing the particular domain of family functioning affected: cognitive, affective, or behavioral. Helpful hints about intervention are offered in Box 7–8.

In choosing interventions, we encourage nurses to attend to several factors to enhance the likelihood that the interventions will focus on change in the desired domain of family functioning. Interventions, offered within a collaborative relationship, are not a demand but rather an invitation to change (Robinson, 1994). Some factors to consider

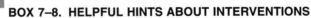

BOX 7–8. HELPFUL HINTS ABOUT INTERVENTIONS

- They are the core of clinical work with families.
- They should be devised with sensitivity to the family's ethnic and religious background.
- They can be offered only to families. The nurse cannot direct change but can create a context for change to occur.
- They may fit family members and be useful to them.
- They may not fit family members, and thus nurses should be open to offering alternative interventions rather than blame themselves or the family because the intervention was not desired by the family.

Adapted from Levac, A. C., Wright, L. M., & Leahey, M. (1997). Children and families: Models for assessment and intervention. In J. Fox (Ed.), *Primary health care of children*. St. Louis: Mosby, p. 12, with permission.

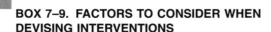

> **BOX 7–9. FACTORS TO CONSIDER WHEN DEVISING INTERVENTIONS**
>
> - What is the agreed-on problem to change?
> - What domain of family functioning is the intervention aimed at?
> - How does the intervention match the family's style of relating?
> - How is the intervention linked to the family's strengths and previous useful solution strategies?
> - How is the intervention consistent with the family's ethnic and religious beliefs?
> - How is the intervention new or different for the family?

when devising interventions are outlined in Box 7–9. First, the intervention should be related to the problem that the nurse and the family have contracted to change. Second, the intervention should be derived from the nurse's hypothesis about the problem and what the family says the problem means to them and their beliefs about the problem (Wright, Watson & Bell, 1996). Third, the intervention should match the family's style of relating. (We have found in our own clinical work that sometimes we are biased toward one particular domain of family functioning, such as cognitive or affective, and that we have thus erred in devising interventions that we are most comfortable with rather than ones that the family may find most useful.) Fourth, the interventions should be linked to the family's strengths. We believe that families have inherent resources and that the nurse's responsibility is to encourage families to use these resources in new ways to tackle the problem. Fifth, the interventions should take into consideration the family's beliefs influenced by ethnicity, spirituality, class, gender, and sexual orientation. Sixth, the nurse should devise a few interventions so that nurse and family can consider their relative merits. For example, are they new ideas for the family or are they "more of the same" solutions of the type that the family has already tried?

We do not believe that there is one "right" intervention. Rather, there are only "useful" or "effective" interventions. In our experience, we have found that a nurse sometimes reaches an impasse, with a family not changing, when the nurse persists in *either* using the same intervention repeatedly *or* switching interventions too rapidly. Kuehl (1995) suggests that clients often fail to notice responses containing possible solutions. The same can be said of nurses. Interventions are successful when constraints are lifted and important aspects of life change are noticed. There is a clearer image of how things can be different in the future.

With the greater availability of computers and telecommunication devices, we believe that nurses will become increasingly creative in finding electronic means to facilitate intervention. Davis (1998) described telephone interventions with caregivers of elders with dementia. Findings from her feasibility study "suggest that telephone-based skill building may increase dementia caregivers' sense of social support, reduce their depressive symptoms, and improve their life satisfaction in the midst of caregiving" (p.265). We believe that, just as the use of computers and telephones for business and education has had dramatic effects on family interaction, so too will their use in health-care profoundly affect nurse-family interaction.

Once the nurse has devised an intervention, he or she must attend to the executive skills (see Chap. 5) required to deliver the intervention. Part of the success of any intervention is the manner in which the intervention is given. The family must feel confident that the intervention will promote change. The nurse also needs to show that the *nurse has* confidence and belief that the intervention or task requested will benefit the family.

However, interventions need to be tailored to each family; therefore, the preamble or preface to the actual intervention will vary. For example, if a family is feeling very hopeless and frustrated with a particular problem, the nurse might want to say, "I know this might seem like a hard thing that I'm going to ask you to do, but I know your family is capable . . ." On the other hand, if the nurse is making a request of a family that tends to be quite formal with one another, then the nurse might preface it with, "What I'm going to ask you to do may make you feel a little foolish or silly at first, but you'll notice that, as you do it a few times, that you will become more comfortable."

Pearson (1998) gives a good example of a generic intervention, the "What are you prepared to do?" question, and how he tailors it with each couple. Typically, he says "(name), I'd like you to tell (partner's name) and me, based on what we've discussed, one specific thing you are prepared to take personal responsibility to do on a daily basis, over the next two weeks with the intention of increasing the happiness of your partner, regardless of what your partner does." (p. 281). In this example, each partner commits to the other and the "thing" chosen is very specific rather than global. The term "prepared" is an important word suggesting a voluntary decision to participate in the change process. The word "intention" is also important because "couples tend to allow each other more latitude in their self-change efforts if they perceive their partner's heart to be in the right place" (p. 282). Pearson also highlights the importance of disconnecting one partner's responsibility for change from the attitudes, actions, and comments of the other partner.

When giving a particular assignment for a family to do between sessions, it is a good idea to try to include all family members. Haley (1987) suggests that one way to make this possible is to think of the assignment as you would any other piece of work. Therefore, it requires some family members needed to do the "job," someone to supervise, someone to plan, and another family member to check to see if the job gets done.

Sometimes it is necessary to review with the family members what the particular assignment is in order to check their understanding of what is being requested. Reviewing the assignment is a good idea, whether it is something to be carried out within the interview or between interviews. If assignments or experiments are given between sessions, the nurse should always ask for a report at the next interview. If the family has not completed or only partially completed the assignment, the reason needs to be explored.

We do not subscribe to the view that families are noncompliant or resistant if they do not follow our requests. Rather, we become curious about their decision to choose an alternate course and try to learn from their response. We believe that family interviewing is a circular process. The nurse intervenes and the family responds in its unique way. The nurse then responds to this response and the process continues.

During the intervention stage, the nurse must be aware of the element of time. How useful or effective an intervention is can be evaluated only after the intervention has been implemented. With some interventions, change may be noted immediately. However, it is more common that changes will not be noticed for a lengthy period. Just as most problems occur over time, problems also need an appropriate length of time to be resolved. It is impossible to state how long one should wait to ascertain if a particular intervention has been effective, but changes within family systems need to filter through the various system levels. Families themselves offer useful observations and feedback about what interventions are most useful. Robinson and Wright (1995), in discussing a study conducted by Robinson, cite that families identified interventions within two stages of the therapeutic change process that they thought were critical to healing: creating the circumstances for change and moving beyond and overcoming problems. (For further elaboration on these stages, see Chap. 1).

More information about devising interventions is provided in Chapters 4, 8, and 10.

TERMINATION STAGE

The last stage of the interviewing process is known as termination or closure. It is critically important for the nurse to conceptualize how to end treatment with the family to enhance the likelihood that changes will be maintained. In Chapter 5, we outlined the conceptual, perceptual, and executive skills useful for the termination stage. In Chapter 10 we address in depth the process of termination and focus on how to evaluate outcome.

■ ■ ■ CLINICAL CASE EXAMPLE

Following is an example of how a nurse conducted family interviews using the guidelines we have given in Chapters 6 and 7. An example of a 15-minute interview is given in Chapter 8.

PRE-INTERVIEW

Developing Hypotheses

The Home Health Agency received a referral on the Auerswald family for home nursing services, physiotherapy, nutrition counseling, and mental health counseling. Mr. Auerswald, 51, was a paraplegic and in a wheelchair because of multiple trauma suffered in an industrial accident. He was unemployed. Mrs. Auerswald, 49, a homemaker, was the primary caretaker. She was reported to be depressed. The homecare nurse hypothesized that Mrs. Auerswald's depression could be related to feeling overresponsible for caring for her husband. The nurse wondered what the husband's role might be in perpetuating this. She was also curious to know what other social and professional support systems were involved and what their beliefs were about the family's health problems. During the course of the family interview, the nurse gained much evidence from both the husband and wife to confirm the usefulness of her initial hypothesis. She used this hypothesis to provide a framework for her conversation with the couple.

Relation to CFAM. The nurse generated her hypothesis based on knowledge of and clinical experience with other families in similar situations (e.g., Robinson, 1998) and with a similar ethnic background. It was also based on the structural category of CFAM (internal and external family structure, ethnicity, gender), the developmental category (middle-aged families), and the functional category (roles, power or influence, circular communication, beliefs).

Arranging the Interview

The wife stated that she did not want to discuss her depression with the nurse while her husband was awake. The nurse requested that for the first home visit that husband and wife be interviewed together. The couple agreed to this.

Relation to CFAM. The nurse elaborated her thinking about family roles and gender. She speculated that Mrs. Auerswald may be protecting her husband from her problem. In terms of the CFAM category of verbal communication, the nurse speculated that there might not be clear and direct communication between the husband and wife.

INTERVIEW

Engagement

The genogram data revealed that:
- The husband and wife are alone in the city; extended families and children live in other cities and visit infrequently.
- The wife had been married previously and had stayed with her first husband for 18 years, although he physically abused her. She thought it was her responsibility to protect her children.
- This was the husband's first marriage.

Relation to CFAM. The above information added some support for the nurse's initial hypothesis in terms of the wife's beliefs about responsibility and an isolated family structure.

Assessment

Problem Definition. Mrs. Auerswald described the problem as "my husband has had such a hard tragedy, but now I'm the one who is depressed. It doesn't make sense." Mr. Auerswald described the problem as his wife's "worrying too much."

Relationship between Family Interaction and Health Problem. By asking circular questions, the nurse elicited the fact that the wife had not allowed herself a break from caretaking for 2 years. The husband encouraged her to "go out and meet people," but she stated that she was fearful he might be too lonely if she met other people. Mr. Auerswald stated that this would not be a problem for him. They both reported that recently Mrs. Auerswald had become depressed. She cried frequently and had difficulty sleeping.

Mrs. Auerswald takes excellent physical care of her husband and bathes him daily. He is appreciative of all her nursing care. She feels guilty about asking for help from his parents.

Attempted Solutions. Mrs. Auerswald had recently visited her family doctor, who prescribed antidepressant medication for her. She had requested homecare services once before, but she said that because "their schedule is unreliable [and she] never know[s] when they are coming," she had discontinued treatment with the nurses. On the advice of her physician, Mrs. Auerswald agreed to try homecare again.

Relation to CFAM. The nurse noted that the Auerswald's problem-solving approaches were directed toward either self-sufficiency or professional resources outside the family. They sought help from the family doctor and from the homecare agency only infrequently, and they were reluctant to call on extended family for assistance.

Goals. Mrs. Auerswald's desire was to "not feel depressed, [to] feel good about myself." The smallest significant change that she was able to describe was to be able to "go out one afternoon a week without feeling guilty." Mr. Auerswald was in agreement with his wife's goals.

Intervention

Consideration of CFIM. Having developed a collaborative relationship with the couple and a workable hypothesis that fit the data from the family assessment, the nurse began to consider interventions with Mr. and Mrs. Auerswald in the cognitive, affective, and behavioral domains of family functioning. The focus of intervention was Mrs. Auerswald's depression.

Interventions and Outcome. Knowing that Mrs. Auerswald had stayed in a physically abusive first marriage for 18 years to protect her children, the nurse asked questions about beliefs and feelings of responsibility. The nurse encouraged change in Mrs. Auerswald's beliefs by asking both husband and wife behavioral effect, triadic, and hypothetical questions about responsibility. She asked the couple to engage in behavioral experiments to try new ways of being self-responsible. Both Mr. and Mrs. Auerswald challenged their own beliefs about depression being a solely biological problem and began to take more responsibility for their own lives. Mr. Auerswald stated that he wanted a bath only three times a week. Mrs. Auerswald requested caretaking help from her mother-in-law and was able to leave her husband alone for 2 hours, three times a week while she played cards with friends. The couple reported significant improvement in her depression. The homecare agency continued to provide nursing and physical therapy services for the family. The nurse and home health aide focused on supporting the couple's new beliefs about responsibility.

▪▪▪ CONCLUSIONS

Guidelines for nurses to consider during initial interviews and during the whole process of interviewing have been delineated. We recommend that nurses use these guidelines as ideas and suggestions for how to maximize the effectiveness of their time with families. We caution nurses, however, to remember the uniqueness of every family situation and encourage them to use guidelines with sensitivity to each clinical situation mindful of the family's cultural and ethnic heritage.

▪▪▪ REFERENCES

Al-Krenawi, A. (1998). Family therapy with a multiparental/multispousal family. *Family Process, 37*(1), 65–81.

Anderson, H., & Goolishian, H. (1988). Human systems as linguistic systems: Preliminary and evolving ideas about the implications for clinical theory. *Family Process, 27*(4), 371–394.

Bell, J. M., Wright, L. M., & Watson, W. L. (1992). The medical map is not the territory; or, "Medical Family Therapy?"—Watch your language? *Family Systems Medicine, 10*(1), 35–39.

Benson, M., Schindler-Zimmerman, T., & Martin, D. (1991). Assessing children's perceptions of their family: Circular questioning revisited. *Journal of Marital and Family Therapy, 17*(4), 363–372.

Cecchin, G. (1987). Hypothesizing, circularity, and neutrality revisited: An invitation to curiosity. *Family Process, 26*(4), 405–414.

Christophersen, E. (1979). Behavioral pediatrics. In D. Hymovich & M. Barnard (Eds.), *Family health care.* New York: McGraw-Hill, Vol. 1, pp. 354–372.

Davis,L. L. (1998). Telephone-based interventions with family caregivers. *Journal of Family Nursing, 4*(3),231–254.

de Shazer, S. (1991). *Putting difference to work.* New York: W. W. Norton.

de Shazer, S. (1988). *Clues: Investigating solutions in brief therapy.* New York: W. W. Norton.

de Shazer, S. (1982). *Patterns of brief family therapy: An ecosystemic approach.* New York: Guilford Press.

Dozier, R. M., Hicks, M. W., Cornille,T. A., & Peterson, G. W. (1998). The effect of Tomm's therapeutic questioning styles on therapeutic alliance: A clinical analog study. *Family Process, 37*(2),189–200.

Fleuridas, C., Nelson, T., & Rosenthal, D. (1986). The evolution of circular questions: Training family therapists. *Journal of Marital and Family Therapy, 12*(2), 113–127.

Fraser, E. (1998). The use of metaphors with African-American couples. *Journal of Couples Therapy, 7*(2/3),137–148.

Freedman, J., & Combs, G. (1996). *Narrative therapy: The social construction of preferred realities.* New York: W. W. Norton & Co.

Furman, B., & Ahola, T. (1988). The return of the question "why": Advantages of exploring pre-existing explanations. *Family Process, 27*(4), 395–410.

Grace, H., & Camilleri, D. (1981). *Mental health nursing: A socio-psychological approach* (2nd ed.). Dubuque, IA: W. C. Brown.

Griffith, M. E. (1995). Opening therapy to conversations with a personal God. *Journal of Feminist Family Therapy, 7*(1/2), 123–139.

Haley, J. (1987). *Problem-solving therapy* (2nd ed.). San Francisco: Jossey-Bass.

Hawley, D. R. & DeHaan, L. (1996). Toward a definition of family resilience: Integrating life-span and family perspectives. *Family Process, 35*(3), 283–298.

Hewson, D. (1991). From laboratory to therapy room: Prediction questions for reconstructing the "new-old" story. *Dulwich Centre Newsletter, 3*, 5–12.

Jaber, R., Trilling, J. S., & Kelso, E. B. (1997). The circle of change: An approach to difficult clinical interactions. *Families, Systems and Health, 15*(2), 163–174.

Kikuchi, J. (1996). Multicultural ethics in nursing education; A potential threat to responsible practice. *Journal of Professional Nursing, 12*(3), 159–165.

Kuehl, B.(1995).The solution-oriented genogram: A collaborative approach. *Journal of Marital and Family Therapy, 21*(3), 239–250.

Leahey, M., & Slive, A. (1983). Treating families with adolescents: An ecological approach. *Canadian Journal of Community Mental Health, 2*(2), 21–28.

Leahey, M., Stout, L., & Myrah, I. (1991). Family systems nursing: How do you practice it in an active community hospital? *Canadian Nurse, 87*(2), 31–33.

Leahey, M., & Wright, L. M. (1987). Families and chronic illness: Assumptions, assessment and intervention. In L. M. Wright & M. Leahey (Eds.), *Families and chronic illness.* Springhouse, PA: Springhouse, pp. 55–76.

Levac, A.C., Wright, L. M., & Leahey, M. (1997). Children and families: Models for assessment and intervention. In J. Fox (Ed.). *Primary health care of children.* St.Louis: Mosby, pp. 3–13.

Maturana, H. R, & Varela, F. (1992). *The tree of knowledge: The biological roots of human understanding.* (Rev. ed.). Boston: Shambhala.

McDaniel, S. H., & Campbell, T. L. (1996). Editorial: Training for collaborative family health care. *Families, Systems and Health, 14*(2),147–150.

McDaniel, S. H., Hepworth, J., & Doherty, W. J. (1992). *Medical family therapy.* New York: Basic Books.

Pearson, D. (1998). The "What are you prepared to do?" question. In T.S. Nelson & T.S. Trepper (Eds.). *101 more interventions in family therapy.* New York: Haworth Press, pp. 280–284.

Prochaska, J. O., DiClemente, C. C., & Norcross, J. C. (1992). In search of how people change: Applications to addictive behavior. *American Psychologist, 47*, 1102–1114.

Rolland, J. S. (1998). Beliefs and collaboration in illness: Evolution over time. *Families, Systems and Health, 16*(1/2) 7–25.

Robinson, C. A. (1998).Women, families, chronic illness, and nursing interventions: From burden to balance. *Journal of Family Nursing, 4*(3), 271–290.

Robinson, C. A. (1994). Nursing interventions with families: A demand or an invitation to change? *Journal of Advanced Nursing, 19,* 897–904.

Robinson, C. A. & Wright, L. M. (1995). Family nursing interventions: What families say makes a difference. *Journal of Family Nursing, 1*(3), 327–345.

Szasz, T. (1973). *The myth of mental illness.* New York: Harper & Row.

Thorne, S. E., & Robinson, C. A. (1989). Guarded alliance: Health care relationships in chronic illness. *Image, 21*(3), 153–157.

Walsh, F. (1996). The concept of family resilience: Crisis and challenge. *Family Process, 35*(3), 261–282.

Weiner-Davis, M., de Shazer, S., & Gingerich, W. J. (1987). Building on pre-treatment change to construct the therapeutic solution: An exploratory study. *Journal of Marital and Family Therapy, 13*(4), 359–364.

White, M. (1991). Deconstruction and therapy. *Dulwich Centre Newsletter, 3,* 21–40.

White, M., & Epston, D. (1990). *Narrative means to therapeutic ends.* New York: W. W. Norton.

Wright, L. M. (1989). When clients ask questions: Enriching the therapeutic conversation. *Family Therapy Networker, 13*(6), 15–16.

Wright, L. M., Watson, W. L., & Bell, J. M. (1996). *Beliefs: The heart of healing in families and illness.* New York: Basic Books.

CHAPTER **8**

How to Do
a 15-Minute
(or Shorter)
Family Interview

The statement "I don't have time to do family interviews" is the most common reason offered by nurses for not routinely involving families in their practice. In numerous undergraduate and graduate nursing courses, professional workshops, and presentations, we have encountered this statement as the resounding declaration for the exclusion of family members from healthcare. With major changes in the delivery of healthcare services through managed care, budgetary constraints, and staff cutbacks, time is of the essence in nursing practice. However, it is our belief that families need not be banned or marginalized in healthcare. To involve families, nurses need to possess sound knowledge of family assessment and intervention models, interviewing skills, and questions. We believe that family nursing knowledge can be applied effectively even in very brief family meetings. We also claim that a 15-minute, or even shorter, family interview can be purposeful, effective, informative, and even healing. Any involvement of family members, regardless of the length of time, is better than no involvement.

But what is time? And what exactly can be accomplished in 15 minutes or less with a family? Perhaps the best portrayal of time, particularly therapeutic time, is Boscolo and Bertrando's (1993) comprehensive descriptions, explanations, and examples of clinical time. They offer three domains of time: individual, cultural, and social. Social or "sociological" time indicates viewing time as a means of social coordination, that is, as having instrumental value (Boscolo & Bertrando, 1993). Much of nursing practice time is socially and culturally coordinated, highly ritualized, and therefore honored. We propose that ritualizing and coordinating meeting time with families, even if it is only 15 minutes, will also become an honored part of nursing practice.

However, for nurses' behaviors to change, they must first alter or modify their beliefs about involving families in healthcare. We have discovered that, when nurses do not include family members in their practice, some very constraining beliefs usually exist (Wright, Watson, & Bell, 1996). Some of these beliefs are:

- "If I talk to family members, I won't have time to complete my other nursing responsibilities."
- "If I talk to family members, I may open up a can of worms and I will have no time to deal with it."

275

- "It's not my job to talk with families; that's for social workers and psychologists."
- "I can't possible help families in the brief time I will be caring for them."
- "If the family becomes angry, what would I do?"
- "What if they ask me a question and I don't have the answer, what would I do? It's better not to start a conversation."

Uncovering these constraining beliefs makes it more comprehensible why nurses may shy away from routinely involving families in nursing practice. We postulate that if nurses were to embrace only one belief, that "illness is a family affair" (Wright, Watson, & Bell, 1996), it would change the face of nursing practice. Nurses would then be more eager to know how to involve and assist family members in the care of their loved ones. They would appreciate that everyone in a family experiences an illness and that no one family member "has" diabetes, multiple sclerosis, or cancer. By embracing this belief, they would realize that, from initial symptoms through diagnosis and treatment, all family members are influenced by and reciprocally influence the illness. They would also come to realize that our privileged conversations with patients and their families about their illness experiences can contribute dramatically to healing and the diminishing or alleviation of suffering (Frank, 1998; Wright et al., 1996).

Therefore, we would like to offer some very specific ideas for conducting a 15-minute (or shorter) family interview. These ideas are the condensed or "Reader's Digest" version of the core elements previously presented in Chapters 5 through 7 about conducting family interviews. The ideas honor the theoretical underpinnings of the Calgary Family Assessment Model (CFAM) and Calgary Family Intervention Model (CFIM) and highlight some of the most critical elements of these models.

■■■ KEY INGREDIENTS

What are the key ingredients of a 15-minute family interview? From our observations and experience, the key and essential ingredients to a successful, productive, and effective 15-minute family interview are manners, therapeutic conversation, family genogram (and in some situations an ecomap), therapeutic questions, and commendations. Of course, all of these ingredients can take place only within the context of a therapeutic relationship.

KEY INGREDIENT 1: MANNERS

Good manners have always been the core of common, everyday social behavior. However, in the last two decades in North America, our social behavior has dramatically shifted from formal to casual social interaction. Even our style of dress has been altered from Sunday Best to Casual Friday. However, not all casualness in our society has been welcomed, and unfortunately much of it is experienced as rude, thoughtless, or uncaring. Judith Martin's (1983) national bestseller on a "guide to excruciatingly correct behavior" offers 700 plus pages of her perspective and humor on manners. Miss Manners, as Martin (1983) is known, gives a thoughtful commentary on what is missing in the core of our interactions with one another and thus what is missing in our society. Manners are those simple but profound courteous acts of politeness, respect, and kindness. Unfortunately, our culture as a whole seems to be undergoing the erosion of manners and thus civility. This erosion has sadly spilled over into the nursing profession.

Nursing has not been immune to the changes in social behavior. In some situations, we can argue that some formal nursing behaviors perhaps inhibited our relations with clients and families. Countless nurses still maintain respectful, polite, and thoughtful relations with their clients. However, we have witnessed and listened to far too many professional and personal encounters between nurses and patients in which manners were pitifully absent.

One of the most glaring examples of the absence of manners in nursing is in the basic social act of an introduction. Numerous stories have been told of nurses who do not introduce themselves to their patients, let alone the patients' family members. For example, a 23-year-old man was seen in an outpatient clinic in a large metropolitan hospital after open-heart surgery. He reported that the nurse did not introduce herself, but began touching his body and adjusting his intravenous pic line without telling him what she was doing or why. He found this experience very invasive, frightening, and rude.

This clinical anecdote is consistent with a study that examined nurse-family relationships in the intensive care unit. Hupcey (1998) found that one of the nursing strategies that inhibits the establishment of therapeutic relationships is the depersonalizing of the patient and family. Examples given were "not referring to the patient by name, labeling the patient or family difficult, providing care without encouraging participation by the patient or family, and not talking or making eye contact" (Hupcey, 1998, p. 187).

Therefore, it is obvious that introduction is an essential ingredient of a successful family interview. Nurses always need to introduce themselves to patients and families. However, introductions by nurses have certainly changed from overly formal to overly casual. Just a few years ago, nurses would introduce themselves as "Miss Sanchez," whereas now a more typical introduction is "Hello, my name is Sasha and I'm your nurse today." Any introduction is better than no introduction, but as one client remarked to us, "Nurses don't introduce themselves any differently from a waiter who says 'Hi, my name is Josh and I'm your waiter tonight.' " We would encourage nurses to introduce themselves by their full names except in unique circumstances when there might be concerns of safety.

Sadly, the most serious sin of omission is the lack of introduction by nurses to their patients' family members. What inhibits or prevents nurses in hospitals, community health clinics and homecare from introducing themselves to persons at a patient's bedside? What prevents nurses from inquiring about their relationship to the patient? Worse yet, what precludes nurses from making eye contact with family members or friends, one of the most expected social norms in our culture? We have discussed this phenomenon with our nursing students and professional nurses. It has been revealed to us that the belief of "lack of time" constrains many nurses from talking with anyone but their patients for fear that visitors may "ask questions" or "require time from me that I just don't have." We would like to counter this belief by offering the suggestion that, in the end, nurses would *save* time if they would use a few manners with family members or friends. Nurses who did this would not be pursued at an even more inopportune time by someone inquiring about a family member. Nurses who have involved family members in their practice have reported that they have enjoyed greater rather than less job satisfaction (Leahey, Harper-Jaques, Stout & Levac, 1995).

Good manners also have the effect of instilling trust in family members. Richardson (1987) described seven ways in which a nurse can build trust with a patient. These seven points could really be described as "good manners" that invite a trusting relationship. They are:

1. Always call a patient by name.
2. Tell the patient your name.
3. Check your attitude.
4. Explain your role for that shift.
5. Explain a procedure before coming into the room with the equipment to do it.

6. If you tell the patient that you will be back at a certain time, keep that appointment.
7. Be honest with the patient.

KEY INGREDIENT 2: THERAPEUTIC CONVERSATION

All human interaction takes place in conversations, and nursing is one of the major networks of conversations. Nurses are always engaged in therapeutic conversations with their clients without perhaps thinking of them as such. No conversation that a nurse has with a patient or family member is trivial (Wright, Watson, & Bell, 1996). Each conversation in which we participate influences change in our own and in family members' biopsychosocial-spiritual structures.

The conversation in a brief family interview is therapeutic because from the start it is purposeful and time-limited, as are the relationships. Therapeutic conversations between a nurse and a family can be as short as one sentence or as long as time allows. All conversations between nurses and families, regardless of time, have the potential for healing through the very act of bringing the family together (Robinson & Wright, 1995; Tapp, 1997). However, it is not the length of the conversation or time that makes the most difference Rather, it is the opportunity for patients and family members to be acknowledged and affirmed that has tremendous healing potential (Tapp, 1997). Nurses are socially empowered and privileged to bring forth either health or pathology in the conversations in which they engage with families.

The art of listening is also paramount. The need to communicate what it is like to live in our individual, separate worlds of experience, particularly within the world of illness, is a powerful need in human relationships (Nichols, 1995). Frank (1998) suggests that listening to illness stories by health professionals is not only an art but an ethical practice. Frequently, nurses believe that when they listen it also entails an obligation to do something to "fix" whatever concerns or problems are raised. More often, however, the most therapeutic move, intervention, or action on the part of the nurse can be showing compassion and offering commendations.

It is the integration of task-oriented patient care with interactive, purposeful conversation that distinguishes a time-effective 15-minute (or shorter) interview. The nurse makes information giving and patient involvement in decision making an integral part of the delivery process. He or she takes advantage of opportunities and searches for opportunities to engage in purposeful conversations with families. These differ from social conversations and can include such basic ideas as:

- Families are *routinely* invited to accompany the patient to the unit, clinic, or hospital.
- Families are *routinely* included in the admission procedure.
- Families are *routinely* invited to ask questions during the patient orientation.
- Nurses acknowledge the patient's and family's expertise in managing health problem by asking about routines at home.
- Nurses encourage patients to practice how they will handle different interactions in the future, such as telling family members and others that they cannot eat certain foods.
- Nurses *routinely* consult families and patients about *their* ideas for treatment and discharge.

KEY INGREDIENT 3: FAMILY GENOGRAMS AND ECOMAPS

Nurses need to make it a priority to draw a quick genogram (and sometimes, if indicated, an ecomap) for *all* families, but particularly for families who will likely be part of their care for more than 3 days. Details for the collecting of genogram and ecomap information were given extensively in Chapter 3 in the discussion about the Structural Assessment category of the CFAM. In a brief interview, the collection of genogram and ecomap information needs to also be brief. This information can be gleaned from family members in about 2 minutes.

The most essential information to obtain includes data about ages, occupation or school grade, religion, ethnic background, migration date, and current health status of each family member. Begin by asking "easy" questions (ages, current health) of the household family members. It is not necessary or time efficient to draw out information relating to, for example, siblings' divorces or grandchildren unless it is immediately relevant to the family and health problem. Once the genogram information is obtained, if indicated, expand the data collection to obtain external family structure information in the form of an ecomap. It may be useful to ask such questions as "Who outside of your immediate family is an important resource to you? Or is a stress for you?" "How many professionals are involved in treating your husband's current heart problems?" Obtaining this structural assessment data through the genogram and ecomap also serves as a quick engagement strategy because families are usually very pleased that a nurse is asking about their entire family rather than just the person experiencing the illness. It quickly acknowledges for the family the nurse's underlying belief that illness is a family affair.

Hopefully, the genogram becomes part of the documentation about the family and patient. In one cardiac unit, the genogram information is collected on admission and the genogram is hung at the patient's bedside. Emergency telephone numbers for family members are listed on the genogram. In this way, the genogram acts as a continuous visual reminder for all healthcare professionals involved with the patient to "think family."

KEY INGREDIENT 4: THERAPEUTIC QUESTIONS

Therapeutic questions are a key, defining element in a therapeutic conversation. Many ideas and examples of linear, circular, and interventive questions were given in the presentation of the CFIM (see Chap. 4) and in the discussion of family nursing skills (see Chap. 5). When a nurse is attempting to have a very brief family meeting, there are key questions that nurses could ask family members to involve them in family healthcare. We encourage nurses to think of at least three key questions that they would routinely ask all family members. Of course, these questions need to fit the context in which the nurse encounters families. For example, the questions that a nurse may ask family members in an emergency or oncology unit in a hospital might differ from the questions that a nurse might routinely ask family members in an outpatient diabetic clinic for children. However, there are some basic themes that need to be addressed, such as the sharing of information, expectations of hospitalization, clinic or homecare visits, challenges, sufferings, and the most pressing concerns or problems. The following are some examples of questions that address these particular topics.

- With which of your family (or friends) would you like us to share information? With which ones would you not like us to share information? (Indicates alliances, resources, and possible conflictual relationships).
- How can we be most helpful to you and your family (or friends) during your hospitalization? (Clarifies expectations, increased collaboration).
- What has been most and least helpful to you in past hospitalizations or clinic visits? (Identifies past strengths and problems to avoid and successes to repeat).

- What is the greatest challenge facing your family during this hospitalization, discharge, or clinic visit? (Indicates actual or potential suffering, roles, and beliefs).
- What do you need to best prepare you or your family member for discharge? (Assists with discharge planning early).
- Who do you believe is suffering the most in your family during this hospitalization, clinic visit, or home care visit? (This identifies the family member who has the greatest need of support and intervention.)
- What is the one question you would most like to have answered during our meeting right now? (Wright, 1989). I may not be able to answer this question at the moment, but I will do my best or will try to find the answer for you. (Identifies most pressing issue or concern).
- How have I been most helpful to you in this family meeting? How could we improve? (Shows a willingness to learn from families and to work collaboratively).

KEY INGREDIENT 5: COMMENDING FAMILY AND INDIVIDUAL STRENGTHS

The important intervention of offering commendations was fully discussed in the presentation of the CFIM (see Chap. 4). We wish to restate that we routinely commend families in each session on the strengths observed during the interview. In a brief family interview of 15 minutes or less, we still endorse the practice of offering at least one or two commendations to family members of individual or family strengths, resources, or competencies that the nurse observed or were reported to the nurse. Remember that commendations are observations of behavior that occur across time. Therefore, the nurse is looking for patterns rather than a one-time occurrence that is more likely to be the offering of a compliment. An example of a commendation is: "Your family is showing much courage in living with your wife's cancer for 5 years." A compliment would be "Your son is so gentle despite feeling so ill." Families coping with chronic, life-threatening, or psychosocial problems frequently feel defeated, hopeless, or failing in their efforts to overcome the illnesses or live with them. Therefore, one can never offer too many commendations. We experience that frequently there is a "commendation-deficit disorder" with most families who are experiencing illness, disability, or trauma.

The immediate and long-term positive reactions to such commendations indicate that they are powerful, effective, and enduring therapeutic interventions. Robinson's (1998) study explored the process and outcomes of nursing interventions with families experiencing difficulties with chronic illness. The families reported the clinical nursing team's "orientation to strengths, resources, and possibilities to be an extremely important facet of the process" (Robinson, 1998, p. 284). Families who internalize commendations offered by nurses appear more receptive and trusting of the nurse-family relationship and tend to readily take up ideas, opinions, and advice that are offered.

By commending families' resources, competencies and strengths, nurses offer family members a new view of themselves. By changing the view they have of themselves, families are frequently able to look at their health problem differently and thus move toward more effective solutions to reduce any potential or actual suffering.

■■■ PERSONAL EXAMPLE OF INVOLVING FAMILY IN NURSING PRACTICE (LMW)

To poignantly illustrate how involving family members in healthcare can be both effective and healing, or ineffective and result in needless increased suffering, Lorraine M. Wright offers a personal story to illustrate the best and worst of family nursing. These experiences occurred during two very brief interactions with nurses in the emergency unit of a large city hospital while accompanying her mother for a possible admission.

> Over the last 5 years, my 77-year-old mother has experienced several major exacerbations of multiple sclerosis (MS), with frequent hospitalizations. Each exacerbation has left my mother more physically disabled. The extreme exacerbations of this last year have now left her a quadriplegic. With each exacerbation she has never returned to the level of either physical or cognitive functioning that she previously enjoyed. Currently, one of the most demoralizing aspects of this disease is the chronic pain my mother suffers in her hands. Despite all of these setbacks, there is tremendous courage on the part of both my mother and my father. Amazingly, my mother's moments of complaining, sadness, or grief have been minimal, which of course buffers other family members' suffering. I have seen my father become a very caring caregiver and "nurse" while his own life has become very constrained.
>
> On one of my mother's recent admissions to the hospital, I encountered two very brief but powerful conversations with nurses in the emergency unit of a large city hospital. One I prefer to call "Naughty Nurse" and the other "Angel Nurse." Both of these nurses had a profound impact on my emotional suffering. Both of

these nurses interacted with me for a very brief time, not more than 5 minutes each.

Before our arrival at the hospital emergency department (ED), a very exhausting few hours had been spent with my mother. My father, mother, and I were enjoying a day at our cottage about an hour out of the city. As the afternoon unfolded, it became apparent that my mother was becoming more wobbly when walking (at that time she was still able to walk a few steps with assistance). As we were packing to leave, she became unable to bear weight. With great difficulty, my father and I lifted her into her wheelchair and headed down the ramp of our cottage to the car. Now the greater challenge lay ahead of us, to get her from the wheelchair into the car. It took all of our strength and ingenuity to accomplish the task, with my mother, of course, frightened that we would drop her. After some 30 minutes and lots of perspiring, we realized our goal with my mother safely in the car. On the way into the city, we made a mutual decision to take her to the hospital where she had been admitted on previous occasions to have her assessed for possible admission. We all believed that she was having another severe exacerbation.

When we arrived at the ED, I was very relieved. It had been a very worrisome and arduous few hours. I now looked forward to my mother receiving nursing and medical assessment and treatment to assist her and us. My father waited with her in the car at the curb of the ED while I entered to seek assistance to lift my mother out of the car. On arriving at the nursing station, I encountered "Naughty Nurse." I explained the current situation to her and requested assistance to lift my mother out of the car and into the ED. "Naughty Nurse" responded in a curt, mistrusting tone by saying, "How did you get her into the car?" This initial brief interaction was shocking to me. Our initial and brief conversation was accusatory, blaming, and mistrusting of one another. No therapeutic relationship was being developed here. This nurse's response invited me to counter with an equally rude, impolite response. I said, "With great [difficulty], so we will need help to lift her out of the car." Our conversation now escalated in terms of accusations and recriminations as "Naughty Nurse" retorted, "Well, I can't lift her out of the car." I suggested that perhaps one of her male colleagues could assist us. As "Naughty Nurse" and the male colleague approached the car to assist my mother, they did not introduce themselves to my mother, nor did they discontinue their conversation with each other. This was the worst example of what family nursing should not be. By now, I was very distressed and upset by our treatment by this particular nurse. Of course, she was completely unaware that, in my professional life, I teach, practice, research, and write about family nursing.

However, all was not lost. Within a short while, we were placed in a room in the ED and, after a brief wait, "Angel Nurse" appeared.

First, she introduced herself to my mother, explained that she would be taking her blood pressure and temperature and that "blood work" had been ordered. This "Angel Nurse" competently and kindly attended to my mother, inquiring about both her medical history and her illness experiences with MS. In a very impressive manner, she reassured my mother that she would probably be admitted for another round of intravenous steroids and that everything would be done to keep her comfortable. Then she came to me, reached out her hand to shake mine, introduced herself, and warmly inquired about the nature of my relationship to the patient. I was softened by this nurse's kind and competent approach. I offered the information that I was the patient's daughter and that I was visiting from another city. Then the nurse offered a possible hypothesis in the form of a statement, "This must be very upsetting for you." In that one sentence, this nurse assessed and acknowledged my suffering. "Angel Nurse" provided comfort and understanding through her very brief interaction with me in probably less than 2 minutes. However, in just those 2 minutes, she had involved me in her practice, and healing of emotional suffering had taken place.

Later, on reflection, I realized that my reaction to this nurse's encounter with me was to make every effort to assist her in caring for my mother because I could see that she was overloaded with patients in the ED. "Angel Nurse's" particular nursing approach had encouraged me to want to be more helpful to her. Kindness invites kindness; accusations invite accusations. Perhaps not all the key ingredients that we have suggested for a brief family interview are evident in this interaction with "Angel Nurse." However, it exemplifies how the context and the appropriateness of the situation determine how much family members can be involved. This nurse beautifully demonstrated that family nursing can be done even in busy emergency units, even in 2 minutes, and still effect healing.

ACTUAL PROFESSIONAL EXAMPLE OF A BRIEF FAMILY INTERVIEW

Greta, a 32-year-old woman, was admitted to a medical unit with a questionable diagnosis of influenza. Her weight had dropped to 82 pounds, a loss of 10 pounds in the week before admission. Greta also had a genetic disease involving weakness and wasting of skeletal muscles. The nursing staff perceived her to be angry and abrupt; they also wondered what the problem was. They felt sorry for Greta and thought of her as "very dependent." A brief interview was scheduled to explore Greta's expectations, beliefs, and resources. Her family was invited to the meeting, which was held on the unit, but they did not come.

In a 15-minute interview with Greta alone, the nurse initially drew a quick genogram. She learned that Greta lived with her two younger brothers and their mother, all of whom had what Greta called "the disease" (wasting of the muscles). She was the only family member who was able to drive, and this was why the others did not attend the meeting. (This was new information for the nurse.)

The nurse then asked Greta about her expectations for the hospitalization and how the nurses could be most helpful. Greta responded to the circular questions by saying that she would know how the staff would care for her "by how they talk with me and other patients, show me respect and trust, and treat her independently." She stated that she needed to be strong to care for her brothers and mother "who depend on me."

The nurse asked Greta what hopes and expectations the other family members had for Greta's hospitalization. She replied that, when her mother had previously been hospitalized, the staff had "pushed her to eat." Greta found this very disrespectful. The nurse asked how the current staff was treating Greta's reluctance to eat. Greta described how they offered her food choices and found this quite satisfactory. The interview concluded with the nurse inviting Greta to talk more with her if she had any concerns about her care.

From this interview, the nurse revised her opinion of Greta being "very dependent" to thinking of her as someone who needed to be commended for her independence and caregiving. She now saw Greta as a "strong person" and passed this message on to her nursing colleagues.

A few days after the 15-minute interview, Greta commented to the nurse during morning care, "Remember when you told me to tell you if something wasn't going right?" She then related that the evening staff was "pushing me to eat and not respecting my choices." She had lost 1 pound. The nurse listened and remembered the morning report, in which Greta was talked about as being "manipulative." The staff members were concerned with her weight loss and therefore "pushed her" to eat more. In turn, Greta ate less.

The nurse conceptualized the problem as a vicious circular interaction (see Chap. 3) between the patient and the evening staff. She decided to intervene by:

- Inviting the dietitian to talk with the staff regarding food groups and choices
- Putting a note in the record system that Greta could "eat on demand"
- Encouraging individual members of the nursing staff to give Greta more choices of various types of food

The outcome of this brief family-oriented interview and interventions was that Greta gained some weight over the course of hospitalization. The other staff nurses said that they felt "less responsible for making Greta eat" and more responsible for offering her choices and promoting her independence. Most significant to the primary nurse was the intervention used in the unit documentation system in which she identified the problem, proved a rationale, and recommended direction for other staff members.

From our perspective, an important outcome was that Greta's skills and competencies to manage and live with her chronic illness were reinforced. She went home stronger both physically and emotionally. In addition, she was able to assist herself and other family members with ongoing health issues. This 15-minute interview also indicates how nurses can include other family members in the therapeutic conversation even if the members are not present. Involving family members in nursing practice includes inquiring about them whether they are present or not.

▪▪▪ CONCLUSION

In conclusion, an overall framework for a 15-minute (or shorter) family interview is:

1. Use manners to engage or reengage. Introduce yourself by offering your name and role. Orient family members to the purpose of a brief family interview.
2. Assess key areas of internal and external structure and function—obtain genogram information and key external support data.
3. Ask three key questions of family members.
4. Commend the family on one or two strengths.
5. Evaluate usefulness and conclude.

We generally find this framework a useful guide when conducting a 15-minute (or shorter) family interview. However, these key ingredients of a brief family interview need to be adapted according to the competence of the nurse, the context in which nurses and families encounter one another, and the appropriateness and purpose of the family meeting. We are confident that, if the interview is suitably implemented, nurses and families will both be satisfied with the usefulness of a brief family interview. Nurses can and do reduce families' physical, emotional, and spiritual suffering by engaging in therapeutic conversations with family members. This can occur in 15 minutes or even in one sentence!

▮▮▮ REFERENCES

Boscolo, L., & Bertrando, P. (1993). *The times of time: A new perspective in systemic therapy and consultation.* New York: Norton.

Frank, A. (1998). Just listening: Narrative and deep illness *Families, Systems, and Health, 16*(3), 197–212.

Hupcey, J. E. (1998). Establishing the nurse-family relationship in the intensive care unit. *Western Journal of Nursing Research, 20*(2), 180–194.

Leahey, M., Harper-Jaques, S., Stout, L., and Levac, A. M. (1995). The impact of a family systems nursing approach: Nurses' perceptions. *The Journal of Continuing Education in Nursing, 25*(5), 219–225.

Martin, J. (1983). *Miss Manners' guide to excruciatingly correct behavior.* New York: Warner Books.

Nichols, M. P. (1995). *The lost art of listening.* New York: Guilford Press.

Remen, N. R. (1996). *Kitchen table wisdom.* New York: Riverhead Books.

Richardson, B. K. (1987, March). 7 ways to win your patient's trust. *Nursing87,* 14–15.

Robinson, C. A., & Wright, L. M. (1995). Family nursing interventions: What families say makes a difference. *Journal of Family Nursing, 1*(3), 327–345.

Tapp, D. M. (1997). *Exploring therapeutic conversations between nurses and families experiencing ischemic heart disease.* Unpublished doctoral dissertation, University of Calgary, Calgary, Alberta, Canada.

Wright, L. M. (1989). When clients ask questions: Enriching the therapeutic conversation. *Family Therapy Networker, 13*(6), 15–16.

Wright, L. M., Watson, W. L., & Bell, J. M. *Beliefs: The heart of healing in families and illness.* New York: Basic Books.

CHAPTER 9

How to Document Family Interviews

It is very important for the nurse to devise a workable, efficient system for integrating, recording, and documenting the large amount of complex data gathered in the family interviews. Such a system provides the nurse with an organized and clear overview of the family. Using this overview, the nurse can decide which are key issues to focus on and which issues are tangential. With an organized recording system, the nurse is able to move back and forth from macroscopic to microscopic data, and the family receives more holistic healthcare. Having an organized documentation system is particularly germane in today's healthcare delivery climate of downsized hospital facilities, increased healthcare networks, and proliferation of managed care ventures. There is an emphasis on capitation, decreased financial resources, decreased beds, shorter hospital stays, and limited staff time. Therefore, there is even more necessity for efficient documentation and useful communication between nurses to achieve helpful family nursing.

The purpose of this chapter is to discuss how to integrate and record data obtained from families and from the nurse's own interpretations and observations. The nurse's impression of a family interview is addressed first. How to examine the data and use both the Calgary Family Assessment Model (CFAM) and the Calgary Family Intervention Model (CFIM) are discussed. A list of strengths and problems, an initial assessment summary, and an intervention plan are also detailed. The use of progress notes for integrating and recording hypotheses, interventions, and family responses is addressed. How to record a discharge synopsis is presented. The issue of confidentiality of records is also discussed.

▪▪▪ INITIAL IMPRESSIONS, OBSERVATIONS, AND RESPONSES

There are usually several factors that affect the nurse's first response to an initial family interview. External factors might include how cold or warm the interview room is, how dirty or clean it is, how noisy the surrounding area is, and so forth. Internal factors have an even more profound influence on the nurse's evaluation. Inherent within each nurse are his or her self-image, beliefs, mores, prejudices, attitudes, and past personal and professional experiences, as well as his or her unique way of perceiving other individuals. These internal factors strongly influence the nurse's response to a family.

The nurse's response must be recognized as important data. Too often in the past, nurses have striven for a purely clinical response to an individual or a family. They were either embarrassed or ashamed, or most likely did not recognize how their personal thoughts and feelings influenced their clinical judgment. We recommend that nurses consciously take a few minutes after an interview to blurt out (to themselves) personal initial reactions to a family interview. These quick "gut reactions" can be dealt with as the nurse formally starts to integrate the data. In our experience, interviewers who are able to quickly acknowledge their personal reactions about a family have a far easier time integrating the data. The *unacknowledged* initial hypotheses or responses, if not addressed, are the most mischievous and can be the seedbed of disrespect and a judgmental attitude toward families.

The following case scenario illustrates a nurse's initial reactions to a family interview. The family is composed of the husband, Leroy Hamilton, age 28, who is a roofer; the wife, Melvina, age 27, who works part-time for a dry cleaner; and the children, Junior, age 3, and Vicki, age 9 months. The couple has been married for 6 years. When Junior was examined in the outpatient clinic, his speech was found to be approximately 8 months delayed and it was noted that he was small for his age. The nurse also noticed the difficulty that the mother had in controlling Junior when he was running up and down the halls. After the clinic session, the interdisciplinary team made the following plans: the physician would continue with the physical investigations; the nurse would arrange for a family interview to discuss Junior's difficulties; and the team would reconvene for a conference in 2 weeks.

Mr. and Mrs. Hamilton, Junior, and Vicki attended the initial interview. During the interview, it was revealed that Mr. Hamilton's parents were interfering with the children's upbringing and that Mrs. Hamilton was upset by this interference. More of the story will unfold throughout this chapter. Immediately after the interview, the nurse said to herself:

- So much crying! I would have been so frustrated with Vicki. I could never have been so nice to her as Mrs. Hamilton was! Mr. Hamilton never once offered to take the baby or help out.
- The poor parents, they have so many problems with their extended family. No wonder they feel "maybe we're doing something wrong as parents."
- They are awfully critical of Junior and never had a good word to say about him.

- But Junior's friendly. Gave me a hug on the way out.
- They jump around a lot in their conversation. I am not sure what really is the issue, Junior's misbehavior or his problem with eating. They never mentioned his delayed speech.

In voicing these initial impressions and reactions, the nurse was able to express her own anxiety and feelings of empathy, compassion, and frustration. She was also reminded of her own family and how her ex-husband, who was Korean, worked excessively long hours and did little to support her when their infant was crying. The nurse also remembered how her Korean mother-in-law was very "controlling" when she tried to be what she called "helpful." The nurse was aware, therefore, that she had to guard against a tendency to feel overly sympathetic toward the wife and overly critical toward the husband.

In summary, we recommend that nurses acknowledge their feelings and immediate reactions, impressions, and observations of family members. After doing so, they can decide to either discard these beliefs or feelings or use them appropriately. For example, the nurse *used* her own initial impressions of the Hamiltons in the following methodical way:

- The baby's prolonged crying may stimulate frustration in the father and Junior. I'll explore this in the future.
- Given the relationship with their extended family, the parents are probably exquisitely sensitive to being blamed. I must watch my tone of voice and choice of words so that I don't inadvertently blame them.
- Junior's hugs may indicate that he's hungry for attention. It would be inappropriate for him to receive much attention from me because I'm not available to him consistently. Also, the parents may feel that I'm usurping their position if I give him lots of praise. I'll try to encourage the parents to do this.
- The parents are quite concerned but seem to be under a lot of stress. Maybe that's why the conversation jumped around a lot. I'll try to keep the next interview more focused.

Having acknowledged her initial impressions, the nurse can proceed to review the content *and* process of the interview by using CFAM. The content of the interview refers to the concrete communication; the "what" is stated. The process refers to the "how," implying movement. Process is a dynamic concept, whereas content is static. The process is not the activity *per se*, but the way in which the activity is carried out. An example of *content* from the Hamilton interview is the description of the grandparents' interfering with the couple's management of the children. The *process* of the discussion was that Mrs. Hamilton became sad and tearful and her husband tried to minimize the problem: "Ah, she gets too emotional with the folks all the time. The best thing is to forget about what they say and live your own life."

▪▪▪ RECORDING SYSTEM

There are many different kinds of tools a nurse can use to record family interviews. Some are fairly specific, whereas others are more general. The ideal recording tool should, above all, be consistent with the nurse's interviewing practice. That is, if the thrust of the family interview is to obtain information about medication compliance, then considerable space should be allocated for this data. Second, the record should provide an integrated picture of family strengths and problems. Too much emphasis on problems or constraints can lead to too much involvement and intrusion by the nurse. It can also foster dependency on the part of the family. Third, an assessment record should be a springboard for developing an intervention plan. Isolated bits of information, such as "the mother is experiencing depression" or "the father is unemployed" need to be drawn together into a composite picture. Strengths need to be linked to the problem so that they can be used as resources for problem solving. From this integrated picture, a plan of action emerges. Without this picture, the deficiencies and gaps in the data are obscured. Last, the recording system should be one that the nurse interviewer can easily use. Most nurses have heavy workloads and become frustrated if they have to fill out lengthy forms.

The recording system that we recommend is fairly general. It can be adapted to almost any agency's or hospital's philosophy and any style of nursing practice, and it can be computerized. The system consists of six parts:

1. CFAM
2. Strengths and problems list
3. Family assessment summary
4. CFIM
5. Progress notes
6. Discharge summary

Before dealing with each part separately, we would like to emphasize strongly the conceptual skills that are involved in integrating the data after an interview. Nurses must think in a critical, analytical, and interpretive fashion to integrate data; that is, they must sort through all the information and generate ideas about its meaning. They must distinguish between observation and inference. They must be willing to entertain hypotheses and equally willing to discard them as new data emerge that are inconsistent with their first hypothesis. In deciding which information to include and which to discard, nurses engage in the processes of deliberation, judgment, and discrimination. The task of integrating and recording the data is not an easy one. It requires intellectual discipline.

HOW TO USE THE CALGARY FAMILY ASSESSMENT MODEL

As we discussed in Chapter 3, the CFAM is an integrated conceptual framework consisting of three major categories: structural, developmental, and functional. Each category contains several subcategories. It is useful to conceptualize the three assessment categories and the many subcategories as a branching diagram (Fig. 9–1 and inside back cover). As nurses use the subcategories on the right of the branching diagram, they collect more and more microscopic data. It is important for nurses to be able to move back and forth on the diagram to draw together all relevant information into an integrated assessment. For example, the nurse may explore boundary issues in depth with a family. The nurse thus obtains microscopic data within the structural category of the assessment model, and needs to be able to integrate this with other data within the diagram. Isolated microscopic statements such as "The parental subsystem has a diffuse boundary" have little meaning and are of limited help in devising an intervention plan. In combination with other data, however, this statement may become particularly rich and meaningful: "The parental subsystem has had a diffuse boundary since Sanjita was born with Down syndrome and the grandmother began to care for her." In this example, structural, developmental, and functional data are combined:

- Structural: parental subsystem diffuse boundary
- Developmental: stage of families with young children
- Functional: grandmother assumes parenting role

After an initial interview, it is important for the nurse to mentally review each category. In this way, the nurse gains a macroscopic view of the family.

After reviewing the family structure outline (the top branch of Fig. 9–1), the nurse should examine the family genogram and ecomap. This will help the nurse to conceptualize *this particular family* and how it differs from or is similar to other families. The Hamilton family, for example, is a young, nuclear, working-class family with the mother working part-time and the father working full-time. The family bound-

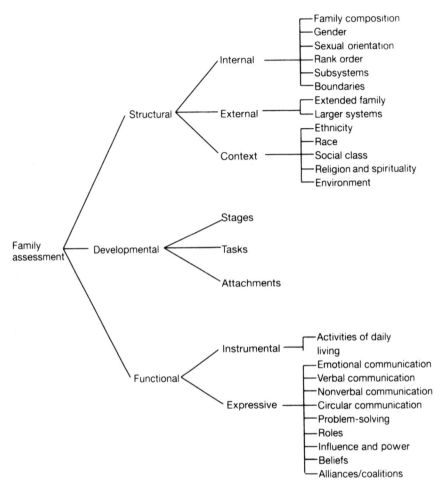

FIGURE 9–1. Branching diagram of CFAM.

ary seems fairly permeable, with much interface with the extended families of origin. Subsystem boundaries are clear.

In addition to an understanding of the family structure, who is in it and how they fit into their context, the nurse requires an understanding of how *this* family came to be at *this* stage in its developmental life cycle (Box 9–1). We recommend that the nurse review the stages and tasks appropriate to the family's specific developmental life cycle (e.g., Table 9–1; see also Tables 3–4 through 3–7). Also, we suggest that the nurse draw a diagram illustrating family attachments. The Hamilton family attachment diagram is given later in this chapter.

BOX 9–1. THE DEVELOPMENTAL CATEGORY OF CFAM: SAMPLE FAMILY LIFE CYCLE VARIATIONS

- Middle-class North American
- Divorce and postdivorce
- Remarried and stepfamily
- Professional and low-income
- Adoptive
- Other types

While reviewing the developmental category, the nurse can identify the normative as well as the crisis issues that the family dealt with during each stage. For example, the Hamilton family is currently in Stage 3 (Families with Young Children). They have adjusted the marital system to make space for children. During Stage 2, they had to deal with the unexpected death of Mrs. Hamilton's brother. This influenced their marital relationship by creating emotional distance between the couple. Also, the relationships with their families of origin were not adequately defined during Stage 2. These past difficulties in Stage 2 are having repercussions for task achievement in Stage 3. Hence, they are of current significance.

After mentally examining the CFAM structural and developmental categories, the nurse can review the family functioning category. This third CFAM category is detailed in Box 9–2.

For the Hamilton family, the nurse can identify strengths as well as difficulties in the area of expressive functioning, particularly emotional and circular communication; influence and power; and coalitions.

The nurse need not be too microscopic in the review of CFAM categories. If the nurse uses too many subcategories, she may become overwhelmed by the complexity of the data. It is important for the nurse to maintain a macroscopic, integrated metaview of the family. After the nurse has used the CFAM several times, the categories will be familiar.

HOW TO DEVELOP A STRENGTHS AND PROBLEMS LIST

Having reviewed the CFAM, the nurse should identify family strengths and problems in the structural, developmental, and functional catego-

TABLE 9–1.
THE STAGES OF THE FAMILY LIFE CYCLE

Family Life Cycle Stage	Emotional Process of Transition: Key Principles	Second-Order Changes in Family Status Required to Proceed Developmentally
1. Leaving home; single young adults	Accepting emotional and financial responsibility for self	1. Differentiation of self in relation to family of origin 2. Development of intimate peer relationships 3. Establishment of self re: work and financial independence
2. The joining of families through marriage; the new couple	Commitment to new system	1. Formation of marital system 2. Realignment of relationships with extended families and friends to include spouse
3. Families with young children	Accepting new members into the system	1. Adjusting marital system to make space for child(ren) 2. Joining in childrearing, financial, and household tasks 3. Realignment of relationships with extended family to include parenting and grandparenting roles
4. Families with adolescents	Increasing flexibility of family boundaries to include children's independence and grandparents' frailties	1. Shifting of parent-child relationships to permit adolescent to move in and out of system 2. Refocus on midlife marital and career issues 3. Beginning shift toward caring for older generation
5. Launching children and moving on	Accepting a multitude of exits from and entries into the family system	1. Renegotiation of marital system as a dyad 2. Development of adult-to-adult relationships between grown children and their parents

(continued)

TABLE 9–1. *(continued)*
THE STAGES OF THE FAMILY LIFE CYCLE

Family Life Cycle Stage	Emotional Process of Transition: Key Principles	Second-Order Changes in Family Status Required to Proceed Developmentally
		3. Realignment of relationships to include in-laws and grandchildren
		4. Dealing with disabilities and death of parents (grandparents)
6. Families in later life	Accepting the shifting of generational roles	1. Maintaining own and couple functioning and interests in face of physiological decline; exploration of new familial and social role options
		2. Support for a more central role of middle generation
		3. Making room in the system for the wisdom and experience of the elderly, supporting the older generation without overfunctioning for them
		4. Dealing with loss of spouse, siblings, and other peers and preparing for own death. Life review and integration

Source: Carter, B., & McGoldrick, M. (Eds.) (1999). *The expanded family life cycle: Individual, family and social perspectives* (3rd ed.). Boston: Allyn and Bacon, p. 2. Copyright © 1999 by Allyn & Bacon. Reprinted by permission.

ries. Using the interview data, the nurse should prepare a strengths and problems list and indicate issues at whatever system level the nurse presently conceptualizes them. Thus, the nurse will have completed three steps in integrating the assessment data:

1. Review the CFAM.
2. Identify strengths and problems.
3. List strengths and problems according to system level.

BOX 9–2. FUNCTIONAL CATEGORY OF THE CFAM FAMILY FUNCTIONING

A. Instrumental
  1. Activities of daily living
B. Expressive
  1. Emotional communication
    a. Types of emotions
    b. Range of emotions
  2. Verbal communication
    a. Direct versus displaced
    b. Clear versus masked
  3. Nonverbal communication
    a. Types
    b. Sequencing
  4. Circular communication
  5. Problem solving
    a. Identification patterns
    b. Instrumental versus emotional problems
    c. Solution patterns
    d. Evaluation process
  6. Roles
    a. Role flexibility
    b. Formal versus informal
  7. Influence or power
    a. Instrumental
    b. Psychological
    c. Corporal
  8. Beliefs
    a. Family expectations or goals
    b. Family beliefs about problems
    c. Family beliefs about change
  9. Alliances and coalitions
    a. Directionality, balance, and intensity
    b. Triangles

Various systems levels are indicated on the strengths and problems list. Community–whole-family system refers to the relationship between the family and its neighborhood or community. A problem at this system level might be, for example, that the family members are isolated and have been made scapegoats by the community because of their race. The professional–whole-family system level depicts the relationship between the family and healthcare providers in particular but also with other professionals such as teachers or clergy. A strength at this system level might be, for example, that the family and the home-care service have developed a cooperative working relationship.

The next system level is that of the nurse and the whole family. This level depicts the nature of the relationship between the nurse and the family. The relationship could be one of naive trust, disenchantment, guarded alliance (Thorne & Robinson, 1989), or one of the other types discussed in Chapter 6. The whole-family system level refers to interactions among all family members. The marital subsystem designates issues pertaining to the couple as marital partners or as parents. The parent-child system level refers to issues between the children and the parents. The sibling subsystem depicts the relationship issues among brothers and sisters. The individual systems level refers to the biological, psychological, and social issues pertaining to individual family members.

Family strengths are very important to note. They can be used effectively to enhance family life. More specifically, they can be linked to problems and used as effective resources in problem solving. It is crucial to ask the family what they believe their particular strengths are versus the nurse arbitrarily categorizing a family's strengths. For example, if during the interview the nurse asked Rajesh, in the presence of his family, what his wife did that was most helpful for him since he had his stroke, the nurse could note this in the documentation. Some typical family strengths include:

- The ability to provide for the physical, emotional, and spiritual needs of the family members.
- The ability to be sensitive to the needs of the family members
- The ability to communicate thoughts and feelings effectively
- The ability to provide support, security, and encouragement
- The ability to initiate and maintain growth-producing relationships and experiences within and outside the family
- The capacity to maintain and create constructive and responsible community relationships
- The ability to grow with and through children
- The ability to perform family roles flexibly
- The ability for self-help and to accept help when appropriate
- The capacity for mutual respect for the individuality of family members
- The ability to use a crisis experience as a means of growth
- The concern for family unity, loyalty, and interfamily cooperation

In developing a strengths and problems list, the nurse should acknowledge major structural, developmental, and functional issues that are presently affecting *family* interaction. The nurse should not try to make a perfect list, but rather strive to identify the major issues. Problems frequently overlap several systems levels. It is often difficult, therefore, to differentiate whole-family problems from marital issues and from individual difficulties. Under which system level a problem is placed is quite arbitrary. It does have significance, however, in that it guides which interventions are chosen. For example, a nurse could identify Mrs. Hamilton's sadness as an individual problem and list it as depression. Most likely, the intervention for this problem would be medication or individual therapy. However, if the problem of sadness is identified as "difficulty with emotional communication" and is listed as a marital issue, the intervention would be different. It would probably involve marital intervention to help both partners meet their needs.

We strongly recommend that beginning nurse interviewers *first* attempt to identify as many *family* strengths and problems as possible. That is, they should initially restrain themselves from listing issues under the individual category level. We find that this helps nurses to "think family." Nurses are often very accustomed to thinking of individual issues, such as the father's alcoholism or the mother's anxiety. They need to reconceptualize these problems at a higher system level if they are to deal with the *family*. Some questions we recommend that nurses ask themselves to assist in this conceptualization include:

- Who is most affected by (e.g., the father's drinking)?
- How does that person attempt to influence the father?
- Who supports that person in attempting to influence the father?
- Who does not support that person's attempts to influence the father?

By thinking through these questions, the nurse will start to conceptualize the father's individual issue as a whole-family system or marital system problem.

Although we strongly recommend family assessment and intervention, we do not subscribe to the view that *all* issues are family centered, however. Major physical, psychological, and social issues that are primarily personal in origin are listed under the individual category level. For example, Junior Hamilton's delayed speech and short stature are listed as individual problems. Mrs. Hamilton's sadness, on the other hand, is conceptualized as a marital issue, "difficulty with emotional communication." It is therefore listed under the marital system level. Her interest and concern about being a good parent are also listed under the marital and parental system levels and not under the individual level.

Table 9–2 shows a sample strengths and problems list for the Hamilton family.

TABLE 9–2.
STRENGTHS AND PROBLEMS LIST FOR THE HAMILTON FAMILY
Family name: Hamilton   Date

Subsystems	Strengths	Problems
Community—whole family system	• Grandparents a possible support	• Unresolved conflict with both families of origin • Isolated—five moves in 3 years
Professionals—whole family system	• Engaged with pediatric clinic	• Reluctant to ask for information concerning Junior's health problems
Nurse—whole family system	• Guarded alliance	
Whole family system	• Strong beliefs: "We're survivors," "special family"	
Marital/parental subsystem	• Care about each other • Concerned about being good parents	• Difficulty with emotional communication—Melvina sad, shows helplessness. Leroy disconfirms.
Parent-child subsystem	• Able to bond with Vicki • Father can be positive with Junior	• Difficulty with behavior controls • Unrealistic expectations of a 3 1/2-year-old with new sibling • Isolation of Junior
Sibling subsystem	• At clinic Junior can be positive with Vicki	• Intense rivalry reported
Individual systems		• Junior—speech delay of 8 months, small stature

When the nurse has identified the strengths and problems of the family, she can begin to analyze the relationship of the family's strengths to its problems. For example, in the Hamilton family's strengths and problems list, the unresolved conflict between the couple and the grandparents is identified. Thus, the nurse should think about the following questions, "What is the relationship between the strengths and the problems?" "Is there a way that the strength can be used to deal with the problem?"

With the Hamiltons, the nurse hypothesized that the grandparents were genuinely concerned about Junior and the family but demonstrated their concern in a way that exacerbated the problem rather than helped it. The grandparents tended to interfere by offering advice, and the couple had not found ways to deal with this.

In evaluating the strengths and problems list, the nurse decided to leave the apparent conflictual data on the list. She reasoned that this would help her to maintain a neutral stance vis-à-vis the grandparents. Furthermore, it would help her to keep a metaperspective on the Hamilton family situation. Should the nurse and the couple decide in the future to invite the grandparents for a joint family interview, the nurse would be aware of the boundary issue between the generations.

Having considered the relationship between family strengths and problems, the nurse should attempt to prioritize the concerns. The nurse and the family will have already collaborated on this during the interview. We recommend, however, that the nurse reflect again after completing the strengths and problems list. In our experience with beginning family interviewers, we have found that they often become overly enthusiastic and "change oriented" when they are integrating and recording the data. Not every family needs intervention. Nor do all problems require resolution. Rather, some problems or illnesses require adjustment and others invite us to accept and "live with them." We therefore strongly urge nurses to concentrate on the *presenting* issue. With the Hamilton family, the parents' priority concern was their difficulty in controlling Junior's behavior.

HOW TO SUMMARIZE THE FAMILY ASSESSMENT

Although the strength and problems list is a useful working tool, it does not provide a sufficient summary of the family assessment. It would probably be too cryptic and fragmented for the rest of the nursing and healthcare team to use in delivering service to a family. Box 9–3 outlines a family assessment summary. Box 9–4 presents a sample family assessment summary of the Hamilton family.

BOX 9–3. OUTLINE OF A FAMILY ASSESSMENT SUMMARY

Family Name: _____ Date: _____
Family Members Present at Interview: _____
Interviewer: _____
Place of Interview: _____

I. Referral Route and Presenting Problem
One or two sentences summarizing reason for referral and referral source.

II. Family Composition
Draw a genogram. Include name, age, and occupation or school grade for each member of the family. Circle those currently living at home.

III. Family Attachment
Draw an attachment diagram. Indicate the strength and nature of the bonding among family members.

IV. Pertinent History (very brief and relevant to presenting problem)
a. Chronological sequence of events leading to current presenting problem. Include previous solutions to cope with the problem and professional help sought.
b. Developmental history of the family, including pertinent information re: families of origin and significant personal, social, vocational, and medical events.

V. Strengths and Problems
Identify family strengths. List family problems (structural, developmental, and functional) and individual problems (physical, psychological, and social) at their appropriate system levels.

VI. Hypothesis/Summary
Summarize the connections between the initial hypothesis, presenting problems, pertinent history, and family strengths. If necessary, refine the hypothesis to provide directions for intervention.

VII. Goals and Plans
Indicate plans for interventions, referral, or discharge. Indicate family's reaction and the outcome.

VIII. Signature

Box 9-4.   FAMILY ASSESSMENT SUMMARY: THE HAMILTON FAMILY

Family Name: <u>Hamilton</u>   Date: <u>1/4</u>

Family Members Present at Interview: <u>Whole Family</u>

Interviewer: <u>Anne Marie Levac, RN, BS</u>

Place of Interview: <u>Children's Hospital</u>

I. Referral Route and Presenting Problem
    Junior Hamilton, age 3½, and his mother were identified at the Pediatric
    Outpatient Clinic by myself and Dr. Carpenter as needing a family assessment.
    The mother had difficulty controlling his behavior (running up and down the halls)
    and appeared extremely upset.

II. Family Composition
    The family is composed of husband, Leroy, 28, a roofer; wife, Melvina, 27, who
    works part-time in a dry cleaners; and children, Junior, 3½, and Vicki, 9 months.

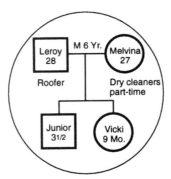

III. Family Attachment

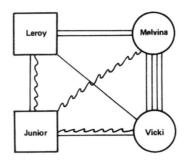

IV. Pertinent History
    Junior: Normal pregnancy and delivery and milestones to age 34 months. Speech
    delay of 8 months and small stature. Complete history on Dr. Carpenter's report.
    Family: When Junior was approximately 1 year old, parents began to have
    difficulty controlling his behavior, that is, spreading feces, refusing to listen, and
    being a picky eater. Tried toilet training him at 13 months and have tried punishing
    him by sending to his room, getting him to help clean up the mess, and spanking.
    Have also visited two other pediatric clinics for the same complaints. Report these
    visits were "not helpful."
      The couple has been married for 6 years, no separations, five moves within the
    past 3 years (two between cities). Mother's brother died when Junior was 1 year old.
    Both families of origin are heavily involved in giving conflicting advice.

Continued

FAMILY ASSESSMENT SUMMARY: THE HAMILTON FAMILY
(Continued)

V. Strengths/Problems
 a. Community–Whole Family System
  1. Strengths
   Extended family interested. The grandparents might be available as a source of support.
  2. Problems
   (a). Unresolved conflict with both families of origin. The paternal grandparents live outside of the city but see the family about once a month. They telephone frequently and, according to both parents, imply that the children are not being raised properly. Melvina in particular feels angry at them for interfering. The maternal grandparents live in the city and, although they do not interfere as much with regard to the children, seem to imply that Melvina is not a competent mother. She apparently was overprotected as a child and feels resentful that her parents now seem to favor her sister-in-law. The couple has not found helpful ways of dealing with their anger toward their parents.
   (b). Isolation. The family has moved five times in 3 years and has no close neighbors or friends.
 b. Professionals–Whole Family System
  1. Strengths
   The family engaged readily with Pediatric Clinic. The father took time off work without pay to attend.
  2. Problems
   The parents lack information about Junior's health problems.
 c. Nurse–Whole Family System
  1. Strengths
   The parents asked about my qualifications and areas of expertise. They responded fairly quickly to a collaborative approach. We developed a guarded alliance given their feelings of mistrust with previous nurses.
 d. Whole Family System
  1. Strengths
   Family believes they are "special." They have overcome adversity in the past (e.g., unemployment, automobile accident) and are proud of being "survivors."
 e. Marital/Parental System
  1. Strengths
   Concerned re: good parenting. The couple cares a tremendous amount for each other and are concerned about being good parents.
  2. Problems
   Difficulty with emotional communication. Since the mother's brother's death, the couple has had difficulty communicating emotionally. Mrs. H. reports that her brother was "the only person we could talk to." She is sad, feels inadequate as a mother, and tends to share this by crying or expressing her helplessness. How this affects her husband is not clearly known at this time. He responds to his wife by overprotecting her, not confirming what she says, or trying to talk her out of it. This perpetuates her feelings of inadequacy. The couple report not having a satisfactory emotional relationship.

Continued

FAMILY ASSESSMENT SUMMARY: THE HAMILTON FAMILY
(Continued)

f. Parent-Child System
   1. Strengths
      Ability to bond. The couple has been able to bond adequately with Vicki. The father can be positive with Junior and seems interested in him. The father is very concrete but seems willing to learn.
   2. Problems
      Difficulty with behavioral controls. Junior seems confused about behavioral limits and tends to act up. When he does test, his father responds by becoming frustrated and ignoring him or withdrawing. His mother feels overwhelmed, and both parents focus on the negative rather than on the positive. They have limited knowledge of normal growth and development.
g. Sibling Subsystem
   1. Strengths
      Sharing. Junior can be positive with Vicki as was evidenced with he gave her an appropriate toy during the family interview.
   2. Problems
      Intense rivalry. Junior has placed feces in Vicki's crib, bites her, pushes her, and so forth. During the family interview, no negative behavior was noticed.
h. Individual System
   1. Strengths
      Peer interaction. Junior has been attending nursery school for 3 months and according to his mother is reported to be doing well although his speech is delayed.
   2. Problems
      Health. Junior has a speech delay of 8 months. He is below the third percentile in height.

VI. Hypothesis/Summary
   Junior Hamilton, $3^1/2$, and his parents present with difficulty controlling his behavior. The problem has existed for $2^1/2$ years. One hypothesis is that the parents, unaware of normal child development, use age-inappropriate techniques. It is also hypothesized that a precipitating factor was the unexpected death of Mrs. Hamilton's brother, a close confidant of both Mr. and Mrs. Hamilton. Although the couple stated that they tried to separate their own feelings and not to displace them onto the children, it is my hypothesis that when Mrs. H. is feeling sad, she handles this by getting angry with Junior. Mr. H. "gets after" Junior particularly when he sees his wife upset. Vicki seems to stimulate and receive positive feelings from the parents while Junior encourages and receives negative feelings. The children seem triangulated into the marriage.

VII. Goals and Plans
   a. The parents and Junior agreed to meet for four sessions to learn how to manage Junior's behavior.
   b. Joint meeting with parents, Dr. Carpenter, and myself set for January 19 to discuss Junior's health, that is, short stature, delayed speech, and normal growth and development.

VIII. Signature: <u>Anne Marie Levac, RN, BS</u>

It is in the family assessment summary that the nurse must synthesize theory and practice. All the isolated questions and answers discussed in the interview are woven into a synthetic pattern. For example, the nurse hypothesized that the Hamilton couple had a helpful symmetrical relationship when they were both able to share emotionally with Mrs. Hamilton's brother. Since his death, they have had difficulty with emotional communication. They are attempting now to have a complementary relationship with each other, whereby Mrs. Hamilton cries and expresses her feelings to her husband. It is her expectation that he in turn should provide her with support. He attempts to do this by joking around with her. However, this does not help to alleviate her sadness. Thus, they are experiencing tension in their relationship. The nurse identified this pattern and discussed it as a problem under the marital system level in the family assessment summary.

HOW TO DEVELOP AN INTERVENTION PLAN

When the nurse has reviewed the CFAM, identified and listed the family's strengths and problems, and prepared an assessment, he or she should develop an intervention plan. We have found the following three steps helpful when we develop intervention plans in our clinical practice:

1. Identify specific problems.
2. Review the CFIM.
3. Choose interventions.

Each of these steps is discussed separately.

Identify Specific Problems

The intervention plan that the nurse creates will depend on the severity and complexity of the family's problems and the richness of their strengths. A problem list that indicates mild problems may reflect a family coping with a normal developmental crisis or a transient situation. If the problem list, however, suggests severe family issues, it is essential that the nurse recognize the gravity of the situation and not offer placebos or unrealistic interim solutions for conditions that require more expert assistance. In these situations, the nurse may wish to refer the family for more specialized assistance. Suggestions for how to refer are given in Chapters 5 and 10.

If the nurse is going to continue to work with the family, however, the nurse and the family should identify specific target problems. Priorities need to be set. It is generally unwise for the clinician to move too quickly to work on marital issues unless the couple has specifically asked for help in this area. A rule of thumb is to start with the presenting issue and try to influence the most change in the system; that is, the nurse should promote change where the maximum benefit will be realized by all family members. With the Hamilton family, the nurse and parents chose to work on controlling Junior's behavior because that was an area that concerned both parents. Also, it would enable the nurse to bring the couple together to discuss their feelings and beliefs about childrearing. In this way, the nurse would be indirectly fostering emotional communication between the spouses. In addition, she planned to have sessions with the father, the mother, and Junior to foster positive feedback. The nurse reasoned that if they had to travel to and from the pediatric clinic by themselves (without Vicki), Junior would be likely to receive more attention. Thus, by choosing to work on behavioral controls, the nurse was stimulating change at several levels: whole-family system, parent-child subsystem, and marital and parental subsystem.

Review the Calgary Family Intervention Model

The nurse reviews the CFIM to stimulate her ideas about change and match interventions to the particular domain of family functioning: cognitive, affective, or behavioral. As we know from our own clinical practice, some interventions work better with some families than with others. It is desirable to address the specificity question: that is, "What intervention will most effect change with this particular problem with this particular family at this particular time?"

We encourage nurses to review the CFIM, the intersection of domains of family functioning and intervention (Fig. 9–2) before deciding on a specific intervention or group of interventions. We have found in our own clinical work that sometimes we are biased toward one particular domain of family functioning (e.g., cognitive or affective) and

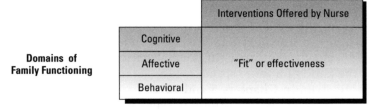

Figure 9–2. CFIM: Intersection of domains of family functioning and interventions.

thus are most likely (as a result of our own biases) to choose certain interventions whether or not they match the family's style of relating. Over the years of clinical practice, we have also become more aware of how ethnicity, race, class and other diversity issues influence the effectiveness of interventions. Thus, we review the following before choosing a particular intervention for a particular family situation:

- Questions as interventions
- Interventions directed at the cognitive domain of family functioning
- Interventions directed at the affective domain of family functioning
- Interventions directed at the behavioral domain of family functioning

When the nurse chooses interventions, we recommend that he or she choose those that best match the problem that the nurse and the family have agreed to change. The nurse and the Hamilton family agreed to meet for three sessions to increase their skill in managing Junior's behavior.

Another consideration in choosing an intervention is to pick one that flows from the nurse's hypothesis. Some interventions are more effective than others in bringing about change. One of the nurse's hypotheses with the Hamiltons was that Junior was negatively triangulated into the marital subsystem. Thus she decided to choose interventions that would establish a more firm marital boundary while at the same time promoting effective parental controls of Junior's behavior.

A further consideration in choosing interventions is to find those that match the family's strengths. We believe that families have tremendous resources to solve their own problems and that intervention by outsiders should be kept to a minimum. The nurse, in working with the Hamiltons, was aware of their belief about themselves as "special." They took pride in the fact that they were "survivors" and had overcome such adversity as unemployment after a serious motor vehicle accident. The nurse decided to build on such strengths in co-constructing the intervention plan with them.

A final consideration when choosing interventions is to pick those that match the nurse's competence level. We have discussed in Chapters 5 and 7 ideas for nurses to consider when evaluating their own competence level.

Choose Interventions

The following is a sample intervention plan for the Hamilton family.

> *Problem: Parent-Child System: Difficulty with Behavioral Control.* The nurse decided to have a meeting with Mr. and Mrs. Hamilton to discuss normal 3-year-old child behavior, how to set limits,

and how to positively reinforce good behavior. The nurse chose interventions aimed at the following domains:

Cognitive Domain. The nurse thought of recommending books to the parents on behavior management skills if they were interested in reading on this topic.

Behavioral Domain. The nurse thought about asking the couple to gather information about the available child-management courses sponsored by local community agencies (e.g., school board, parent-teacher groups, daycare centers, and so forth).

Affective and Behavioral Domain. The nurse decided to invite Mr. Hamilton and Junior to a session with the hope of increasing positive feedback and attachment between them. Mrs. Hamilton and the nurse planned to sit behind a one-way mirror and coach Mr. Hamilton in improving his behavior management skills with Junior. Vicki would be left at the grandparents' home during this session. In this way, the nurse hoped to draw forth more positive experiences of unique outcomes for father, son, and mother. At the same time, the nurse hoped that the grandparents, by babysitting Vicki, would be supportive of Mr. and Mrs. Hamilton but not critical of their parenting abilities.

Use of Questions as Interventions. Every time the nurse met with the Hamiltons, she asked *difference questions* that invited the family to comment on the differences between their past, present, and future behavior management skills. She also used *behavioral-effect questions* to stimulate more solution-focused conversation about the positive effects of appropriate behavioral control of Junior. That is, when Junior responded to the parents' appropriate behavioral limits, the nurse hoped that the parents would recognize this.

We wish to emphasize that the nurse and the couple could have devised many other intervention plans to deal with the Hamiltons' difficulty with behavioral control of Junior. For example, the nurse could have decided to focus more specifically on teaching the parents to control Junior's eating patterns. Had the nurse chosen to do this, she might have invited Mrs. Hamilton to meetings to discuss nutrition for a 3-year-old child. During such sessions, the nurse would provide support for the mother. There is the danger, however, that the nurse, by having interviews only with the mother, might assume the role of "surrogate husband." The nurse would then exacerbate the difficulty between the husband and wife. This type of intervention would not match the nurse's hypothesis, although it could conceivably match the contracted problem. Instead of choosing to work only with the mother, the nurse elected to work with both parents. In this way, she was choosing an intervention consistent with her hypothesis and hoped to exert maximum influence on the "problem-determined system."

HOW TO RECORD PROGRESS NOTES

After the nurse has developed an intervention plan and has continued to have contact with the family, he or she must maintain a record of the evolution of work with the family. In particular, it is important to record the specific work around the contracted presenting problem. A sample progress note is shown in Figure 9–3. The ideal progress note provides a structure for the nurse to identify his or her hypothesis, connect the assessment and intervention components, and maintain a sense of the evolving nature of the work with the family through time. Many hospital and agency progress notes are blank sheets of paper. They are not easily conducive to stimulating the nurse to connect his or her hypothesis with the assessment and intervention plan, let alone providing an opportunity for the nurse to connect the family's responses to the intervention.

We have found it helpful to address the areas listed in Box 9–5 when writing progress notes.

Some nurses have found it useful to co-construct notes with family members. Some families and nurses each keep a record of the meeting. Other nurses have sent letters to families after a meeting outlining the content of the session. We do not have a particular preference for sharing or not sharing notes with families. What we believe is most essential is for the nurse and family to work collaboratively to solve problems, bring forth strengths, and promote health. If sharing records aids this endeavor, it is useful to do so.

When learning how to work with families, it is important for nurses to conceptualize problems within a systems framework. Learning both the "thinking" and "doing" can be facilitated by an integrated approach to record keeping (Bernstein & Burge, 1988). The progress note presented in this chapter structures interview recording in a manner that facilitates systems thinking. It reflects the evolving connections between assessment and intervention. Hypothesizing, session planning, intervention, and family response are inextricably connected. The nurse reviews the previous hypotheses, questions, content and process themes, interventions, and family responses before each meeting with the family. By carefully recording the evolution of the therapeutic conversation, the nurse is more likely to remain focused on change in the presenting problem. This effectively leads toward closure with the family.

Family name: _____ Interview date: _____

Participants: _____ Interview place: _____

Nurse interviewer name and signature: _____

Hypothesis or plan pre-interview:

New information:

Content/process of interview (including interventions and family's responses):

New hypothesis:

Plan for next meeting:

Figure 9–3. Sample progress note.

HOW TO RECORD A DISCHARGE SUMMARY

Some nurses, particularly those in community health settings, have an opportunity to synthesize their work with families by doing a discharge summary. Other nurses, particularly those in hospital settings, have less of an opportunity to synthesize, in a written manner, their work with families. Nevertheless, we believe that where the opportunity exists, synthesizing information into a termination sum-

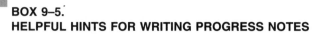

BOX 9–5.
HELPFUL HINTS FOR WRITING PROGRESS NOTES

1. **We note the family members and the professionals who were present at the meeting, as well as the date and place of the meeting.** This is particularly important if the interview takes place in a hospital setting because frequently health professionals other than the nurse interviewer may be involved.

2. **We record our hypotheses or plan for the interview before the meeting with the family.** We have found this invaluable in focusing ourselves for the meeting. It does not mean that we are slaves to, or become married to, the plan. For example, if the family comes in with a new crisis, we can alter the plan, but it does mean that we have an idea of how we will approach the meeting before the interview.

3. **We record the new information on what the family tells us has happened since the last meeting.** We are most interested in new information pertaining to changes in interaction around the presenting problem. These changes could be at the cognitive, affective, or behavioral domains of family functioning. For example, with the Hamilton family, the nurse recorded the father's report that he and his wife had gone to a parenting class the previous week. After the class they had stopped for a quick meal, which he said was "the first time we were out together in 6 months without the children."

4. **We record the content and process of the meeting.** We include the interventions and the family's responses to them. For example, the nurse used future-hypothetical questions to follow up on the information that Mr. Hamilton reported about their going to the parenting class and out for a meal. The nurse asked the couple, "If you were to continue having time for yourselves to focus on parenting issues, what effect might this have on Junior's behavior?" The parents' response that they thought Junior would continue to be more compliant with them was recorded by the nurse.

5. **We record a new hypothesis or a refinement of an old one.** For example, as the Hamiltons progressed in achieving their goals, the nurse abandoned her hypothesis that the children were triangulated into the marriage. Rather, she developed a new hypothesis that focused on their strengths. She integrated the couple's previous history of positive coping (with the effects of a motor vehicle accident) and their need to deal with the effects of Junior's health problems (delayed speech and short stature).

6. **We address the plan for the next meeting.** We jot down any ideas that we have for the next meeting and aim to review them just before or when we meet with the family.

Family name: _____ Date of first meeting: _____
Nurse's name: _____ Date of last meeting: _____
Nurse's signature: _____ Number of meetings: _____

Presenting problem and referral route:

Interventions and outcome:

Prognosis and recommendations:

Figure 9–4. Sample discharge summary.

mary is a useful and meaningful event for both the family and the nurse. A sample discharge summary is shown in Figure 9–4. We highly recommend that nurses take advantage of this opportunity. There are many ways in which one can record a discharge summary. In Chapter 4, we presented examples of some closing letters to families. In our own clinical work we have found the areas listed in Box 9–6 useful to include in a discharge synopsis.

BOX 9–6. HELPFUL HINTS FOR WRITING DISCHARGE SUMMARIES

1. **We include the presenting problem or illness and referral route information in one or two sentences.** We find that this focuses the report so that all the information written is relevant to the identified problem.

2. **We focus on the interventions used and the outcome.** By identifying the interventions used, we are able to learn more about what worked and what did not work to effect change in the presenting issue. For example, in working with the Hamilton family, the nurse had recommended that the couple read books about effective behavioral management of children. She found that this intervention triggered a limited amount of change because neither the husband nor the wife was very interested in reading the material.

   Rather, they did benefit from the intervention in which the nurse asked them to "poll their friends, work colleagues, and relatives" about effective behavioral management strategies for young children. The couple enjoyed "survey research" and found time to discuss the results together. They reported that they enjoyed discarding some of the ideas. However, they retained and used the ones that were most consistent with their own childrearing beliefs. They also offered the nurse some information about web sites that offer helpful parenting tips.

3. **We address the area of prognosis and recommendations.** Given the limited resources in our healthcare delivery systems, we find it useful to make recommendations that may be helpful if the family should come back for additional assistance. For example, the nurse who worked with the Hamilton family recommended that, if they should ever need assistance in the future, it would be useful to inquire what was most useful and least useful about this series of contacts with the pediatric clinic.

   In the future, the nurse most likely would not try to use bibliotherapy as an intervention without reassessing with the family whether this type of intervention might be useful. Rather, the nurse might recommend that the couple try experiments in soliciting others' ideas about how to handle the new issue. Once having done that, the couple could then come back and discuss with the nurse the advantages and disadvantages of adopting these solutions. By recommending such ideas, the nurse builds on the information gathered in working with the family this time. It does not prevent the new nurse interviewer from trying different ideas; it merely provides a tentative guide.

▪▪▪ ISSUES IN RECORDING, STORING, AND ACCESSING RECORDS

Nurses are continually faced with issues about confidentiality. Who should have access to the family assessment summary or the discharge synopsis? Is it a family record or an individual record? Which family members can legally give consent for its release to another agency? Can the nurse talk to one family member about a meeting with another member when the first member is not present? These issues of confidentiality are becoming more numerous with the continuing advancements in communications technology. For example, if the family meeting was videotaped, family members sometimes request a copy of the video so that they can play it on their own videocassette player at home.

In the last decade, the subjects of human rights and confidentiality have increasingly come to the fore. In the areas of record content, release, consumer access, informed consent, records of minors, and compulsory reporting, nurses and other professionals have become increasingly more knowledgeable.

Guidelines regarding confidentiality exist in federal, state, and provincial regulations. Hospitals, clinics, and agencies also have guidelines for specialty areas. In the area of mental health, there is a great variety of age designation and conditions under which minors, for example, may receive care.

In family nursing, confidentiality is a particularly complex issue. Data concerning more than one person are included in the file. Some of the family members are usually minors and some are adults. When children and adults are in treatment as a unit, care must be taken to protect the privacy of each person. Nurses must be acquainted with the relevant legislation in their jurisdiction as well as the agency's or hospital's policies on confidentiality of family records.

Another practical issue concerning confidentiality is often raised. Family members sometimes try to obtain special attention by making telephone calls between sessions or by asking for private meetings with the nurse. The meaning of such behaviors should be carefully considered in the context of the nurse's understanding of the family system. For example, a nurse may be working with a family whose 25-year-old daughter, Puja, has a diagnosis of manic depression. The father, mother, and daughter may agree during a family interview that the young woman should follow the physician's advice and take lithium. If, however, the father calls the nurse after the family session to discuss why he believes his daughter should *not* take lithium, the nurse should hypothesize about the meaning of the father's call. Could he fear disagreeing with his wife and daughter in front of them? Could he want the nurse to align with him against his wife and daughter? Generally, we recommend that nurses tell family members who request a private session that they bring their concerns to the family interviews. In this way, the nurse avoids becoming triangulated between two or more family members.

■■■ CONCLUSIONS

A particular format has now evolved in the process of family interviewing. Box 9–7 also provides some helpful hints for organizing and documenting family assessment data. The nurse ascertains whether a family assessment is indicated. If it is indicated, a family assessment is conducted. After the nurse has assessed the family, we recommend that the nurse review the CFAM categories and delineate a strengths and problems list. The nurse should then write a family assessment summary. A decision to intervene is based on a consideration of the family's level of functioning, the nurse's competence, and the work context. If intervention is indicated, the nurse has to decide, in collaboration with the family, which are the key issues to focus on and which are tangential ones. We recommend that the nurse review the

---

■■■■ BOX 9–7. HELPFUL HINTS TO ORGANIZE AND DOCUMENT FAMILY ASSESSMENT DATA

- Identify and document a list of presenting problem(s) and family strengths.
- Create a CFAM document that lists each category and subcategory. Enter reported and observed data in relevant (sub)categories. Note gaps to be filled at a future date.
- Include a genogram, an ecomap, brief family life cycle and family development data, and an attachment diagram for significant family relationships.
- Formulate systemic hypotheses.
- Formulate an intervention plan.
- Continue to update the family assessment, using progress notes to document family changes and the impact of family nursing interventions.

Source: Reprinted with permission from Levac, A. M., Wright, L. M., & Leahey, M. (1997). Children and families: Models for assessment and intervention. In J. Fox (ed.), *Primary healthcare of children.* Baltimore, MD: Mosby, p. 11.

CFIM. The nurse must also consider with the family which members are to be seen and what is the frequency and length of treatment. An intervention plan should then be devised. The decision as to which interventions will be used to facilitate change within this particular family is a critical one. The nurse then records on a progress note a record of his or her therapeutic conversations with the family, and at the time of discharge synthesizes the work in a discharge summary.

■■■ REFERENCES

Bernstein, R., & Burge, S. (1988). A record-keeping format for training systemic therapists. *Family Process, 27,* 339–349.

Thorne, S., & Robinson, C. (1989). Guarded alliance: Health care relationships in chronic illness. *Image, 21*(3), 153–157.

CHAPTER **10**

How to Terminate
with Families

To end professional relationships with families in a therapeutic fashion is one of the most challenging aspects of the family interviewing process for nurses. Termination has been the least examined of the treatment phases in clinical work with families (Roberts, 1992). An important aspect of the termination stage is not only to end the nurse-family relationship therapeutically but to do so in a manner that will sustain the progress that has been made. Nurses often establish very intense and meaningful relationships with families and, therefore, frequently feel guilty or fearful about initiating termination. This is especially evident in nursing practice where the relationship has been a long-standing one over months or even years such as in nursing homes, extended-care facilities, and clients' homes.

This chapter reviews the process of termination by examining the decision to terminate when it is initiated by the family or the nurse, or as a result of the context in which the family members find themselves. Often the nurse's decision to terminate with a family does not necessarily mean that the family will cease contact with all professionals. Therefore, we will discuss the process of referring families to other health professionals. Specific suggestions for how to phase out and conclude treatment are given, as well as suggestions for evaluating the effects of the treatment process.

▪▪▪▪ DECISION TO TERMINATE

NURSE-INITIATED TERMINATION

It is important to emphasize that it is not necessary that a total "cure" or complete resolution of the presenting problem or illness be evident. Rather, it is the family's ability to master or to live alongside problems or illness, not eliminate them, that is the most important indicator for the decision to initiate termination. The termination stage evolves easily if the beginning and middle stages of treatment have concluded successfully. However, the most difficult decision for any nurse to make in regard to termination is the question of time. *When* is the right time for termination? The question of when one should begin to think about termination is directly related to what new views, beliefs,

323

ideas, or solutions have been generated by the family and nurse to re-solve current problems. If new solution options have been discovered and consequently the family functions differently, it is time to termi-nate because change has occurred. The skills necessary for nurse-initiated termination are given in a later section of this chapter (i.e., Phasing out and Concluding Treatment) and in Chapter 5.

When we have decided that additional meetings are not necessary and the family agrees, we enter the termination phase of treatment. First and most importantly during this phase, we prefer to help fami-lies to expand their perspective to focus on strengths and positive be-haviors that have occurred or re-emerged rather than an exclusive fo-cus on troublesome behaviors. We try not to have the families tie these new behaviors to our work with them but rather to their own work. For example, we ask them what positive changes they have noticed over the last 3 months rather than asking what positive changes they have noticed since working with the nurse.

Another useful clinical idea when terminating is one generated by White and Epston (1990) in which they recommend that the inter-viewer "expand the audience" to describe and acknowledge the fami-ly's unique outcomes and progress. For example, we often ask a family to tell us what advice they would have for other families confronting similar health problems. Sometimes we have families write letters to other families to offer their suggestions of what has or has not worked in coping with a particular illness. One woman, who was experiencing MS but was successfully living alongside her illness, wrote a letter to a young woman who was as yet not as successful. The letter gave hope and encouragement to this young woman. In the writing of the letter, the older woman expressed the thought that it was a very "cathartic" experience for her. She also went on to say, "MS is still here, but it does not dominate our lives and occupies only a small space over in the cor-ner. I did experience a minor flare-up after Christmas but it cleared quickly. I remain optimistic." The nurse highlights and becomes en-thusiastic about the family's ideas and advice as a way of both reinforc-ing their positive ideas, new beliefs about themselves and of generating useful information for other families. Thus, the family's competencies and strengths are overtly acknowledged.

The emphasis throughout the termination process when initiated by the nurse is to identify, affirm, amplify, and solidify the changes that have taken place within family members. Consequently, it is es-sential that change be distinguished to become a reality (Wright, Watson, & Bell, 1996). One way to distinguish change is to obtain the perspective of others. The nurse can ask such questions as "What changes do you notice in your wife since she has adopted this new idea that 'illness is a family affair?'" or "what else would your family or friends notice that is different in you since your anger about experiencing cancer has dissipated?"

Termination rituals can also emphasize change and give families courage to live their lives without the involvement of healthcare professionals (Roberts, 1992). If the initial concerns have been with children, we often have a party (balloons, cake, and all) to celebrate a child mastering a particular problem such as enuresis. In addition, the child is given a certificate indicating that he or she has overcome his problem, whether it is enuresis, fighting fears, or putting chronic pain in its place. This helps families to acknowledge change through celebration.

Other families have been given something by the clinical nursing team to symbolize their progress. For example, one family was given a feather to indicate that their problems now only require "the touch of a feather" to be able to keep them in place. It is essential to mark family strengths and problem-solving capabilities as families fully integrate back into their daily lives (Roberts, 1992) without the involvement of nurses.

At the Family Nursing Unit, University of Calgary (Wright, Watson, & Bell, 1990; 1996), a closing letter is routinely sent to each family highlighting what the clinical nursing team has learned from the family and what ideas the team offered the family. These therapeutic letters serve as a closing ritual. They provide the opportunity to highlight the family's strengths, and the reciprocal influence of the relationship between the family and the clinical nursing team. The letters document in a personal way the family and individual interventions that were offered.

FAMILY-INITIATED TERMINATION

When a family takes the initiative to terminate, it is very important for the nurse to acknowledge this and then to gain more explicit information regarding their reasons for wanting to terminate. This information will help the nurse to understand the family's responses to the interviewing process. For example, has the family discovered new solutions to their problems? Are the family and nurse able to identify and agree on significant changes that have occurred in individual and family functioning? Is the family also aware of how to sustain these changes? Segal (1991), in discussing the Brief Therapy approach of the Mental Research Institute, Palo Alto, California, suggests three criteria in the client's, or family's, report that indicate readiness to terminate. These three criteria are: (1) a small, but significant, change has been made in the problem; (2) the change appears to be durable; and (3) the client or family implies or states an ability to handle things without the therapist.

If the family specifically states that they wish to terminate, but the nurse believes this would be premature, it is important for the nurse to take the initiative to review the family's decision. In so doing, the nurse reconceptualizes the progress that has been made by the family and recognizes what problems remain and what goals and solutions might yet be achieved. One way to do this is to have family members discuss with one another their desire to continue or discontinue sessions and explore who is most in favor of which opinion. Also, the specifics of the decision may be helpful, such as when the family decided and what prompted them to decide on termination. After establishing who is most keen to continue, the nurse can invite that family member to share with the other family members the anticipated benefit of further sessions. It is helpful for families to be specific and emphasize the benefits that could be achieved if family interviewing were to continue. However, there are times when termination is inevitable. At such a point, it is reasonable and ethical to accept the family's initiative to terminate and do so without applying undue pressure even though the nurse may disagree with their decision (Tomm & Wright, 1979).

We strongly urge nurses not to engage in linear blame of either families or themselves when they believe that families have prematurely left treatment. Rather, we encourage nurses to hypothesize about the factors that may have contributed to the termination. These factors may include such nurse-related behaviors as being too aligned with children, too slow to intervene, and so forth. Family-related behaviors such as involvement with other agencies and so forth should also be considered.

There are times, however, when the family states that they want to continue treatment but initiate termination indirectly. Indications may be late arrivals for the sessions, missed appointments, and the absence from sessions of certain family members who were asked to attend. Another indicator that families are perhaps considering termination is their expression of dissatisfaction with the course of treatment or complaints about the logistical difficulties of attending or the loss of time from work. Again, we suggest that the same steps be taken as when the family initiates termination directly.

The challenge of family-initiated terminations is to determine if they are premature or not. In the nursing literature, there is a dearth of research to provide insights into reasons for premature terminations. However, the family therapy literature does have a few studies that suggest some of the reasons for premature termination by families. Gaines and Stedman (1981) evaluated 97 families over a 4-month period in a mental health clinic. They found that families who missed the first treatment session are at high risk of dropping out over the course of treatment. The implication of missed appointments refers back to the importance of the engagement stage and even to the initial contact with families on the telephone.

In that same study, they discovered that failure of the family to bring all members to the first session (when the entire family was requested) is also a poor prognostic sign. Another interesting finding was that the nature of the referral source had a direct correlation with the family's continuing in treatment. Families who were referred by institutions (e.g., school, court) tended to discontinue treatment more frequently before achieving treatment goals than families who were individually referred (e.g., physicians, mental health professionals). Most of the families who continued in treatment were those who were self-referred.

A relationship between families with chronic problems and attendance in therapy was also found (Gaines & Stedman, 1981). Families with chronic problems attended more treatment sessions than families with acute problems, but they tended to discontinue treatment more frequently before the treatment goals were reached.

It is critically important to help families understand the nature of the treatment contract. Many families have no real understanding of what takes place in family interviewing. Therefore, they may relate to the nurse as they do to physicians or clergy; whereby, they use the services as they wish and discontinue when they so desire.

CONTEXT-INITIATED TERMINATION

In some settings, particularly managed healthcare systems, it is not the nurse or the family who initiates termination but the healthcare system or insurance company. Ideally, some continued contact would be possible if family needs remained the same. In these situations, it is very important for the nurse to assess whether the family needs further treatment or can continue to resolve problems and discover solutions on their own. If the family needs to be referred, the nurse requires some specific skills in this area. The referral process will be discussed in a later section of this chapter.

PHASING OUT AND CONCLUDING TREATMENT

In Chapter 5, we highlighted some of the specific skills required for therapeutic termination in the form of learning objectives. We will now expand on these particular skills.

REVIEW CONTRACTS

For families seen on an outpatient basis, we strongly encourage periodic review of the present status of the family's problems and changes. The use of a contract for a specific number of sessions provides a built-in way not only to set a time limit to the meetings but also to ensure periodic review. The contract also helps nurse interviewers to be mindful of the progress and direction of their work with families rather than seeing them endlessly and without purpose beyond the vague good intention of "helping." We prefer a designated number of sessions to open-ended sessions. However, nurses need to be flexible as to the frequency and duration of sessions. Normally, the frequency decreases as problems improve. Periodic reviews allow family members to have the opportunity to express their pleasure or displeasure with the progress that is being made.

DECREASE FREQUENCY OF SESSIONS

If adequate progress has been made, this is an ideal time to begin to decrease the frequency of sessions. In our experience, we have found that families are able to work toward termination more readily and with more confidence when they recognize the improvement in their own ability to solve problems. Many families, however, find it difficult to acknowledge changes. In these circumstances, Tomm and Wright (1979) suggest the use of a question such as, "What would each of you have to do to bring the problem back?" to elicit a more explicit understanding or statement from family members regarding the changes that have been made.

Another very significant time to decrease the frequency of sessions is when the nurse has inadvertently fostered undue dependency. We have had many family situations presented to us in which nursing students or professional nurses provide "paid friendship" with mothers. These nurses have become the mother's major support system because they have not mobilized other supports, such as husbands, friends, or relatives. In situations in which this dependency has occurred and is recognized, we strongly suggest that the nurse help foster other supports for the family and decrease the frequency of sessions.

If a nurse encounters hesitancy or reluctance to decrease the frequency of sessions or to terminate completely, the nurse should encourage a discussion of the fears related to termination and solicit support from other family members. It has been our experience that family members frequently fear that if there are fewer sessions or if sessions are discontinued, they will not be able to cope with their problems or their problems will become worse. Thus, asking a question such as "What are you most concerned would happen if we discontinued sessions now?" can get to the core of the matter very quickly. By clarifying family members' fears openly, other family members (who may be less fearful) have an opportunity to provide support.

GIVE CREDIT FOR CHANGE

Nurses have frequently chosen the profession of nursing because they have a strong desire to be helpful to individuals and families in obtaining optimal health. Their efforts are usually helpful, and they are often given all or much of the credit for the changes and improvements. However, it has been our experience in family work that it is vitally important that the *family* receive the credit for change. There are several reasons for this necessity of stressing to the family they are responsible for the change:

1. Families experience the tension, conflict, and anxiety of working through problems and therefore deserve the credit for improvement.
2. If the identified patient is a child and the nurse accepts credit, the nurse can be seen to be in a competitive relationship with the parents.
3. Perhaps the most important reason for giving the family credit for change is that this increases the chance that the positive effects of treatment will last. Otherwise, you may inadvertently convey the message that the family cannot manage without you and they will become indebted or too dependent. Termination provides an opportune time to comment on the positive changes that have already happened during the course of treatment.
4. Praising the family for their accomplishments in having helped or corrected the original presenting problem will provide them with confidence in handling future problems. Specific statements such as "You did the work" or "You people are being far too modest" can re-

inforce to the family members the idea that their efforts were essential in making the change.

It is never possible to really know what precipitated, perturbed, or initiated the change that occurs within families. Often nurses create a context for change by helping family members to explore solution options to their difficulties or suffering. Wright, Watson, and Bell (1996) suggest that creating a context for change "constitutes the central and enduring foundation of the therapeutic process" and further suggest that "it is not just a necessary prerequisite to the process of therapeutic change, it is therapeutic change in and of itself" (p.129). Sometimes the very effort of bringing a family together in a room to discuss important family concerns can be the most significant intervention (Robinson & Wright, 1995).

If families present themselves at termination with concerns about progress, we must express our appreciation for their positive efforts to solve problems constructively even when there has been no significant improvement. When such is the case, we strongly recommend that nurses discuss with their clinical supervisors some hypotheses about why the interview sessions do not seem to have been effective. Perhaps the goals of the family or the nurse have been too high or demanding. If the family does not progress, this is usually the result of our inability to discover an intervention that is a fit with the family. Too often, we excuse ourselves from making further efforts to intervene when we label families as noncompliant, unmotivated, or resistant (Wright & Levac, 1992). It is very important, however, that the nurse believe that the family has worked hard despite minimal progress, and it is important to praise them for having done so.

We do not mean to imply, however, that because we are encouraging nurses to give families the credit for change that the nurse cannot enjoy the change. Family work can be very rewarding, and certainly the nurse is part of the change process.

EVALUATE FAMILY INTERVIEWS

It is important to provide a formal closure to the end of the treatment process with a face-to-face discussion whenever possible. During this final session, it is very valuable to evaluate the effectiveness of the treatment process and the effect of changes on various family members. We recommend evaluating the impact not only on the whole family system but also on various subsystems, such as the marital subsystem and individual family member functions. Such questions as

"What have you learned about yourself and MS?" and "What have you come to appreciate about your marriage?" invite reflection from the family about its changes. An even more dramatic evaluation can occur by having each family member and the nurse write about their reflections on the family meetings, emphasizing what they learned, what has changed, and what new ideas or beliefs they have about their problems or illness. One such family clinical nursing team wrote poignant descriptions about dealing with their grief (Levae, McLean, Wright, "Ann," & "Fred," 1988).

We also suggest asking family members the following questions: "What things did you find most and least helpful during our work together?" and "What things did you wish or were hoping would happen during our work together but did not?" In this way, it demonstrates that the nurse is also open and receptive to feedback. It is important at this time that the nurse not become defensive to any of the feedback. Rather, the nurse can express appreciation to the family and inform them that this feedback will assist and educate him or her to be even more helpful in work with future families. "For too long evaluation has been a one-way process—from the dominant to the dominated. Participatory evaluation research turns the traditional evaluation process on its head. Outsiders are no longer the 'experts' but instead empower the consumers of services to become leaders in evaluation and change" (Piercy & Thomas, 1998. p. 165). We strongly concur.

EXTEND AN INVITATION FOR FOLLOW-UP

Nurses often place themselves or are placed in situations of "follow-up." However, the follow-up is often a negative experience for both the nurse and the family. For example, community health nurses (CHNs) have reported that they are frequently requested to "check" on family members to assess their functioning. But those who request the visit (e.g., physician, Department of Child Welfare) have made no clear statement to the family about the purpose of the visit. Therefore, the nurse is in a very awkward position. We strongly discourage nurses from placing themselves in these kinds of situations unless there has been clear, direct communication with the family by the requesting party. Follow-up in this manner can give a very unfortunate and unpleasant message to the family that we anticipate further problems. It is better to make clear to the family that progress has been made and that the sessions are finished. However, if they would like input again in the future, indicate that you would be willing to see them. Families usually appreciate knowing that backup support by professionals is available to them in times of stress.

For nurses employed in hospitals, a follow-up session is usually not possible, but referral can be made to a CHN or homecare if deemed appropriate. Our experience has been that families do appreciate knowing whether they will have future contact with the nurse who has worked intimately with them.

CLOSING LETTERS

Another way to positively punctuate the end of treatment is to send the family a letter giving a summary of the family sessions. This letter provides the opportunity to highlight the family strengths, reinforce the changes made, offer the family a review of their efforts and what they have accomplished, and list the ideas (interventions) that were offered to them. At the Family Nursing Unit, University of Calgary, closing letters are routinely sent to each family on completion of treatment (Wright, Watson, & Bell, 1996). Many families have commented about how much they appreciate the letters and how they frequently refer back to them. An example of an actual closing letter follows. The names of the family members have been changed for purposes of confidentiality.

> Dear Family Barbosa:
>
> Greetings from the Family Nursing Unit. We had the opportunity to meet with various members of your family on eight occasions. I have also had several phone conversations with both Venicio and Fatima in recent months.
>
> *Clinical Impressions.* Throughout our work together, our clinical nursing team has been very impressed with your family. Although a great many challenges have been presented to all of you over the past years, your family was able to overcome many obstacles and search for ways of helping each other through these difficult times.
>
> *What Our Team Learned from Your Family.* Our experience with your family has taught our clinical nursing team a great deal. The following is a synthesis:
>
> 1. Families dealing with a life-shortening illness in one of its members have the strength to deal with unresolved issues of blame, guilt, and shame. Even though there has been a great deal of pain and hurt in a family, they can heal their relationships and move on.
> 2. Although it can be a common response for family members to distance themselves from the possibility of death with a life-shortening illness and to be afraid of dying, it is possible for

them to make peace with each other and find peace in themselves, giving them the courage to go on.

3. Although a mother and son may reside in different places and may not see each other often, they can still play a significant part in each other's lives. No matter how old a child and parent are, the knowledge that they love and accept each other for what they are can make a significant difference in their lives.

4. The uncertainty involved with a life-shortening illness can be the most difficult thing for families to handle. Family members can help each other with the uncertainty by discussing the situation openly among themselves.

5. Grandparents and grandsons have very special relationships that are different from those of parents and sons.

As you all continue to face the many challenges that are ahead, we trust that you will draw on your own special strengths as well as on more open communication to help you meet these challenges. It was truly a privilege to work with you. We wish you continued strength for the future.

Should you desire further consultation at any time, you can arrange this by contacting the Family Nursing Unit's secretary. A Research Assistant will be in contact with you in approximately 6 months to ask you to participate in our outcome study to ascertain your satisfaction with the Family Nursing Unit.

Sincerely,
Jane Nagy, R.N. Masters   Lorraine M. Wright, R.N., Ph.D.
Student   Director, Family Nursing Unit
                                              Professor, Faculty of Nursing

Therapeutic letters, whether sent during clinical work with families or at the end of treatment, have proven to be a very useful and often potent intervention to invite families to reflect on ideas offered within the session as well as to reflect on changes they have made over the course of sessions (Levac, McLean, Wright, Bell, "Ann," & "Fred," 1998; Watson & Lee, 1992; White & Epston, 1990; Wright & Nagy, 1993, Wright & Simpson, 1991; Wright & Watson, 1988; Wright, Watson & Bell, 1996).

■ ■ ■ REFERRAL TO OTHER PROFESSIONALS

Referrals to other professionals may be advisable for a variety of reasons. We will list some specific tasks that are required to make a smooth transition for the family from one professional to another. First, however, we will discuss some of the more common reasons for nurses to refer families to other professionals.

With the expanding specialty areas within nursing, it is becoming impossible and totally unrealistic to expect nurses to be experts in all areas. Therefore, there are times when it is most appropriate for nurses to seek the input of additional professional resources when problems are quite complex. A nurse may refer families or specific family members for consultation or ongoing treatment. For example, if a senior within a family is experiencing temporal headaches, it is very important that any organic or biologic origin of this problem be ruled out. Therefore, a nurse might refer the family for consultation with a neurologist and may suspend treatment until the consultation is complete.

In other instances, the nurse may discover that a particular child has a learning disability that is out of the realm of the nurse's expertise. The nurse may suggest referring the child to an education center where personnel have greater expertise in dealing with children with learning difficulties. Nurses need to be open to referring individuals or entire families for consultation. It is inappropriate to perceive this as an inadequacy in their repertoire of skills. To refer wisely, nurses need an extensive knowledge of professional resources within the community.

Another reason for referring to other professionals, but not as common as the one above, is when the family moves or is transferred to another setting or is discharged before treatment is over. It is very important that the nurse, especially in hospital settings, maximize the opportunities to do family work. A beautiful illustration of this was given by one of our graduate nursing students. After some university seminars on the importance of family involvement, this student, who was working part-time in a rural hospital, invited the parents of an asthmatic child to a family interview. The student obtained much valuable information regarding the interrelationship of the child's asthmatic problem with other family dynamics. Shortly thereafter, the child was discharged. The nursing student ascertained that the family was interested in changing the recurring problem of frequent admissions for this young child. The student made an appropriate referral to the mental health services within the community. This highlights the point that with only *one* family interview, an assessment can be made and a significant intervention completed through referral for a recurring problem.

Some of the specific skills required in making appropriate referrals are described in the following paragraphs.

PREPARE FAMILIES

It is most important to adequately prepare families so that they understand the nature of the referral to a new professional. This can be done by explaining directly to families the reason for the referral and why the nurse feels that they would benefit from such a referral. Another method that can be useful for ensuring openness and clarity about the nature of the referral is for the nurse to write a summary and then to review this summary with the family. This summary can then be sent to the new professional and a copy made available for the family. In this way, the family is not left wondering what information will be shared with the new professional. Also, an important implicit message is given that this information is confidential and private *about them* and, therefore, they have a right to know what is shared.

Selecting a new professional can sometimes pose a challenge. If a nurse is known in the community, it is wise to solicit the help of colleagues for ideas and advice on which agencies or professionals are best for the type of treatment needed, or to seek information from community information directories and booklets.

MEET THE NEW PROFESSIONAL

It has been our experience that the transition to the new professional is much more effective and efficient if the nurse can be present with the family at the first meeting. In this way, a more personal referral is made. It often reduces the fears and anxieties that families may have about starting "fresh" with someone new. Before the referral, opportunities should be given to the family to express concerns or ask questions about the referral. At the first meeting, the family may wish to clarify with the new professional their expectations and understanding of the referral. The new professional can also clarify the nurse's understanding of the reason for the referral and any misconceptions can be dealt with at that time. A conjoint meeting with the family, nurse, and new professional can also serve as a "marker" for the end of the nurse's relationship with the family.

KEEP APPROPRIATE BOUNDARIES

When a family has been referred but the nurse continues providing care for the family's physical needs, it is extremely important that boundaries of responsibility be clear. Otherwise, there is a potential for the nurse to inadvertently become triangulated between the family and the new professional.

For example, a homecare nurse regularly visited an elderly patient who lives with her adult daughter. The purpose of the visits by the homecare nurse was to assist with colostomy care. The nurse observed and assessed the interaction between the elderly parent and the adult daughter as a severe and long-standing conflict. This conflict was having a negative effect, deterring the elderly patient from assuming more responsibility for her physical care. Because of her family assessment skills, the nurse was able to make an important referral to a family therapy program where more in-depth work on the intergenerational conflict began. However, in future visits with the elderly patient, the nurse was listening to complaints about the adult daughter that the patient was not discussing in the family meetings. Also, the family therapist called the nurse and asked the nurse to apply pressure on the elderly parent to be more cooperative in attending sessions. Thus, very quickly the nurse had become "caught in the middle" between the family and the therapist. The nurse dealt with the situation by requesting to join in a meeting with the family and the therapist to clarify expectations of all parties. In this one session, the nurse was able to "de-triangulate" herself by clarifying her present role with the family and the new professional.

TRANSFERS

In our more than 25 years of clinical experience, we have not found the practice of transferring families from one nurse to another to be very successful. We view the process of transfers as very different from referrals. A referral is usually made to another healthcare professional with different expertise. A transfer, on the other hand, is usually made to another colleague of similar expertise and competence. We recommend, if possible, that nurses conclude treatment with the families they are working with rather than transfer them to another colleague. In our experience, families frequently disengage with the new nurse through missed appointments, not showing up, or not stating any particular concern. It is understandable that families do not wish to "start over" with another nurse. We hypothesize that transfers are frequently made to assuage the nurse's feelings about leaving versus the family's desires about continuing treatment.

If, however, a transfer is necessary, we recommend that the "old" nurse use language indicating an ending of her relationship with the family. For example, she can say, "Now that my work with you is coming to an end, what would you like to work on with Sanjeshna (the "new" nurse)?" In addition, we encourage the new nurse to directly ask the family about their relationship with the previous nurses. Questions such as "What do you anticipate will be different in our work together versus your work with Li?" are useful. This type of conversation punctuates a change rather than a continuance of the same work. It fosters engagement and is important for the new nurse and the family in establishing a collaborative relationship.

Another way to increase engagement is for the current nurse to ask the family to take a break between contacts before setting up an appointment with the new nurse. This again emphasizes the change in the working relationship, and encourages the family to be self-directive in initiating the new contact rather than simply responding to the professionals.

▓▓▓ SUCCESS OF TREATMENT IN FAMILY WORK

Although interventions may obtain positive and possibly dramatic results *during* treatment, the real success of family work is the positive changes that are *maintained* or continue to evolve weeks and months after nurses have terminated treatment with particular families. We strongly encourage professional nurses and nursing students to make it a pattern of practice to obtain data from the family as to outcome. When there is a focus on outcome, it directs the nurse to orient her work toward change, focus on problems that can be changed, and think of how the family will cope without the nurse in the future. We also suggest that in any follow-up with families, the nurse can explain that this is a *normal* pattern of practice (e.g., "We normally contact families with whom we have worked within 6 months to gain information on how things are evolving"). It is also important to use this follow-up with specific goals in mind. Thus, a very useful reason for follow-up can be for research purposes. In our experience, beginning family nurse interviewers tend to be more focused on what is going on in the family, whereas more experienced nurses focus on quite specific goals for treatment. Carter (1986) also suggests that "the criteria for 'success' change over the course of a career, and that it is not so much one's view of success that changes as one's view of what is possible" (p. 19). Therefore, outcome is important.

To facilitate evaluation, we suggest formalizing follow-up of families, particularly those seen on an outpatient basis, by live interview, questionnaire, or both. At present, we favor the use of a questionnaire that is answered by all available family members.

At the Family Nursing Unit (FNU), University of Calgary, families are routinely interviewed 6 months after the last session by a research assistant who has had no previous contact with the families (Wright, Watson, & Bell, 1990; 1996). This outcome study is designed to evaluate the services provided by the FNU. The variables examined by this study are the family's satisfaction with the services provided, satisfaction with the nurse interviewer, and change in the presenting problem and family relationships. A semi-structured questionnaire designed for this study asks for each family member's perspective on each of the variables. Questions are asked in relation to two periods: at the conclusion of the family sessions and at the time of the survey. Results from the survey indicate that the most helpful aspects of family sessions were the opportunity to ventilate family concerns thereby increasing communication among family members and to obtain support from the FNU clinical nursing team. Families ranked the interview process and the suggestions from the FNU clinical nursing team as the second most helpful aspects (Bell, 1993).

Family members reported satisfaction with the nurse interviewer, who was a Master's or doctoral student or a faculty member specializing in family systems nursing. They indicated that the friendly, professional, and nonthreatening manner of the graduate nursing students made them comfortable.

Seventy-seven to 86 percent of the family members reported the presenting problem was better at the time of the survey. Regardless of the presenting problem, 56.7 percent of fathers and 47.5 percent of mothers reported positive changes in the marital relationship, such as increased communication, improved relationships, and decreased tension (Bell, 1993), suggesting support for the systems theory tenet that change in one part of the system affects change in other parts.

This type of outcome study suggests that assessing change should be evaluated at the individual, parent-child, marital, and family system levels. We believe that a higher level of positive change has occurred when improvement is evidenced in systemic (total family) or relationship (dyadic) interactions than when it is evidenced in individuals alone. That is, individual change does not logically require system change, but stable system change does require individual change and relationship change, and relationship change requires individual changes.

Family treatment does appear to be having creditable success as reported by outcome studies in family therapy. Specifically, marital and family therapy has shown to be significantly and clinically more effective than no psychotherapy or individual treatments for adult schizophrenia, adult achoholism and drug abuse, adult hypertension, elderly dementia, cardiovascular risk factors in adults, adolescent conduct disorder, adult obesity, anorexia in young adolescent girls, chronic physical illnesses in adults and children (asthma, diabetes, and so forth), child obesity, and cardiovascular risk factors in children, and depressed outpatient women in distressed marriages (Campbell & Patterson,

1995; Pinsof & Wynne, 1995). Nurses could contribute significantly to family outcome research by focusing on follow-up with families in which particular family members experience a health problem. This area of family work is just beginning to be researched and lends itself beautifully to the active involvement of nurses in its evolution.

■■■ CONCLUSIONS

In reading this chapter, it can be seen that the matter of concluding treatment in a therapeutic and constructive way is a challenge for any nurse working with families. Unfortunately, much more has been written in the literature about how to begin with and treat families than how to effectively and therapeutically terminate with them. However, we want to emphasize the extreme importance of terminating contact with families in a manner that will increase the likelihood of change being maintained, celebrated, and expanded.

■■■ REFERENCES

Beck, M. (1981). Therapist-initiated termination from family therapy. *American Journal of Family Therapy, 9*, 94–95.

Bell, J. M. (1993). Personal communication.

Campbell, T. L., & Patterson, J. M. (1995). The effectiveness of family interventions in the treatment of physical illness. *Journal of Marital and Family Therapy, 21*(4), 545–583.

Carter, B. (1986). Success in family therapy. *Family Therapy Networker*, July–August, 10, 17–22.

Gaines, T., & Stedman, J. M. (1981). Factors associated with dropping out of child and family treatment. *American Journal of Family Therapy, 9*, 45–51.

Guldner, C. A. (1981). Premature termination in marital and family therapy. In A. S. Gurman (Ed.), *Questions and answers in the practice of family therapy*. New York: Brunner/Mazel, pp. 510–512.

Levac, A. M., McLean, S., Wright, L. M., Bell, J. M., "Ann," & "Fred" (1998). A "Reader's Theatre" intervention to managing grief: Post-therapy reflections by a family and a clinical team. *Journal of Marital and Family Therapy, 24*(1), 81–94.

Piercy, F. P., & Thomas, V. (1998). Participatory evaluation research: An introduction for family therapists. *Journal of Marital and Family Therapy, 24*(2), 165–176.

Pinsof, W. M., & Wynne, L. C. (1995). The efficacy of marital and family therapy: An empirical overview, conclusions, and recommendations. *Journal of Marital and Family Therapy, 21*(4), 585–613.

Roberts, J. (1992). Termination rituals. In T. S. Nelson & T. S. Trepper (Eds.), *101 Interventions in family therapy*. New York: Haworth.

Robinson, C. A., & Wright, L. M. (1995). Family nursing interventions: What families say makes a difference. *Journal of Family Nursing, 1*(3), 327–345.

Segal, L. (1991). Brief therapy: The MRI approach. In A. S. Gurman & D. P. Kniskern (Eds.), *Handbook of family therapy*, volume II. New York: Brunner/Mazel, pp. 171–199.

Stanton, J. D. (1981). Who should get credit for change that occurs in therapy? In A. S. Gurman (Ed.), *Questions and answers in the practice of family therapy*. New York: Brunner/Mazel, pp. 519–522.

Tomm, K., & Wright, L. M. (1979). Training in family therapy: Perceptual, conceptual and executive skills. *Family Process, 18*, 227–250.

White, M., & Epston, D. (1990). *Narrative means to therapeutic ends*. New York: W.W. Norton & Co.

Watson, W. L., and Lee, D. (1993). Is there life after suicide?: The systemic belief approach for "survivors" of suicide. *Archives of Psychiatric Nursing, 7*(1), 37–42.

Wright, L. M., & Levac, A. M. (1992). The non-existence of non-compliant families: The influence of Humberto Maturana. *Journal of Advanced Nursing, 17*, 913–917.

Wright, L. M., & Nagy, J. (1993). Death: The most troublesome family secret of all. In E. Imber Black (Ed.), *Secrets in families and family therapy*. New York: W.W. Norton & Co., pp. 121–137.

Wright, L. M., & Simpson, P. (1991). A systemic belief approach to epileptic seizures: A case of being spellbound. *Contemporary Family Therapy: An International Journal, 13*(2), 165–180.

Wright, L. M., & Watson, W. L. (1988). Systemic family therapy and family development. In C. J. Falicov (Ed.), *Family transitions: Continuity and change over the life cycle*. New York: Guilford Press, pp. 407–430.

Wright, L. M., Watson, W. L., & Bell, J. M. (1990). The Family Nursing Unit: A unique integration of research, education and clinical practice. In J. M. Bell, W. L. Watson, & L. M. Wright (Eds.), *The cutting edge of family nursing*. Calgary, Alberta: Family Nursing Unit Publications, pp. 95–109.

Wright, L. M., Watson, W. L., & Bell, J. M. (1996). *Beliefs: The heart of healing in families and illness*. New York: Basic Books.

Index

Page numbers followed by f indicate figures; page numbers followed by t indicate tables; page numbers followed by b indicate boxed material.